TALK ABOUT SEX

# TALK ABOUT SEX

*The Battles over Sex Education in the United States*

With a New Preface

Janice M. Irvine

University of California Press   Berkeley   Los Angeles   London

University of California Press
Berkeley and Los Angeles, California

University of California Press, Ltd.
London, England

First paperback printing 2004
© 2002 by the Regents of the University
of California

Library of Congress Cataloging-in-Publication Data
Irvine, Janice M.
    Talk about sex : the battles over sex education in
the United States / Janice M. Irvine
        p.    cm.
    Includes bibliographical references and index.
    ISBN 0-520-24329-3 (pbk : alk. paper)
    1.  Sex instruction—United States.
2.  Community and school—United States.
I.  Title.

HQ57.5.A3 178    2002
613.9'07'073-dc21                    2001058500

Manufactured in the United States of America
12   11   10   09   08   07   06   05   04
10   9   8   7   6   5   4   3   2   1

*To my father,*
*William A. Irvine*

# CONTENTS

# ACKNOWLEDGMENTS

Certain films speak to writers. Although I resisted watching *The Shining* again while working on this book, I could not help mentally replaying parts of *Julia*. There is a scene in which Lillian Hellman's character—pacing and smoking—finally grabs her typewriter and hurls it out the window. It is an immensely satisfying gesture. Shortly after the film's release, I heard Hellman speak at Radcliffe College, where someone asked her about that particular scene. "Garbage," she snapped, adding that no self-respecting writer would throw her typewriter out the window—she would throw herself out first. That, of course, would be the truer impulse (although I am sure that if Hellman had been writing in the computer age, her certainty about this might have weakened). In the end, nothing went out my study window, for which I have the pleasure of thanking many colleagues and friends.

I am particularly grateful to all the local and national activists who agreed to be interviewed for this book. In many cases they welcomed me into their homes, spent hours talking with me, and often gave me stacks of their files. Especially generous was Bobbie Whitney, a leader in the sex education field, who had just taken sick leave from her job at the Board of Education of the City of New York when I phoned her about this project. She returned to work in order to meet with me, giving me access to files on the *Children of the Rainbow* teacher's guide. Her enthusiastic support at this early phase of my research was crucial, and her death has left a void among advocates for young people.

Deb Tolman, who conducted an extended oral history in the late eighties with Mary Calderone, founder of the Sexuality Information and Education Council of the United States (SIECUS), generously gave me access to those transcripts. This book is much richer as a result. Chip Berlet, Sarah Cunningham, Mike McGee, Renee Romano, Marc Steinberg, Brian Wilcox, and Susan Wilson all kindly sent me their own unpublished manuscripts on related topics. Mary Bonauto, Liz Galst, Barbara Huberman, Konstance McCaffree, Louise Rice, and Gayle Rubin gave me key documents that enriched this book. Jeanne Blake provided me with a copy of her video *What Works: Sexuality Education.* Jo Ann Gasper mailed me the entire file of her newsletters, *The Right Woman.* Harold Shurtleff of the John Birch Society gave me important Society documents from the sixties.

The staffs at the Schlesinger Library, SIECUS (in particular Martha Kempner, William Smith, and Leslie Kantor, who is now at Planned Parenthood of New York City), the Reproductive Freedom Project of the American Civil Liberties Union (ACLU), and the Center for Reproductive Law and Policy were all extremely helpful and patient throughout my research. Thanks also to William Martin at Rice University and to Lumiere Productions for making available to me interviews conducted for the documentary *With God on Our Side: The Rise of the Religious Right in America.* The staff at Political Research Associates provided invaluable information and support during this project. Jean Hardisty, Chip Berlet, Surina Khan, and Jude Glaubman were consistently responsive to my interruptions.

I was fortunate to have received a Rockefeller Fellowship for 1994–95 from the Center for Lesbian and Gay Studies (CLAGS) at the City University of New York. My thanks to Martin Duberman for his vision and to the others at CLAGS for their support. Valerie Barr and Susan Yohn provided far more than housing that year, offering friendship, food, and those crucial subway directions.

I am extremely grateful for the generosity of colleagues and friends who read all or parts of the manuscript, in some cases several times: Chip Berlet, Peggy Brick, Barbara Cruikshank, Naomi Gerstel, Jean Hardisty, Margaret Hunt, Carolyn Stack, Jackie Urla, Carole Vance, Nancy Whittier, and Robert Zussman. Their insights and criticisms were vital. Each of them knows, I hope, how much I value our particular conversations. Thanks also to Lauren Berlant for helpful comments on the chapter, "Doing It with Words," a version of which appeared in *Critical Inquiry*. I presented this work several times at my faculty seminar on sexuality studies. I am fortunate to have been part of wide-ranging discussions (and pool parties) with Lee Badgett, Barbara Cruikshank, Lisa Henderson, Margaret Hunt, Lynn Morgan, Kathy Peiss, and Jackie Urla. Thanks also to Martin Duberman, Kathy Peiss, and Margaret Hunt for crucial help at the last minute.

Special thanks to my agent, Sydelle Kramer, of Frances Goldin Literary Agency, for her sound advice and unwavering support for this book. I would not want to be without her guidance and humor. I appreciate Naomi Schneider's belief in the book and Annie Decker's help in navigating the inevitable snares of production. Randy Stokes and Gene Fisher repeatedly saved me from my computer, printer, and disks, none of which seemed to work as they should. During five years of writing, no problem was ever too trivial for me to call Judith Levine, who has been smart, funny, and consoling throughout. Cindy Cohen has been a sharp listener and a loving friend. Finally, all my love to Sam.

# PREFACE TO THE PAPERBACK EDITION

In 1992, as I began my field research into conflicts over sexuality education, I was riveted by what I found: community discussions that morphed into disagreements, then flared into furious public displays of feeling. I heard neighbors scream at each other and saw angry shoving outside of public meeting halls. School board members told me about receiving death threats. After a sex education foe collapsed from an anxiety attack while addressing an especially rancorous meeting, the tense minutes in the hushed school auditorium as he was carried out rank among the most dramatic in my research career. The adrenaline that buzzed throughout public meetings, all of us alert to what might trigger the next outburst, also kept me up into the night poring over my field notes. These were the sights, sounds, and feelings of community controversies, local dramas played out in the shadow of national politics.

Throughout the nineties, Americans fought long and hard over sex education, and the conflict was particularly visible at the local, community level. The Sexuality Information and Education Council of the United States (SIECUS), an advocacy organization that follows these debates, tracked more than eight hundred local controversies during the final decade of the twentieth century.[1] Like all acute emotionality, however, the intensity of these community battles waned. Consequently they dropped from the front pages of daily newspapers in the early years of the new century. Some journalists have asked me if sex education has become a non-issue. It has not; even though intense debate has cooled in some communities, controversies over sex education are not resolved. In fact, the actual number of local disputes vacillated through these years. SIECUS documented one hundred and twenty-two conflicts during the 1999–2000 school year. There were seventy-five in 2000–2001, sixty-two in 2001–2002, and the number jumped again to one hundred controversies throughout thirty-nine states during the 2002–2003 school year.

However, the number—or even ferocity—of local conflicts has never been the measure of sex education's progress in the United States. As *Talk about Sex* argues, local disputes about sex education have always been inextricably linked to national politics, in particular the nation's political shift to the right since the sixties. It is a shift that was, in fact, partially accomplished through a cultural politics of sexuality. In this book I describe the political transformations, cultural dynamics, and affective rhetorics that together helped ignite the passionate conflicts over sex education on both the national and local levels in the United States.

*Talk about Sex* links the last four decades of community controversies to the rise of the Christian Right through its emphasis on issues of sexuality. Although the emergence of the Christian Right is commonly dated at the late 1970s with the founding of groups like the Moral Majority and the rise of the pro-family movement, I tell the story of a powerful conservative and right-wing Christian presence in sexual politics a full decade earlier. The controversies over sex education in 1968–69 served as a bridge issue from the Old Right to the New Right.

Leaders of the early New Christian Right recognized that sexuality would prove a crucial tool for political mobilization. Since the sixties, religious conservatives have viewed sex education as a powerful vehicle by which to agitate parents, recruit constituents, raise money, and ultimately consolidate political power through election to school boards and other political positions. While local sex education debates revealed that there was a movement to be built around sexual politics, in turn, national Christian Right organizations shaped both the form and content of local discussions. *Talk about Sex* shows the ways in which discursive strategies designed to evoke intense public affect through provocative and stigmatizing sexual rhetoric have played an important role in igniting community battles.

The cultural power of secular and religious conservatives in sexual politics has only intensified in the early years of the twenty-first century. The efforts of national evangelical organizations such as the Traditional Values Coalition, Concerned Women for America, the American Family Association, and Focus on the Family—all of which oppose comprehensive sex education, abortion, sexual representation in the media, and gay rights—gained momentum on legislative and policy fronts during George W. Bush's administration. In the final chapter of this book, I discuss the myriad successes of these religious conservatives throughout the nineties in establishing abstinence-only sex education programs and opposing comprehensive programs. Since 2000, with conservative Republicans in control of both houses of Congress and the White House, advocates of abstinence-only sex education have advanced even more significantly on two related fronts: control over dissemination of sexuality information to the public; and control of federal funding for sexuality education and research. Both of these expansions of power have helped consolidate conservative control over the terms of public debate about sexuality.

Access to sexual knowledge shrank in the public domain during the first years of the new century. For example, only 2 percent of public school teachers in 1988, compared with 23 percent in 1999, taught abstinence as the sole means for control of pregnancy and sexually transmitted diseases. A poll of schools in September, 2003 indicated a sharp increase to 30 percent among instructors who taught abstinence only and did not provide information about condoms and other contraceptives.[2] Moreover, the Bush Administration's control over sexuality information reached beyond the public schools to include federal Websites. For example, the Centers for Disease Control removed a posting it had run since 1992—"Programs That Work"—listing sex education curricula of proven effectiveness. All were comprehensive programs. In October, 2002, the CDC replaced an online fact sheet on the effectiveness of latex condom use for disease prevention with one that deleted instruction on condom use and efficacy. Significantly, the revised sheet also omitted data that showed that sex education does not lead to increased sexual behavior.[3] In addition, the Website for the National Institutes for Health (NIH) removed the widely substantiated finding from the National Cancer Institute that abortions do not increase the risk of breast cancer.

Sexuality research also came under attack. In May 2003, the *New York*

*Times* reported that Health and Human Services (HHS) might apply "unusual scrutiny" to grants with key words such as *gay, sex worker, anal sex,* and *men who sleep with men.*[4] By fall, 2003, NIH launched a review of 160 academic studies, most of them peer-reviewed projects involving HIV/AIDS and sexuality research, after the evangelical organization, the Traditional Values Coalition, and a few Republican Congressmen complained that the research was a waste of taxpayer money.[5] These initiatives prompted anger and opposition from many scientists, politicians, and activists. For example, U.S. Representative Henry Waxman (D-CA) investigated what he termed the Bush Administration's promotion of ideology over science. Waxman, as Ranking Member of the Committee on Government Reform, wrote to Tommy Thompson, the Secretary of Health and Human Services stating that the administration was censoring government Websites to conform with its own moral stance.[6] Waxman also called the NIH investigation into sexuality and HIV/AIDS research "scientific McCarthyism."

During the Bush administration, the allocation and monitoring of federal funds became a vehicle by which conservatives advanced their vision of appropriate sexuality education and research. Government funding for abstinence-only-until-marriage programs massively increased. The Adolescent Family Life Act, which had launched the abstinence-only movement in 1981, was a small demonstration project that was never fully funded. Congress appropriated $10.9 million for it in 1982. By contrast, Congress spent over $120 million in 2003 for abstinence-only-until-marriage programs, with an additional $37.5 million in state matching funds funneled to these programs. In a related appeal to social conservatives in the 2004 election year, Bush earmarked $1.5 billion in his 2005 budget, to be spread over five years, for marriage-promotion projects, mostly aimed at the poor. As of this writing, the Family Life Education Act, a bill introduced in 2001 to allocate $100 million for comprehensive sex education, has failed to pass.

While allocating disproportionately greater funding for abstinence-only compared with comprehensive sex education, the Bush administration scrutinized the latter far more scrupulously and often than the former. Non-profit organizations dedicated to comprehensive sexuality and AIDS education, such as SIECUS and Advocates for Youth, found themselves subjected to multiple government financial audits in the early years of the decade. SIECUS, for example, was audited twice in 2003, while Advocates for Youth was audited three times in under a year. Neither organization had ever been audited before, despite ten and eighteen years, respectively, of receiving federal funds. The San Francisco organization STOP AIDS underwent three federal audits in ten months. The media reported suspicions that such audits were politically motivated. For example, the *Washington Post* published a leaked email in which an ordained Catholic deacon working in the Department of Health and Human Services suggested that HHS Secretary Tommy Thompson might object to Advocates for Youth's programs, saying, "You should know that the secretary is a devout Roman Catholic."[7] The email message described Advocates as "ardent critics of the Bush Administration," apparently because of the organization's criticisms of administration policies prohibiting funding to international agencies that discuss abortion.[8] Salon.com reported that STOP AIDS was repeatedly audited after activists booed HHS Secretary Tommy Thompson at an AIDS conference, while SIECUS was audited after creating an educational Website (No New Money) urging an end to the sharp increase in federal funding of unproven abstinence-only programs.[9] No irregularities were found in any of these audits of comprehensive programs. However, the *Washington Post* reported that a number of abstinence-only grantees illegally used federal money for programs that taught scripture and funded prayer vigils at abortion clinics.[10]

*Talk about Sex* shows a national dimension in the ways by which communities fought about sex education. Conservative religious activists on the national level came to dominate the public conversation on sex education through discursive strategies that triggered the fierce emotionality of local political debates. My perspective on these local battles shifted during the course of this project. Initially the fighting and vitriol struck me as spontaneous irruptions of community disagreement. Then I began to discern striking similarities in both form and content of local sex education arguments. It was as if there were a national script for sex education debates, rendering every unhappy community unhappy in precisely the same way. I had anticipated, and found, the same eerie uniformity in the cognitive dimension of my field research, for example in some routinized interview accounts by social movement activists of their beliefs and motivations.[11] I had been less alert to the affective dynamics of communities in conflict until I heard so many citizens expressing the same feelings in precisely the same ways. Whereas early on I had thought volatile emotions were inconsequential compared to the rational terms of political debate, gradually I understood that the affective dimension was significant in its own right, requiring analysis and theorization. I began to recognize community battles as the fruit of political strategy and tactics. The political dimension of collective emotionality, and the affective qualities of sexual discourse, became central research questions, the themes of this book.

This book shows that the discursive strategies of national Christian Right organizations acted as a key trigger of volatile sex education controversies in the late sixties and throughout the nineties. National discourses of sexual danger and depravity shaped the ways citizens in localities throughout the U.S. spoke and felt about sex education. The vocabularies and symbols of sex education discourses are crucial to the production of bitter public conflicts. Provocative sexual language and graphic symbols could exacerbate anxieties, amplifying local confusion about a sex education program into civic brawls.

Social conservatives continue to employ the rhetorical strategies that I detail in this book, such as inflammatory terms and images, misleading information, and depravity narratives—all designed to play on broad public anxieties about sexuality. For example, in 2002 the allegation by Hal Wallis of the Physicians Consortium that comprehensive sex education programs "promote all kinds of deviant sexuality—bondage and all types of bizarre sexual behavior" was widely promulgated by prominent national evangelical organizations like Focus on the Family.[12] The terms by which national organizations describe safer-sex and comprehensive-sex education, such as "pornography" and "vulgar,"[13] continued to appear in local conflicts, for example when parents in Kohala, Hawaii criticized a brochure from the *Weekly Reader* series *Current Health* used during the 2002–2003 school year as "lewd," "licentious," and "pornographic."[14] Finally, further evidence surfaced for my argument that it is religious conservatives themselves who disseminate the explicit material they attempt to censor. For example, in December, 2003, a Roman Catholic diocese in Pennsylvania ordered one of its own priests to stop distributing the anti-gay sex brochure, "Medical Consequences of What Homosexuals Do," saying that it "borders on the pornographic."[15] The pamphlet, which was authored by Paul Cameron of the Family Research Institute (whose controversial and methodologically problematic research I discuss in chapter 8), graphically describes sexual activities such as contact with urine and feces.

Dynamic transformations in the sexual culture fuel conflicts over sex education, so it was not surprising that sexual orientation was the subject of intense controversy in public schools during the early years of the new century. By 2003, two historic court decisions moved gay rights to ground zero in the culture wars over sexuality. In June, 2003, in *Lawrence v. Texas*, the Supreme Court struck down Texas sodomy laws, establishing important new protections for private sexual behavior. Likewise, the Massachusetts Supreme Judicial Court ruled in November, 2003 that same-sex couples are legally entitled to wed under the state constitution. Conservative Christian political organizations promptly condemned both decisions, taking actions consistent with their initiatives against sex education discussed in this book. Again, national Christian Right organizations entered local debates. For example, the Colorado-based evangelical group Focus on the Family launched a major campaign in Massachusetts to organize clergy in overturning that state's gay marriage ruling.[16] As they did in the sexuality education debates, conservative activists threatened that children would be harmed by access to sexual information or expansion of sexual rights. After *Lawrence*, Robert Knight, of the Culture and Family Institute and the Heritage Foundation, warned that the court's decision would result in schoolchildren being taught "that homosexual sodomy is the same as marital sex."[17] Not surprisingly, SIECUS found that sexual orientation was at the epicenter of school controversies during the 2002–2003 school year.[18]

This book's central question is: how and why do public conversations about sex education become so divided and turn so furious, when most citizens repeatedly express overwhelming support for comprehensive public school programs? Intensely emotional community battles over sex education, I suggest, are prompted by the feeling rules and expression rules[19] that in part constitute the provocative discourses of sex education's religiously conservative opponents. They manifest the social and political roots of collective emotional performativity. These conflicts are not random or spontaneous, but rather are extremely responsive to discursive cues. Sex education battles are not incidental to the political regulation of sexuality. They are central. Far from irrational, these episodic hostilities reveal the deep normativity of emotion and its expression, an ideal feature for its collective mobilization in moral politics. In short, citizens through the 1990s fought with each other over sex education in public affective displays that themselves operated as part of the social control of sexuality.

*Talk about Sex* recounts the success of a movement of social and religious conservatives at limiting comprehensive sex education through discursive strategies that include misrepresentation and distortion of sexual information. In these pages, conservative sex education foes voice their own arguments and points of view. Sometimes they sound unpleasant—they use inflammatory language, they make sexually stigmatizing accusations against their opponents, and they are caught in misrepresentations and lies. These strategies are not unique to sex education debates; rather, the broader political landscape has always shaped the discursive politics of sex education. Since this book's initial publication, public concern about the integrity of government discourse spiked as a result of allegations involving possible cover-ups, distortions, and lies by the George W. Bush administration concerning issues of public significance such as those about the war in Iraq and the economic impact of deep tax cuts. Amid dozens of popular books released in 2003 on the veracity of current political discourse, several of them by progressives—for example Joe Conason's *Big Lies: The Right-Wing Propaganda Machine and How It Distorts the Truth* and Al Franken's *Lies and the Lying Liars Who Tell Them*—alleged serious deceptions by conservatives in government and the media.[20] Non-partisan organizations also weighed in, such as the Carnegie Endowment for International Peace, which issued a report concluding that the Bush administration systematically misrepresented the threat from Iraq and the existence of weapons of mass destruction.[21] In addition, a broad range of citizens, including scientists, academics, and health activists and researchers, decried political interference with scientific research and manipulation of research data by the Bush administration.[22]

This book raises similar issues about sexual knowledge, politics, and discourse, with their attendant consequences for democracy and citizenship. *Talk about Sex* recounts the history of how conservatives have used volatile sexual rhetoric—rhetoric that I show is often misleading and sometimes deceptive—in order to build a movement, capture the terms of public debate, and reshape the sexual culture according to their own vision. In many respects, this political transformation has reached its culmination in the early years of the twenty-first century under the Bush administration. However, one of the most powerful lessons of the sex education controversies concerns the unpredictability of political speech. This book is about political dominance, but it is also about resistances, reversals, and backlashes by citizens on both the local and national levels, which suggests that conservative control over sexuality education is formidable but not inevitable or irrevocable.

## NOTES

1. The "actual" number is most likely much higher. SIECUS did not track debates in the early nineties, plus once it began following local conflicts it largely relied on media coverage of such controversies.

2. "Sex Education in America." A poll jointly conducted by the Kaiser Family Foundation, National Public Radio, and Harvard University's Kennedy School. Released in January, 2004. See www.kff.org.

3. See "Condom Effectiveness," www.house.gov/reform/min/politicsand science/.

4. Erica Goode, "Certain Words Can Trip Up AIDS Grants, Scientists Say," *New York Times*, 18 April 2003. A10.

5. Jeffrey Brainard, "NIH Begins Review of Studies That Were Questioned at a Congressional Hearing," *The Chronicle of Higher Education*, 7 November 2003, A24. The Traditional Values Coalition document, titled "HHS Grant Projects," listed some of its specific objections next to the studies it condemned, such as "endorses sexual behavior and condom use among teens," and "awarded to abortionist." NIH contacted all of the 160 researchers to inform them of potential congressional investigation. Subsequently, the House Energy and Commerce Committee claimed it had never intended to scrutinize this entire group of researchers and had only intended an investigation into ten studies. Thirty-five scientific organizations, such as the American Public Health Association, the American Association for the Advancement of Science, and the American Sociological Association, signed a statement supporting the peer-review process at NIH and criticizing ideological interference with research on sexuality and HIV/AIDS.

6.  See "Politics and Science in the Bush Administration" a report and website by Henry A. Waxman, investigating the Bush Administration's interference with scientific research: www.house.gov/reform/min/politics andscience/.

7.  Ceci Connolly, "Administration Promoting Abstinence; Family Planning Efforts Are Being Scaled Back," *The Washington Post*, A01.

8.  Ibid.

9.  Christopher Healy, "No Sex, Please—Or We'll Audit You," Salon.com.

10.  Ceci Connolly, "Judge Orders Changes in Abstinence Program; LA Groups Found to Be Promoting Religion," *The Washington Post*, 26 July, 2002, A03.

11.  Over several years I visited communities, conducted interviews, attended public meetings, maintained telephone connections with contacts in several cities, combed media reports, and analyzed film clips of distant town meetings. Both seasoned activists and neophytes not uncommonly repeated national Christian Right rhetoric right down to the exact same stories, sentences, and even phrases. Often I recognized material as verbatim quotes from the documents of national Christian Right groups. At times, reading the local documents from widely diverse communities was like grading papers from a course in which every student had plagiarized from the same text, right down to the typos. This is a not uncommon experience of field research with social movements, and Kathleen Blee has also discussed this phenomenon in relation to her work with organized racist groups in the U.S. (Kathleen M. Blee. *Inside Organized Racism: Women in the Hate Movement*. Berkeley: University of California Press, 2002). Such homogenization of discussion about sexuality education is an important indication of how national organizations can authorize particular ways of thinking and talking through discourses. Significantly, I argue that these national discourses can also evoke routinized feelings and emotional expressions in local community debates.

12.  Stuart Shepard and Pete Winn, "Vulgar 'Safe-Sex' Programs Threaten Abstinence-Funding," Citizen Link, a Web Site of Focus on the Family, 10 April, 2002.

13.  Ibid; also see Robert E. Recotor, "When Sex Ed Becomes Porn 101," The Heritage Foundation, 27 August, 2003.

14.  Myra Batchelder, "Trends 2002–2003: A Tug-Of-War Between Abstinence-Only and Comprehensive Sexuality Education," *The SIECUS Report*, Vol. 31, 2003, 6.

15. "Priest is Told to Discard an Antigay Pamphlet," *The Boston Globe*, 11 December, 2003, A2; The Associated Press, "Diocese Tells Priest to Stop Distributing Anti-gay Sex Pamphlet," NEPA News, 10 December, 2003.

16. Raphael Lewis, "Christian Group Sets Mass. Clergy Sessions Against Gay Marriage," *The Boston Globe*, 16 December, 2003, B5.

17. "Supreme Court Strikes Down Texas Sodomy Law," CNN.com, November 18, 2003.

18. Myra Batchelder, "Trends 2002–2003: A Tug-of-War Between Abstinence-Only and Comprehensive Sexuality Education." *SIECUS Report*, Vol. 31, Fall, 2003, 5–14.

19. Arlie Hochschild's research on the commercialization of feeling has been indispensable to my work on the politicization of emotion. For a discussion of feeling rules and expression rules, see Arlie Russell Hochschild, *The Commercialization of Intimate Life* (Berkeley: University of California Press, 2003).

20. These also include Jim Hightower's *Thieves in High Places: They've Stolen Our Country—And It's Time to Take It Back* and Molly Ivin's *Bushwacked: Life in George W. Bush's America*. It was striking that so many books by progressives inhabited the best-seller lists after years of dominance by conservatives.

21. See www.ceip.org.

22. In an anonymous essay released in October, 2003, a senior scientist at NIH called for public scrutiny of alleged Bush administration "frontal attacks" on NIH and "science itself." See Henry A. Waxman's site, www.house.gov/reform/min/politicsandscience/. See also Jeffrey Brainard, "How Sound Is Bush's 'Sound Science'?: Leading Scientists Say the White House Distorts Research Data to Meet Its Policy Goals," *The Chronicle of Higher Education*, 5 March, 2004, A18.

In December 1994, Surgeon General Joycelyn Elders was fired for suggesting that it might be beneficial to teach children about masturbation as part of sex education. Elders, who did not raise the issue herself, replied to a question at an AIDS forum about whether she thought masturbation could be more openly discussed: "I think that it is something that's part of human sexuality and it's part of something that perhaps should be taught. But we've not even taught our children the very basics. And I feel that we have tried ignorance for a very long time and it's time we try education."[1] She was asked to resign almost immediately. Although Elders might easily have been dismissed for any one of her other controversial statements about welfare or drug policy, she was instead fired for speaking about sex education. This is not simply coincidence. Elders's dismissal was widely understood as President Clinton's conciliatory gesture to hardline conservative Republicans who had just swept Congress, a group for whom "family values" has been an important organizing theme. It is a political cohort which, since the sixties, has made it risky to speak out on behalf of sexuality education.

Initiatives to protect children from exposure to allegedly corrupting sex talk, whether from sex education programs or the media, are central to conservative cultural politics. A few years after Elders was fired, however, the Republican "managers" of Clinton's impeachment made public the sexually explicit details of the president's affair with White House intern Monica Lewinsky. Significantly, they posted the Starr Report on the Internet. Suddenly sexual narratives about the cigar, fellatio, and masturbation were widely available to young people at the simple click of a mouse. The irony was heightened by the fact that in 1996 a coalition of legislators, including House Judiciary Committee Chairman Henry Hyde, who oversaw the impeachment, and major Christian Right leaders such as Ralph Reed of the Christian Coalition, had advocated legislation that would impose strict criminal penalties against anyone using computer technology to distribute "obscenity to anyone or indecency to children."[2] Had this legislation stood, those responsible for placing independent counsel Kenneth W. Starr's report on the Internet might have been arrested and imprisoned. Even so, their support of Starr left social conservatives in an awkward position. It did not go unnoticed that the movement that called for restoring "traditional" sexual morality through restricting what can be said to young people was itself responsible for the widespread public dissemination of frank sexual detail.

During these years, meanwhile, sex education conflicts raged throughout the nation. Hundreds of American communities suffered acrimonious battles over what to teach in the public schools about sexuality. Mistrust and anger suffused these communities. During fiery debates, neighbors accused their opponents of "fascism" or "McCarthyism." Sometimes violence erupted. Like implacable Hollywood screen monsters, these conflicts would not die. They have, in fact, persisted since the late sixties. In part, sex education battles reflect different moral visions of the sort that have divided Americans over issues such as abortion and gay rights. However, volatile sex education conflicts cannot be wholly explained as the result of polarized worldviews, for, as we shall see, most Americans claim to support comprehensive sexuality education.

This book will show that recursive sex education battles are of a piece with a major transformation of national American politics, rooted in the sixties, wherein the right wing came to dominate the political arena by the end of the century. The rise of the Right did not simply trigger bitter conflicts over sexuality; it was partly accomplished through them. I approach these contemporary debates over sex education as a form of discursive politics[3]—national and local contests over how we think, talk, and feel about sexuality. Their history is the subject of this book.

Critic Samuel R. Delany has said, "To explore a discourse is inevitably to tell a story: at such and such a time, people did this and that; thus they thought and felt one thing and another."[4] In that tradition, this book tells a story of contemporary sex education controversies, a story about individuals, their communities, political movements, and national organizations (see On Methods and Terminology at the end of this book). In particular, this story explores how battles over sex education have been central in the rise to political power of an amalgam of conservative Catholics and right-wing evangelical Christians. It describes a paradox by which social conservatives, who advocate the restriction of sexual speech, have themselves heavily relied on public talk about sex in order to build a movement and mobilize supporters. In so doing, they now figure as one of the most visible and vocal cohorts in our national sexual culture.

Conservative opponents of comprehensive sex education have scored an impressive political victory. They have paralyzed countless community debates and constrained programs nationwide, despite widespread support for sex education, public discomfort with political extremism, and mistrust of Christian fundamentalism. By popularizing a public vocabulary framing sex education as radical, dangerous, and immoral, they have fostered the climate in which Elders, along with scores of professionals before and after her, have suffered reprisals for speaking in support of sexuality education.

Like Elders's firing, this is a story about sex, politics, and words. It examines the historical evolution of national Christian Right sex education discourses and how they shape local community debates. It is also a story about emotions, for if ways of talking help turn community debates into pitched battles, they do so through evoking passionate feelings. I will argue that emotional conventions are a crucial aspect of discursive politics and that local conflicts over sex education are highly volatile events in which emotions are politicized. While acknowledging the important particularities of grassroots politics, this story nonetheless suggests a nationalizing influence on local public arguments about sexuality. As a school board chair in one community said about a disruptive sex education opponent, "Somebody's giving him words." It turned out that she was right. And as we shall see, those words—and the feelings they can evoke in community debates—have shaped the history of sex education in the United States.

.    .    .

Sex education breaks a silence. It introduces talk about sex into the regulated public space of the school. Classroom discussion of sexuality unfolds in a historical context, and ours is one of unprecedented access to sexual representation. There has been perhaps no more profound change in our sexual culture over the past century than the increasing openness of sexual speech and the visibility of sexual images. Restrictions on what can be spoken publicly have eroded. When a pundit in the early twentieth century proclaimed it "Sex O'Clock in America,"[5] he was lamenting a new era of the public discussion of prostitution and venereal disease; by the late twentieth century, conservative critics of popular entertainment were decrying expressions such as "fuck" in movies and "piss off" on television.[6] Rob and Laura's twin beds on the sixties' *Dick Van Dyke Show* are quaint nostalgia in an era in which one in ten television programs includes portrayals of sexual intercourse.[7] Formerly invisible sexual minorities—such as bisexuals, gay men, lesbians, and transpersons—now occupy prominent media roles. The emergence of new communication technologies like the Internet has further expanded the boundaries of public sexual speech, a development subject to much debate.

However, talk about sex in the public realm is consistently met with ambivalence and outright efforts to contain and silence it. After all, Elders was fired for a speech act, not a sexual act, which is significant in Washington, D.C., a town with so many sex scandals that it is wryly dubbed Sodom on the Potomac. Elders did not masturbate in public; she was fired for discussing how teachers might talk about masturbation. The fear that sexual language will trigger social chaos has historically fueled initiatives to regulate sexual speech. Sex education has been at the center of these conflicts.

Since the sixties, as openness about sexuality in popular culture has intensified, U.S. communities have fought over whether to allow discussions about sexual topics in the classroom. At stake is what is in the best interest of young people. Recently, a young woman was arrested in Massachusetts, my home state, for abandoning the newborn she delivered in a ladies' room stall at Boston's Logan Airport. The baby was found in the toilet, barely alive. Although the case was eventually settled out of court, she had faced seven years in prison if convicted at trial. A former high school honors student, she at first claimed she did not know she was pregnant. Although untrue, her claim was not improbable. A recent study of teenagers between ages twelve and sixteen found a striking lack of knowledge about sexuality.[8] (For example, almost three-quarters of them believed that letting semen drip out of the vagina after intercourse prevents pregnancy. Almost one-quarter believed that a girl does not need birth control if she only has occasional intercourse. Seventy percent did not know that douching is not a contraceptive method. Of the seventy-five test items, the teenagers scored, on average, only 40 percent correct.) At the young woman's arraignment, the prosecutor argued that her actions were completely preventable, by which he meant that she should have called airport security after delivering the baby. Many people would claim that prevention might better have taken place much earlier. But consensus breaks down over the question of how best to prevent such tragedies: More comprehensive education about reproductive sexuality and broader access to birth control? Or an emphasis on abstinence until marriage with few other details—especially details about contraception—so as not to give young people a mixed message? More or less talk with young people about sexuality?

Given the opportunity for open discussion, young people display an indefatigable sexual curiosity. In the sixties, two sex educators compiled a sample of anonymous questions written by public school students in sex education programs. They ranged from the physiological ("How long before [a] boy's period? How long does it last . . . ?"); to the hygienic ("When boys have wet dreams, do they use such things like napkins of some sort? If it happens during the day, what do they do?"); to the familial ("Why are parents so stupid?"); to technique ("I read in a medical book that during sexual intercourse that the woman's conclusion takes longer than mens', also that during the time you should change the subject and talk about the walls or curtains in the room. What does this mean [especially the conclusion]? And how do you know when the end comes?"); and finally, to the existential ("Why do you ever need sex?").[9] The pragmatic educators knew that adults might be shocked by such questions but, they insisted, "the shock is of reality and the teacher must prepare himself to deal with it."[10] Decades later, teenagers' anonymous questions reflected sweeping cultural and stylistic changes ("Is oral sex better with a tongue piercing?"[11]), while others were seemingly timeless ("How do you have sex?"[12]). At the turn of the twenty-first century, broad civic arguments persist over the appropriateness of answering—even giving young people the opportunity to ask—such sexual questions.

Talk about sex has a long history of trouble in America. Sex education's story is part of long-standing efforts to regulate sexual morality through control of sexual speech.[13] Since at least the mid nineteenth century, coalitions of evangelical Protestant clergy and middle-class women activists have crusaded for social purity. At that time, concerns over prostitution and venereal diseases renewed calls for a spiritual, romanticized sexual bond between husband and wife, an elimination of the double standard, and curbs on male lust and out-of-control sexuality. The first calls for school sex education came in the early twentieth century from a disparate group of moral reformers including suffragists, clergy, temperance workers, and physicians dedicated to eliminating venereal disease. While disagreeing among themselves about the content and purpose of sex education, they nonetheless comprised a relatively unified front arguing for public speech against the restrictive measures of vice crusaders such as Anthony Comstock. Unlike Comstock, who sought state restriction of virtually all public sexual discourse including sex education and contraception information, social purity activists advocated an end to the conspiracy of silence—physicians' phrase for the Victorian propriety that made public discussion of sex impossible. Nineteenth-century activists argued that women should openly teach their children "the sanctities and the terrors of this awful power of sex,"[14] while social hygienists in the early twentieth century endorsed sex education in the schools as a way to combat venereal disease. As historians John D'Emilio and Estelle Freedman make clear, regulation of sex was central to both vice crusaders and social purity activists. They disagreed profoundly, however, over whether this was best achieved through the restriction or expansion of public sexual speech.[15]

Contemporary debates about sex education echo this tension between opening or restricting public sexual discussion. In the early sixties a loose coalition of professional advocates, educators, parents, and others constituted a movement for "getting troubling concepts into the open."[16] The Sex Information and Education Council of the United States (SIECUS), founded in 1964, has since been the institutional voice of this perspective. SIECUS has pioneered a model for comprehensive sexuality education in which young people would receive, from kindergarten through high school, age-appropriate information on a range of topics such as human reproduction, anatomy, physiology, and sexually transmitted infections as well as issues including masturbation and homosexuality. Comprehensive sexuality education would offer young people the opportunity to discuss sexual values and attitudes in the classroom.[17] Advocates of comprehensive sex education endorse what they consider the therapeutic potential of frank sexual discussion in the classroom. They believe, like Joycelyn Elders, that silence has fostered ignorance, shame, and social problems like teen pregnancy. Supporters of comprehensive sexuality education view sexuality as positive and healthy, and they typically support gender equality and acceptance of sexual diversity. Comprehensive sexuality education stresses abstinence for youth, and it also provides information on contraception and abortion.

Conservative critics decry this openness as misguided and irresponsible. Sexual intercourse, in their opinion, should be confined to marriage. They favor restrictions on other sexualities, such as masturbation or homosexuality, and they often oppose feminism and the gay rights movement. Sexual discussion with young people about topics like contraception, in their view, has led to high levels of adolescent sexual activity, teenage pregnancy, and sexually transmitted diseases. These critics believe, therefore, that if we talk to young people about sexuality, it should be restricted so as not to lead to destructive and immoral thoughts and behavior. Controlling or eliminating sexual discussion best allows for the protection of young people and the preservation of sexual morality. Not surprisingly, this group has fought comprehensive sexuality education. Conservative Catholics, along with Christian evangelicals and fundamentalists, have founded myriad political organizations to regulate sex education as one route toward restoring "traditional values" of sexuality, gender, and the family. These activists and their institutions comprise part of the Christian Right, and opposition to sex education has, since the sixties, helped build their movement.

These two positions represent very real differences in moral vision among some Americans. Sociologist James Davison Hunter describes these competing worldviews as "the impulse toward orthodoxy and the impulse toward progressivism."[18] Yet there is a large and complicated middle ground. Many scholars of political attitudes agree that Americans tend to know little about public affairs, and quickly forget what, for a time, they do know.[19] So too, regarding sex education in local communities, some people have not thought very much about it and have no idea what their schools are teaching. Others might be religiously or politically predisposed toward one point of view but are confused about a particular program. Some parents I spoke with held seemingly incongruent opinions, for example, favoring instruction about homosexuality but not contraception. Personal experiences can shape such disparities, as, for example, the mother of a gay son who supports the inclusion of gay issues in the curriculum but not abortion. Attitudes about sexuality and sex education, like political attitudes in general, are frequently fluid, changing according to circumstances in local debates.[20] This book is not a community study about how average parents negotiate a path through this highly fraught terrain. Rather, it shows how national advocacy organizations have scripted the public conversation on sex education through rhetorical frames which organize ambivalence, confusion, and anxieties into tidy sound bites designed for mass mobilization. Nuanced argument drops out of this process.[21]

Local sex education politics, then, pose an intriguing dilemma. On the one hand, most people tell pollsters they broadly support sex education. On the other hand, communities across the country have divided in angry struggles over the issue. Indeed, the degree of consensus that citizens publicly report about their attitudes toward sex education is striking, even in embattled communities. Public opinion polls since the sixties have consistently shown widespread support for sex education.[22] A 2000 poll sponsored by the Henry J. Kaiser Family Foundation indicated that by a large majority, parents want their children to have *more* classroom hours of sex education that covers more "sensitive topics" than such programs currently do.[23] A 1998 national poll found that 87 percent of Americans supported sexuality education in the public schools, and a poll commissioned by SIECUS and Advocates for Youth found that 89 percent believe that, along with abstinence, young people should also have information about contraception and STD prevention.[24] Given this popular consensus about sex education, how then can we understand the bitter controversies that have swept communities throughout the nation? How is it that comprehensive sexuality education, which has always been a quite moderate enterprise in public schools, has come to be portrayed as dangerous and immoral?

The answer is that the organized move for sex education in the public schools emerged at the exact moment in which American political life was beginning what would be a profound restructuring. Sex education would play a significant role in that transformation. In 1964, the year SIECUS was founded and Barry Goldwater was defeated, it seemed that Americans agreed on such basic political axioms as the role of the federal government in ensuring the economic welfare, health, and civil rights of its citizens. By the end of the decade, however, the divisions were becoming clearer; the liberal consensus had collapsed. The bitter disputes nationwide over sex education in 1968 and 1969 were evidence of those fault lines. Since the seventies, the nation's political center has shifted to the right, as conservative Republicans, the New Right, and the Christian Right have captured political power.[25] Along with traditional right-wing interests such as global anti-communism and protection of free market capitalism, issues related to sexuality have been at the center of political battles. Opposition to sex education was a bridge issue between the Old Right and the New Right.

National culture wars erupted on the local level in such forms as community conflicts over sex education. The term "culture wars" refers to a bruising set of conflicts launched by secular and religious conservatives in the eighties.[26] They are the now familiar battles over issues such as multiculturalism, school prayer, and homosexuality. Culture wars are efforts at moral regulation, as expressed by Pat Buchanan in his address to the 1992 Republican National Convention: "There is a religious war going on in this country. It is a culture war as critical to the kind of nation we shall be as the Cold War itself, for this war is for the soul of America."[27] Rooted in a longer history of social traditionalism, the strategy of organizing around values and lifestyles rather than economics and foreign policy was explicitly articulated back in the mid-eighties by Paul Weyrich of the Free Congress Research and Education Foundation, who called for a new politics of "cultural conservatism."[28] Reform of key social institutions such as the family, the media, and education became the cornerstone of cultural conservatism, most important for the Christian Right and neoconservatives who want to "recapture the culture" from what they see as the corrupting influence of liberalism.[29] Conservative activists built a vast infrastructure of think tanks, political organizations, media centers, legal groups, and, as I shall show, even their own alternative sexuality industry to advance their social and moral vision. By the end of the twentieth century, conservative efforts at restriction of sexual speech had targeted areas including pornography, the public funding of art with sexual themes, discussions of abortion in federally funded health clinics, sexual content on television, and sexuality and AIDS education. Sex education is a site on which social conservatives have vigorously fought for the establishment of their own programs and policies in public education.

The discursive politics of sex education come alive in how Americans debate what young people should learn in the public schools. Passionate local debates tend to be read as though they are spontaneous, indigenous uprisings of outraged citizens. But they are not simply that. Rather, they are profoundly shaped by national political rhetorics. Conservative national advocacy organizations and political movements, as this book shows, have been actively committed to shaping sexual values and influencing educational policies in communities across the country. When the right wing came to dominate the political arena by the end of the twentieth century, it captured the terms of debate about a range of sexual issues through strategic use of culturally powerful language and images. Although opponents of sexuality education are not all conservative or evangelical Christians, these ways of talking became idiomatic and were adopted by local activists for a range of reasons. In her study of local debates over gay rights, for example, sociologist Arlene Stein shows how residents adopted profoundly anti-gay rhetoric as an expression of a range of concerns, including fears of diversity and economic decline.[30] National vocabularies operate as scripts which are repeated at town meetings, school board hearings, and local media debates, and reproduced in locally produced materials. Although they are political arguments, these national rhetorics take on lives of their own to become accepted "facts." The successful establishment of a public vocabulary framing sex education as evil and salacious has been crucial to a process by which conservative Catholics and evangelical Christians have curtailed such programs nationwide.

A focus of this book is how conservative sex education opponents talk about sex in these debates. It matters how a social movement talks. In part, words, phrases, narratives, and symbols comprise the expressive elements of discursive politics. They are culturally powerful because they naturalize particular sets of meanings and because they are central in constituting our sense of a social world. Language is increasingly recognized as critical to political movements because ways of talking exercise a powerful effect on the process of social change.[31] Capturing the terms of debate diffuses a movement's own political worldview as common knowledge. Once a social movement establishes its own terms in public discourse, as sociologist William Gamson notes, it is exceedingly difficult for even opponents to avoid using them without risking confusion in listeners.[32]

Moreover, vocabularies of protest can inspire and mobilize supporters. They can persuade the indifferent or the reluctant by scaring or outraging them. Social movements can also shape individuals' action through reshaping cultural codes, so that people can be mobilized not necessarily because they have been persuaded to adopt a worldview that animates them, but rather because they understand the codes by which their actions will be interpreted by others.[33] The establishment of a public vocabulary is crucial to this process. Battles over sex education take place within language; their outcomes are shaped by language. Language practices are, therefore, an important domain of political and social change.

There are two rhetorical modes through which the Christian Right engages in sex education debates. The first is oppositional. Oppositional speech dates back to the late sixties, when newly organizing conservative and evangelical Christians opposed the early efforts of sex educators. In oppositional speech, conservatives seek to eliminate a sex education program or a particular curriculum by associating it with a specific set of negative and frightening meanings. This discourse frames sex education and sex educators themselves as dangerous or depraved and plays to historical anxieties about sex. By secularizing their claims about sex education, opponents have both sidestepped public suspicion of religious incursions into public schools and helped foster the acceptance of national political rhetoric as common, taken-for-granted knowledge. Oppositional speech is paradoxical. While I refer to it as evocative or even inflammatory, it incites public arguments while at the same time flattening their complexity. Community debates, even when explosive, come to sound formulaic and scripted.

The second mode of the Christian Right's engagement in sex education debates is participatory. As I show in Chapter 4, the Christian Right has launched its own sexuality industry. Since the seventies, evangelical and fundamentalist Christians have created a commercialized venture involving sexual counseling, research, education, and self-help services. These have resulted in an expansive infrastructure of organizations, media outlets, and sexual commodities such as books, videos, sex education curricula, and workshops. The Christian Right discovered the magnetic pull— the therapeutic appeal—of explicit sexual discussion. Through the creation of a sexuality infrastructure, in which sex education materials occupy a central place, these opponents have actively positioned themselves as sexual experts. By creating alternative sex education curricula, conservative and evangelical Christians shifted the terms of conflict from *whether* sex education would be taught in the school to *which curriculum* would be taught. Both oppositional and participatory strategies proliferate public sexual speech, despite the movement's many calls for regulation and censorship. This is not simply because the censor inevitably repeats the material to be censored, although there is that dynamic. It is because the culture wars depend on more speech that shapes both what people think and, significantly in local battles, how they feel.

I have referred to sex education conflicts as local culture wars, and wars have at least two sides. But in my analysis I focus more attention on the rhetorical strategies of one side: the conservative Catholics and evangelicals who comprise the Christian Right, particularly their national organizations. This is for a compelling reason—quite simply, they say more. This is the book's main story. Since the late sixties, conservative sex education opponents have been more culturally powerful than sex education advocates. Conservatives speak more about sex while simultaneously trying to restrict it. Although they do not always win, their ability to slow the progress of comprehensive sex education has been striking, especially given its widespread popular support. Their advantages are many.

As I show in Chapter 3, conservative national advocacy organizations are bigger, better organized, and richer. Beyond infrastructure, the disparity in the two sides' rhetorical opportunities is palpable. Sex education opponents say more because they *can* say more. Opponents of comprehensive sex education have access to a much more culturally powerful repertoire of negative sexual language and images. Sex-aversive language trumps the barely existent language of sexual affirmation. In matters related to sex, it is easier to accuse than to defend. As Joycelyn Elders found, there is little safe ground for those who speak out in support of sexuality. They can be easily discredited and shamed. Oppositional rhetorics have, since the sixties, consistently overpowered the responses by sex education advocates, who, as we shall see in Chapters 2, 5, and 8, have little available save silence, denials, and complicated clarifications.

This power of the Christian Right's affective vocabularies depends on specific webs of meanings and emotional conventions in the broader sexual culture. Sexual language is not inherently provocative; rather, it *becomes* provocative through history and culture. Sexual language itself bespeaks the way in which sexuality for our society has historically been a negative domain of danger and immorality.[34] Hierarchies regulate sexualities into those which are respectable or disreputable, healthy or unhealthy. Affective conventions of sexuality—in particular, the normativity of sexual shame, fear, disgust—reinforce this regulatory system and are therefore political. The "politics of sexual shame"[35] shapes the type of languages and images available to social movements and potentially enhances the power of rhetoric. We have an extensive sexual vocabulary imbued with negative affect and no comparably strong language of positive sexuality. We use sexual terms as epithets, not blessings. Moreover, nearly all sexual words can conjure anxiety; they are tainted by their association with actual sexual practices. Even seemingly straightforward, descriptive terms such as "oral sex" and "masturbation" can act as an accelerant on a simmering school board debate about sex education. The Right did not create this sexual tradition, but it benefits from it and keeps it alive. Conservative activists anticipate, often correctly, that their rhetoric will resonate with, and be amplified by, this broader climate in which sexuality is bound up with highly negative meanings and affect. The affective vocabulary of the sex education opposition is even more powerful because it fuses cultural anxiety about sexuality with panic about childhood sexuality.

Sex education debates are particularly volatile because they concern children. Indeed, the ideal of what historian Anne Higonnet calls the Romantic child—our modern image of a naturally asexual, pure childhood—is at the heart of century-long conflicts over sex education.[36] By definition, the Romantic child's innocence depends on protection from sexuality—shielded from all information and knowledge. Since the initial calls for sex education in the public schools at the turn of the twentieth century, the phantasm of the innocent child being dangerously corrupted by sexual talk has provoked controversy. Even those early sex education advocates invoked the Romantic child to justify their efforts. Sexual innocence, they claimed, would best be preserved through basic instruction that would thwart the child's sexual curiosity and dampen the imagination. Moreover, these debates over talk versus silence are particularly charged because our determination to preserve the sexually innocent child is infused with such heated emotions. Embedded in the ideal of the Romantic child is the emotional expectation to feel uneasy, at best, when sexual speech is in any way connected to childhood.

However, the myth of childhood innocence, with its tangled fantasies and demands, is a legacy from the late eighteenth century. Although deeply familiar to us, the Romantic child is but one version of the many different narratives we might tell ourselves about the nature and meaning of childhood. Furthermore, it is an image that is in crisis, collapsing under the impossibility of idealizing the asexual child in a culture suffused with sexual representations of all types, including those of childhood sexuality. Higonnet argues that the Romantic ideal is giving way to one more complex.[37] The late twentieth century, she argues, was marked by the gradual emergence of the "Knowing child," who although both pure and deserving of fierce protection is nonetheless in possession of a sensual body and complicated emotions. This new version of childhood acknowledges children's awareness about sexuality and refuses to equate sexual innocence with ignorance. As we shall see in Chapter 1, this is a version of childhood sexuality espoused by the controversial founder of SIECUS, Mary Calderone. Just as the eighteenth-century invention of the Romantic child provoked cultural anxieties and controversies in its time, so too the contemporary reinvention of childhood prompts resistance. Sex education debates, which fuse the highly emotional domains of sex, childhood, and sexual speech, reflect the enormous tensions of this shifting ground. We are not easily letting go of the Romantic child, who meanwhile serves as a powerful political icon in sex education conflicts.

Reflecting on her termination, Joycelyn Elders expressed no regrets and said, "Words are strange things. Once they are out, you can't get them back."[38] As Elders found, words assume a public life. The words with which conservatives have denounced comprehensive sex education came to comprise a vernacular that has significantly shaped the scope of sex education in this country. Chapter 9, for example, shows how sexual discussion in public school classrooms has narrowed over the years. However, the import of these battles extends far beyond the significant question of whether and how young people are able to learn about sexuality in the public schools. Civic dialogue about sex education is one important public arena for the negotiation of sexuality, morality, and citizenship. These troubled spaces of debate involve our logics about children and sexuality, the relationship between sexuality and gender, and the nature and purpose of sexuality itself. Public conversations about sex education involve negotiation about which sexualities will be recognized and valued, about what is spoken and what remains excluded and silenced. This book underscores the power—and the unpredictability—of language and emotion in the cultural politics of sexuality.

# Chapter 1 | REDEFINING SEX, 1964

*A Prologue*

Mary Calderone sat on the dais at a Vassar Club reception filled with her former schoolmates. It was a few short years after she had cofounded the Sex Information and Education Council of the United States (SIECUS). An old friend responsible for the introduction recited Calderone's various academic degrees and titles and then stumbled awkwardly over the title of her current organization. The moderator "haltingly read out, 'The Educational and Informational—' and then gave up, looking miserable. Dr. Calderone, who sat in a chair near her, majestically raised her chin, and, turning to her friend, said in her most dignified tone, 'Say, *Sex.*'"[1] Founded in 1964, SIECUS occupies a unique status as the only single-issue, national advocacy group dedicated to promoting sexuality education.[2] Calderone was the most visible early SIECUS activist. As such, SIECUS and Calderone herself both became symbols of change and magnets for controversy. Getting people to "say sex" was Mary Calderone's mission at SIECUS in the later part of her life.

SIECUS was a study in contrasts. It represented both consistency with, and discontinuity from, an earlier tradition of highly moralistic, social hygiene education.[3] On the one hand, it stressed sexual abstinence and regulation, insisting that open sexual discussion would foster socially responsible sexuality. It might well be seen as a contemporary example of Michel Foucault's claim that sex is put into discourse as a mechanism for the control of the child's sexual body.[4] On the other hand, SIECUS activists condemned many traditional sexual restrictions, such as the guilt imposed by certain religious doctrines. They supported sexual fulfillment and pleasure for all, including children. In many respects, the organization embodied the tensions of its historical time, entering the cultural conversation on childhood sexuality at a moment of instability. As it happened, SIECUS was founded on the cusp of a right-wing revitalization in which speaking against sex education would become a powerful vehicle for political mobilization. Its commitment to the sexual rights of young people would soon make the organization the focus of backlash. In the complex debates over sexuality and children, SIECUS, an essentially moderate group of educational advocates, nevertheless came to symbolize radical transgression among religious conservatives who were just reawakening politically.

## TRADITION AND CHANGE: MID-SIXTIES SEXUAL CULTURE

Public school sex education in the early sixties was, as historian Jeff Moran puts it, "virtually moribund."[5] There were some ambitious programs, to be sure, in cities such as Anaheim, California; Cleveland; Detroit; Evanston, Illinois; Los Angeles; University City, Missouri; and Washington, D.C.[6] Still, a 1965 U.S. Office of Education report criticized most schools for fragmented and uncomprehensive instruction. One survey of administrators in all fifty states reported that 43 percent of them described their programs as "too spotty" or otherwise inadequate.[7] In many towns, the parents, teachers, and administrators alike were wary of introducing sex education. Sally Williams, an Anaheim nurse and sex educator, recalled that in 1964 school programs were "mostly showing the Walt Disney film of the story of menstruation to sixth- and seventh-graders—girls."[8] Another early sex education activist recalled, "It was, you know, the coach, and he divided up boys and girls and then talked to you about physiology or masturbation for the boys and menstruation for the girls."[9] And yet few coaches and teachers were being trained in sex education. At the time a mere twelve graduate programs were preparing future teachers in family life education.[10] Doctors and nurses admitted to ignorance and discomfort in discussions of sexual issues,[11] and as sixties sex educator Esther Schultz recently told me, "Doctors didn't know from diddly-doo."[12] One educator in Michigan observed in the mid-sixties that "in too many places the children's textbooks are the lavatory walls."[13]

Those walls were perhaps more enlightening than the sex education books of that period, however. Although texts by the mid-sixties had become more direct and less prohibitive than in the immediate postwar era, most of them maintained a focus on dating and what the authors considered appropriate gender role behavior. For example, Bernhardt Gottlieb's 1961 book, *What a Girl Should Know about Sex,* said of a mature young woman, "her feminine trait of self-effacement is ever present. It gives her satisfaction."[14] Most authors condemned premarital sex and homosexuality, rarely mentioned sexual pleasure, and cautioned against masturbation. Educator Patricia J. Campbell has written that "while the youth of the sixties were exploring the outer limits of reality with LSD, protesting the Vietnam War, marching in civil rights demonstrations, and making love not war, the sex educators of that decade wrote dozens of books that attempted to keep the lid on a sexual revolution that already was well underway."[15] Such texts, however, risked being simply irrelevant because of their vast disparity with a more vibrant sexual culture. SIECUS emerged not only as a challenge to the inadequate sex education of the times, but also as a response to rapid social changes.

In a cover story on sex at the dawn of 1964, *Time* magazine proclaimed a sexual revolution in the land. With the baby boom swelling the ranks of what would come to be called the youth culture, teenage sexuality was a subject of widespread concern. Historians John D'Emilio and Estelle Freedman point out that although in the mid-sixties the incidence of premarital intercourse held constant from the 1920s, there was by then a major change in attitudes, so that "what was daring and nonconformist in the earlier period appeared commonplace a generation later."[16] The number of out-of-wedlock births was high among both black and white women. Broad resentments about welfare, especially for unmarried black women, led to public debates about providing preventive services such as sex education and birth control.[17] In those pre–*Roe v. Wade* days, pregnant women were adept at finding illegal abortions, which police considered among the most prevalent criminal activity in the nation.[18] Approved by the Food and Drug Administration in 1960, the birth control pill would sharply influence the sexual culture by the decade's end. By that time, the question of whether or not to provide students with information about contraception and abortion would be hotly contested.

Visibility, conflict, and change were hallmarks of mid-sixties sexual culture. Social inequalities loomed large in a turbulent time. For example, racism and homophobia shaped the ways in which sexualities were accepted or demonized. Social historian Ricki Solinger notes the racially specific responses to unmarried women who bore children. By the mid-sixties, public reaction transformed the white unwed mother "from a species of mental patient into a sexual revolutionary," while the caricature persisted of black women as sexually deviant burdens on the taxpayer.[19] People were stigmatized not only on the basis of race, but also because of sexual identity. Homosexuals braved the punitive climate of the mid-sixties to publicly demonstrate at government sites, achieving unprecedented cultural visibility through print journalism and television coverage. Yet just as a flamboyant youth counterculture was emerging, the picketers took care to dress conservatively—"skirts and stockings for the women, suits and ties for the men"[20]—to challenge widespread stereotypes that homosexuals were perverted and sick. Rampant discrimination persisted as gay people in the mid-sixties were hounded out of the military, government service, and the private sector. Gay men and lesbians of color had, in addition, to navigate the intersecting currents of racism and homophobia. Still, public debates and picketing helped bring sexually stigmatized groups into the public eye, although it would be years before such issues were broached in the classroom.

While *Time* magazine lamented the "crisis of virginity," it was the "wide-open atmosphere" of public sexual representation that its cover story denounced.[21] Indeed, historians of sexuality have challenged the popular mythology of the sixties sexual revolution.[22] Youthful sexual behavior changed to some extent, especially by the end of the decade. But as *Time* accurately noted, it was the public discussion about sex that was markedly different. In venues from pornography to the theater to women's magazines, the media in the early to mid-sixties screamed sex. As another newsweekly pointed out, "Whatever they have not already learned from their peers, today's students can learn from the sex manuals that crowd the racks at almost every college bookstore."[23] Or they could turn to *Playboy*, which had commenced publication in 1953, frank novels like

*Naked Lunch* and *Tropic of Cancer*, or the lesbian pulp novels easily found even at small-town newsstands and drugstores.[24] In 1964 the lesbian magazine *The Ladder* left the closet when its editor, activist Barbara Gittings, added the subtitle "A Lesbian Review" so that the word "lesbian" "was no longer unspeakable."[25]

Much was no longer unspeakable. A series of legal changes fueled a striking increase in the sexual content of mid-sixties mainstream media. The Supreme Court, starting in the thirties, issued a range of decisions that relaxed legal prohibitions against printed sexual material.[26] The crucial 1957 decision *Roth v. United States* legally separated sexual explicitness and obscenity, and by 1966, the Supreme Court in the *Fanny Hill* case (*Memoirs v. Massachusetts*) ruled that material must be "utterly without redeeming social value" to warrant a definition of obscenity. One pundit noted that "the nine no-longer-so-old men" had become "a force for broad-mindedness."[27] In the fifties and sixties, movie producers challenged the production code that had been formally adopted in 1927 which had banned even silhouette nudity, "profanity" including "hell" and "gawd," and scenes of childbirth.[28] These policy changes helped ease a chilling climate of self-censorship and thereby helped foster the growing media explicitness. Conversely, the decisions themselves reflected increased social tolerance for public representations of sexuality.

Explicit speech proliferated in print and on the screen, yet it was likely in a different arena that sexual display most reached young people. In the early sixties it was not television (then in its timid infancy) but rock 'n' roll that was arguably the period's most powerful cultural influence. Rock was sexual from its birth. It was 1956 when censors refused to show Elvis Presley below the waist the third time he performed on the *Ed Sullivan Show*.[29] By the mid-sixties, popular music had become a well-nigh unstoppable force—and it was becoming unabashedly sexual. One top song of 1964 was the Animals's mournful ode to a New Orleans brothel, "House of the Rising Sun." That year also marked an event that would have far-reaching effects both on rock 'n' roll and on sexual expression: the Beatles came to the United States. An estimated seventy-three million Americans watched the British performers sing "Love Me Do" on the *Ed Sullivan Show* on February 9. Critic Barbara Ehrenreich dubs Beatlemania "that huge outbreak of teenage female libido"[30] as thousands of adoring, screaming teenage girls created a rebellious, sexual space.

Early sixties media reflected a discontinuous culture. While themes of incest, prostitution, and out-of-wedlock pregnancy proliferated in the movies during that time, the Legion of Decency of the Roman Catholic Church condemned Billy Wilder's *Kiss Me, Stupid* and other films, exerting a censorious effect on Hollywood. Popular music was giving young people a sexual voice, but television's top shows were the saccharine *Ozzie and Harriet* and *Lassie*. Helen Gurley Brown's *Sex and the Single Girl* (published in 1963) touted premarital sex, while Evelyn Duvall's classic *Love and the Facts of Life,* which came out the same year, cautioned against petting. As media critic Susan Douglas put it: "In the early 1960s, the voices of the schoolmarm, the priest, the advice columnist, and Mom insisted, 'Nice girls don't.' But another voice began to whisper, 'Oh yes they do—and they like it, too.'"[31] In this complex moment in which tradition was destabilized daily, a widely quoted survey showed that the schools were a significant source of sexual information for only 8 percent of young people.[32] And so it was onto this unstable turf that a group of crusaders for comprehensive sex education stepped in May 1964.

## EARLY SIECUS: SEX, SCIENCE, AND VALUES

It has been said that if Mary Calderone and her colleagues had not founded SIECUS, someone else would have. The organization was as much a part of the zeitgeist as hula hoops, and it reflected some of the strains in the sexual culture of its time. Calderone's mission, through SIECUS, was to change the sexual culture, a purpose she described years later when reminiscing about her husband, Frank: "Once in a while he'd say, in a puzzling way, 'What are you *doing,* Mary, what are you doing?' And I didn't know how to describe what we were doing, except change the atmosphere. Very difficult."[33] Cultures, of course, are not easily changed. Nor are contemporary sexual cultures as monotone as the portrait of silent repression that Calderone and other SIECUS activists sometimes painted of that historical moment. Viewed from one angle, SIECUS simply gave voice to prevailing cultural tendencies; from another angle its vision was boldly challenging. Had SIECUS been founded in the nineteenth century, it would have been revolutionary. As it was, its birth in 1964 was simply another dimension of the sexual liberalism of the times.

The initiative for SIECUS emerged at an early forum to discuss sexuality and religion, the first North American Conference on Church and Family in 1961. Educator Lester Kirkendall met Calderone and both discovered that they had each been contemplating the need for a national organization to promote sex education. A tall, commanding, gray-haired Quaker fond of describing herself as "a mother and a grandmother and a great-grandmother,"[34] Calderone resigned her post at Planned Parenthood to assume executive directorship of the fledgling SIECUS. She was blunt and brilliant; she could be imperious and difficult. One reporter described her as "an independent Republican, a gourmet cook, an adept horticulturist and an accomplished sailor."[35] A former associate complained that "her main goal in life was to have more and more awards."[36] For years Calderone toured the country speaking bluntly about sex. The public's reaction to her was like a Rorschach of sexual attitudes. In one letter, an exuberant fan addressed her as "the High Priestess of Orgasm."[37] To her religious critics, she became "Typhoid Mary." Calderone was the president of SIECUS from its founding until her retirement in 1982.

In light of SIECUS's later notoriety among conservative Christians, it is significant that from the outset the organization had close ties to religious groups. But again, SIECUS reflected its specific historical moment. By the early sixties, mainstream Protestant Christian thinking was being shaped by broader changes in the sexual culture. The "new morality" in Christianity challenged rigid sexual prohibitions and encouraged a more flexible and expansive approach to sexual ethics.[38] Calderone's own religious institution, the Quakers, issued a document criticizing traditional teachings that condemned premarital and extramarital sex and homosexuality.[39] The enormous momentum among mainstream denominations in the sixties to take up questions of sexuality fostered an affinity between them and SIECUS. An early SIECUS associate said of this time: "It was all over the landscape. People in seminaries were talking about sexuality. You would go and have weekends and workshops. The sixties brought out a lot of people into the sexual arena from religious groups. So it was really going both ways."[40] Calderone firmly believed that "the churches have to take the lead in this area of sexuality,"[41] and so SIECUS founders actively courted the clergy and sought to involve them in the organization. One of the five founders, William Genné, was a minister with the National Council of Churches. SIECUS maintained congenial relationships with many religious denominations and has remained sympathetic to a spiritual approach to sexuality. And yet it also staunchly challenged what it saw as the restrictive and guilt-inducing aspects of religion.

SIECUS sought to effect what Calderone deemed a complete redefinition of sex. SIECUS activists claimed to have popularized the term "sexuality," broadening its definition beyond genital sex. They emphasized that sexuality is far more than simply the sex act; rather, it is part of one's life and personality from birth to death. This was not a new argument, but was consistent with a much broader discursive shift from sex acts to sexual identity, which predated but consolidated in the late-nineteenth century. Disparate cohorts of sex theorists and reformers had helped effect a modern conceptualization of sex as central in defining the core, individual self. Still, changes in sexual meaning systems are gradual and partial. SIECUS spoke to a persistent cultural tendency to split off and marginalize sex from everyday life, especially with relation to young people. Their argument that sexuality is part of the total personality was another way in which SIECUS activists tried to normalize and legitimize sex.

SIECUS valued sexuality and sexual pleasure and vehemently condemned sexual ignorance and guilt. It opposed any social, religious, medical, familial, or other influence that stifled sexual openness. But in many ways the organization was not radical or libertarian. Calderone's emphasis on pleasure within the context of marriage, responsibility, and commitment was consistent with the tension between freedom and containment that is characteristic of sexual liberalism. For example, although she avoided a blanket condemnation of it, she frequently voiced personal disapproval of premarital sex. By contrast, the New York League for Sexual Freedom, also founded in 1964, demanded decriminalization of oral and anal intercourse, interracial marriage, and bestiality and called for reformation of a range of restrictive laws against censorship, public nudity, divorce, contraception and abortion, and statutory rape laws.[42] They were much more radical than the moderate SIECUS. As Calderone would later say, "The loosening up of all of the standards in this country, we didn't cause it, believe me. . . . We don't like what we see any more than the Moral Majority does."[43] All the SIECUS position statements tried to chart an alternate path between on the one hand what Calderone called "dirty-mindedness"[44] and on the other hand a toxic moralism. Still, SIECUS broke from the more traditional sex hygiene programs of the first half of the century in its emphasis on sexual pleasure, its refusal to impose moralism on young people, and its critique of the corrosive power of sexual guilt.

Like sex researchers, SIECUS educators sought to capitalize on the cultural authority of medicine by defining sexuality as a health entity. And scientific inquiry was their preferred tool to evaluate all things sexual. The first "SIECUS Purpose" declared their intent:

> To establish man's sexuality as a health entity: to identify the special characteristics that distinguish it from, yet relate it to, human reproduction; to dignify it by openness of approach, study and scientific research designed to lead towards its understanding and its freedom from exploitation; to give leadership to professionals and to society, to the end that human beings may be aided towards responsible use of the sexual faculty and towards assimilation of sex into their individual life patterns as a creative and re-creative force.[45]

And so in the tradition of sexual modernism as represented by sexologists Havelock Ellis to Alfred Kinsey to Masters and Johnson, the SIECUS ideology expressed a quintessentially rationalist faith that scientific information would ease cultural anxiety and individual guilt about sex. This emphasis on science and health was not unanimously accepted among sixties educators, and individuals around the country adopted other frameworks which de-emphasized health.[46] But Calderone's health approach to sex education was not surprising given her medical training and in light of the legitimating power of biomedicine.

Calderone had a love affair with science. Although she certainly never went to the lengths of researchers Masters and Johnson, who used to conduct their public presentations in white lab coats, she constantly invoked the cultural authority of scientific medicine, especially in controversial domains. For example, she reassured parents that even very young children were sexual beings by explaining that researchers had discovered erections in fetuses. "All I was interested in was finding out the truth, finding out what we could establish by science, scientifically. That's why I was so incredibly excited when I heard about the fetal erection."[47] Although this simple physiological reaction could hardly be interpreted as sexual, especially in the broad definition of sexuality newly promulgated by SIECUS,

Calderone thrilled in using science to assuage anxiety and challenge restrictive sexual morality. She once wrote a letter to the Pope telling him that he should not condemn masturbation because studies had shown it was not harmful. Sociologist John Gagnon said of his correspondence with Calderone: "So I wrote Mary a letter and I said, 'The Pope doesn't care.' I said, 'Masturbation could, in fact, improve everybody's mental life and cure schizophrenia, and he would not approve of it. You're talking past each other.'"[48] Still, Calderone retained an unswerving faith that moral prohibitions concerning sex could crumble under scientific scrutiny.

Her own sexual politics reveal the tension between the conservatizing scientific rationalism she doggedly pursued and the radical political movements of the times. For example, even in 1970, Calderone adamantly insisted she was not a feminist, that she supported human rights not women's rights.[49] Certainly by the late sixties in New York, feminism had achieved widespread visibility by, among other things, voicing criticism of the many ways in which women were oppressed sexually. But it would have betrayed Calderone's sense of objectivity for her to champion the rights of women separate from men. She was also out of step with the modern gay and lesbian rights movement that arose at the end of the decade. In 1987, Calderone recollected, "So many people took it for granted that I was for homosexuality, when it was just very simple—I was not against it. How can you be against something nobody knows the cause of? And I certainly wasn't for it. People are miserable if they're homosexuals."[50] While this sentiment was not uncommon when SIECUS was founded in 1964, it was a good deal less likely to come out of the mouth of a sexuality professional when she said it in the late eighties. And yet it was consistent with Calderone's refusal to embrace or condemn any sexual behavior about which she thought there was little scientific data.

Given this dedication to scientific truth, SIECUS advocates had a complicated relationship to the question of values. Like sexologists, they criticized traditions of sexual condemnation, guilt, and silence. They believed that individuals suffered deeply because of strictures against extremely common behaviors like masturbation. In response, they were loath to judge any behavior, preferring to err on the side of sexual tolerance rather than sexual prohibition. So they took what they considered a determinedly nonjudgmental position toward a broad range of sexualities. As Debra Haffner, a later SIECUS president, remembered, "In the seventies I was taught you were supposed to be non-judgmental, which really translated into you were supposed to present no values at all."[51] An early SIECUS board member noted, "Thirty years ago we were still saying we were going to be objective because what we were against were those people who were preaching values that we didn't endorse. And so one way of being against them and not getting blown out of the water is just to say, 'We want to be neutral.' I don't think we knew that was a clever tactic, but it was."[52] SIECUS's insistence on a scientific, biomedical approach was its tool for claiming neutrality.

Scientific medicine easily masquerades as objective and value-free. As Calderone exclaimed, "We put sexuality into the field of health rather than the field of morals."[53] From today's vantage point, it is clear that science, and certainly sexual science, are highly politicized.[54] But this was well before those critiques had been widely articulated, and SIECUS activists were certainly not alone in their faith in the value-neutrality of scientific rationality. A scientific approach to sex education, then, seemed to allow SIECUS precisely the nonjudgmental stance it so desired. And once again, SIECUS's position was consistent with the rise of sexual relativism in the sixties. As cultural critic Susan Douglas described the times: "Imposing one's own sexual standards on others was now as anachronistic as a Jonathan Edwards sermon; sophisticated tolerance was in."[55] But while it might have been "in," it sometimes got SIECUS in hot water. Once, for example, after the *SIECUS Report* ran an article written by a medical school professor calling for a scientific approach to incest, swift and furious reactions in a range of popular periodicals condemned SIECUS and other researchers as "pro-incest."[56]

Ultimately, the most vehement opposition to SIECUS came from newly politicized evangelicals and their secular and religious allies. And, of course, these groups were on to something they considered very real and dangerous about SIECUS's moral position. SIECUS was not value-free. Individual sex educators themselves were clearly aware of the necessity of values education,[57] and SIECUS consistently addressed the question of teaching morality. Calderone, in fact, insisted that all education must be values-based,[58] and educators associated with SIECUS stressed what they thought of as "family values."[59] However, SIECUS largely espoused values despicable to the conservative Catholics, evangelicals, and fundamentalists who would later comprise the Christian Right. As Calderone said, "We cannot talk about human sexuality without talking about values, but they're not the 'no' values, they're the 'yes' values."[60] It was precisely this affirmation of freer sexual expression that was anathema to conservative religious critics. Calderone herself was religious and commonly spoke of the link between sexuality and the divine. But her view of God's wishes for human sexuality was very particular: "What I'm trying to do is to free people—free a society, really, not people, a whole society—from the horrible incubus that we've been carrying for years of looking upon sexuality as evil instead of a gift from God."[61] It is not difficult to see how SIECUS and Calderone would have been problematic for evangelicals, who relied heavily on the sanctioning of sex to discourage what they considered inappropriate expressions of it.

But even worse than this seeming permissiveness was that, to Christian evangelicals, SIECUS was the embodiment of secular humanism. The organization, they complained, placed individuals themselves, not God, at the heart of a sexual morality system. They were right, of course, and Calderone gave them ample ammunition for this charge. In reflecting later in her life about her many presentations to young people, she said, "I had been asked, 'What do you think of premarital sex?' And I'd give them the standard answer—'Nobody can judge that but yourself. But here are the facts about it.'"[62] By encouraging individuals to develop their own sexual value system, by refusing an arbitrary imposition of the "no" values, SIECUS was flouting what evangelicals and fundamentalists believe to be the divine word. Calderone later complained that conservative Christians criticized her "because I did not come out and mouth the values, the morals; 'thou shalt not do this, thou shalt not do that. . . .' [I believed individuals] are being moral when they are being true to themselves."[63] She encouraged young people to establish their own value systems free from the internalized voice of a punishing God.

It did not matter that SIECUS had widespread religious support; it did not matter that Calderone repeatedly spoke of sexuality as God's gift. SIECUS repudiated evangelical sexual morality simply by encouraging sexual tolerance and a nonabsolutist approach to values. And Calderone was a virtual fountain of secular humanist sound bites. Her claim that "it's the highest morality to live up to the best in you, whether you call it God or whatever"[64] was to opponents an egregious example of humanist philosophy. Cal Thomas of the Moral Majority would later decry SIECUS as "a beehive of so-called secular humanists who deny God."[65] The SIECUS elevation of scientific fact over God's word was unbearable for the enemies of secular humanism. Calderone's glee when she heard about fetal erections expressed her love of citing "facts"—not opinion, rumor, or religious dictate—in this case about how babies are sexual from birth or before. She said, "The fact is there, what you do about it is your business. So I'm talking from strength, I don't have opinions. The only opinion I have is that people should find out the truth, the real truth, not what it says in the Bible, because they didn't have ultrasound in those days."[66] Her fierce reason could itself be a form of literalism and, with respect to her deeply conservative opponents, allowed for many instances of talking past each other.

## SIECUS, SEXUAL SPEECH, AND THE POLITICS OF RESPECTABILITY

By the mid-sixties, as I have shown, public discussion of sexuality was growing. SIECUS was out to change a culture already moving in its direction. But cultural change is uneven, and even amid these transformations, SIECUS activists could recognize—rightly—the overpowering sexual shame and guilt borne by so many. Early SIECUS activists were fueled by their belief in the transformative power of talking openly about sex. The SIECUS philosophy might well have been "and speaking the scientific truth shall set you free." While Calderone's view of the yawning cultural silence about sex was like her portrait of stark sexual repression—oversimplified and hyperbolic—SIECUS's efforts to break sexual silences yielded both wild gratitude and vicious condemnation. The intensity behind both responses speaks to the complicated cultural power of talking, and hearing, about sexuality.

SIECUS was met with a public outpouring of sexual misery and confusion. In those early days the founders must have felt not merely like crusaders but somewhat like saviors. The response was immediate; the demand seemingly endless. The second SIECUS newsletter reported a thousand requests for services in the first six months of 1965.[67] Letters poured in from around the country, especially from young people, sometimes scrawled on index cards or scrap paper. After *Coed* magazine mentioned SIECUS's name in an article, fifteen hundred letters flooded the office.[68] Many of the letter writers were anguished young people struggling over questions about abortion, premarital sex, and masturbation. One young woman who had gotten Calderone's name from a friend who had also written to SIECUS, wrote: "My question is this: I have heard that ejaculation occurs all during intercourse, not just at orgasm. Is this true? Also could you send me any information you have available on methods of contraception, especially the rhythm method. I will appreciate this all very much. It is really great to know that there is someone you can trust, someone you can ask questions without feeling afraid or stupid."[69] Although it is impossible to verify Calderone's claim that she answered all her correspondence personally, there is evidence that she responded to much if not all of the mail. To a long, rambling, and somewhat muddled letter from a young man in New Hampshire who was worried about masturbation, she replied with elegance and reassurance: "I am very much honored that you should have the confidence to write to me as openly as you have. You make it very easy for me to comment. . . . Masturbation is normal and useful, and totally harmless."[70] As the first executive director and only professional staff person of SIECUS at the time, Mary Calderone had emerged not just as the figurehead of this bold new organization, but also as a sexual confidant to people across the nation.

Calderone's profound commitment to the time-consuming task of personal correspondence also fit with SIECUS's mission of direct talk about sex. She decried contemporaneous sex education texts for young people and saw herself as a corrective to such lamentable efforts. In 1965 she wrote, "Have you read recently the tripe and drivel about sex that is written with the adolescent in mind? It is for the most part dishonest and hypocritical."[71] She argued that in its euphemism and ambiguity, sex education material failed to teach teenagers not only about their own sexuality but also "about anybody's sexual behavior." She accused educators of hiding the fact that sexuality is "an attribute of life that lends the variety and color and excitement and creativity that we as adults know" because they were afraid that explicit information about sex would stimulate young people to experiment. She continually refuted this logic, claiming that it was ignorance, not communication, that prompted adolescent sexual experimentation.[72]

With that in mind, Calderone was even willing to consider pornographers as allies in fighting sexual ignorance through direct sex talk. And indeed, in light of the flimsy sex education material available to teenagers at the time, the sentiment was not wholly unreasonable. In later years Calderone seriously considered an invitation by *Hustler* magazine to pen a regular SIECUS column. One can almost see the gray-haired Calderone poring with earnest optimism over an issue of the magazine that was already infamous for its cover of a woman being put through a meat grinder. She wrote to the articles editor, "I've just been looking over the February issue of *Hustler* and trying to figure out where the kind of article you are thinking of might fit."[73] The advantages of spreading sound information clearly outweighed, in her mind, the questionable reputation of the magazine and its publisher, Larry Flynt. It is not difficult to see why. Media critic Laura Kipnis says of the magazine, "You looked to *Hustler* for what you wouldn't get the chance to see elsewhere, for the kind of visual materials the rest of society devotes itself to not portraying and not thinking about."[74] Flynt himself would later become somewhat of a folk hero for championing free speech. It is not surprising that Calderone would see him as a potential fellow crusader against the sexual restriction she so despised.

Free sexual speech, however, requires a sexual language. Calderone complained, "Well, people don't have much of a vocabulary. Or a concept of anything, except fucking."[75] And so the SIECUS vision included the establishment of an appropriate sexual language. For example, sexuality, as Calderone repeatedly lectured, was not about "fucking" and it was not about gender:

> I had a little script. Sexuality means everything that you are, that you were born with, that you experienced, that you thought about, that happened to you, that relates to your being a sexual person. And that is your sexuality at any given moment. What you remember and what you've learned and what you do or decide not to do, whatever. And they would say, "Oh." And then they add a new word to their vocabulary. . . . And that I suppose is really a great achievement. To have put that word [sexuality] into common usage.[76]

Sexual speech, she thought, should be scientific, not euphemistic. Calderone disavowed slang. "I never used cock or cunt, the four-letter words," she insisted.[77] Still, her reputation for blunt sexual language was at least partially responsible for the nickname she was given on a *60 Minutes* segment, "Dirty Old Woman."[78] But Calderone saw herself as a role model: "I wasn't doing it to shock, but to make it easier for people to say the words themselves. If you don't say the right words, if you keep dealing in euphemisms, you're not going to get very far with your thinking. You really have to be very, very clear-cut on that. So I had to set an example. So I did."[79] When she did, depending on one's perspective, she was plain-talking or vulgar.

Like the sixties homosexual activists who picketed in suits and dresses, SIECUS activists were sensitive to their public presentation. As Calderone admitted, "We had to be extremely respectable."[80] One early board member noted the need to publicly differentiate SIECUS from a psychologist who was well known for the number of "frankly hedonistic" profanities that peppered his talks.[81] Board member Isadore Rubin asserted that SIECUS was not a "reform organization," adding, "I think that we should clearly establish at the outset the fact that we are an 'information and education' council, not an 'indoctrination' one."[82] And so as early SIECUS activists hammered out a professional identity, they also articulated what they thought they were not: revolutionaries, hedonists, or even sexual reformers. Yet of course they *were* reformers. To some they were revolutionaries who, at the very least, supported a right to sexual pleasure. Ultimately, as with so many others who are stigmatized on the basis of sexuality, strategies of respectability did not help SIECUS.

The history of SIECUS underscores irresolvable tensions. On the one hand, SIECUS-style sex education can rightly be considered yet another mechanism by which sex is policed through the speech and silences of discourses. Convinced that talking about sex would liberate us, Calderone is part of a long tradition in which schools, psychiatry, religions, and the law all regulate sex through speaking about it.[83] On the other hand, SIECUS and its associates were viciously attacked and marginalized. Despite their religious commitments, their admonitions for responsibility and moderation, their rejection of sexual sensationalism, their disavowals of sexual revolution, and their fit with the changes afoot in the sexual culture, SIECUS nonetheless became notorious. This apparent paradox bespeaks the complicated fields of power that circulate in regard to sex, especially concerning young people. SIECUS was not a singular agent of social control. Regardless of its general compatibility with other social agents committed to regulating sex, SIECUS was at the same time vulnerable to demonization for some of the ways in which it challenged that control. For example, Calderone's wholehearted celebration of sexual expression and pleasure prompted antipathy even when espoused on behalf of adults. She recollected: "I remember one angry woman who said, 'Do you mean to say that you would think it was all right for your mother, if she was 70 or so, to have an affair with someone?' And I said, 'Darned right. She's earned it. Do you want her to sit and knit all day? And not have any kind of life for herself?' Well, that didn't go down very well. It was dirty."[84] Such advocacy was even more outrageous, however, in relation to young people.

In the end, SIECUS did not redefine sex, since the sexual culture was already shifting. Its more enduring impact was its implicit challenge to the Romantic ideal of childhood. Calderone's bold pronouncements about sexuality and young people were a direct affront to the image of the Romantic child. Not only are children not asexual, she proclaimed, but fetal erections also prove they are sexual even before birth. Moreover, she believed that this childhood sexuality and its different expressions are deeply innocent. Young people should not be prohibited from touching themselves, and they should not be shielded from straightforward information about sexuality. They are entitled to bodily sensual pleasures, and adults should not impose on them guilt and shame. In all these assertions, SIECUS advocates broke from the long tradition of sex education designed to stifle sexual curiosity and reinforce the asexual ideal of childhood. Not only did they encounter the resistance of a culture disinclined toward reinvention of the Romantic child; but they also became the target of a movement that found itself able to politically capitalize on the ideal of childhood innocence.

The political climate of 1964 seesawed between revolution and reaction. The most volatile student anti-war protests were still some years off, but the Free Speech Movement that erupted at Berkeley in October of that year presaged later campus upheavals that would lay bare cultural fault lines. In the collective memory, it is these liberation movements, the counterculture, and an ethos of questioning authority that linger about the sixties. However, the country also took a swing to the right, as conservatives of varying stripes effected a significant consolidation of power that continues to today.[85] Right-wing groups like the John Birch Society and the Christian Crusade were tireless in attacking as subversive such developments as the newly passed Civil Rights Act and the early sixties Supreme Court decisions banning prayer and Bible reading in public schools. Their leaders decried the godless hand of communism in everything from race riots and the civil rights movement to changing sexual mores and rock music. In 1964, the year of Freedom Summer, the revenues of both the John Birch Society and the Christian Crusade rose substantially.[86] SIECUS emerged in the thick of these tensions, and sex education would ultimately become the site for stark political conflicts.

The stage was set. The birth of SIECUS was to the sixties what *Roe v. Wade* was to the seventies: a symbol of change amid deep resistance. SIECUS made visible an increasingly sexualized society at a moment in which a new right-wing movement was gathering steam. In their own unique ways, each cohort discovered how sexuality galvanized a constituency, and, with a sense of shock, they discovered each other. Sex educators did not immediately recognize the nature of their opposition, however. John Gagnon, then a SIECUS board member, later recalled, "You ask anybody from the sixties what the role of the Christian Right would be and none of us had an understanding of that."[87] It was not naïveté; the political distance America traveled between 1964 and 1968 was enormous. In 1964, it was possible for SIECUS to imagine transformations in how we talk with young people about sex. Calderone later said about those times, "So everything went on very well and I think we were having a real impact in getting what I call the civilized concepts of human sexuality over." And then, she finished, "suddenly a sour note began to creep in."[88] By 1968, it became clearer that sex education would occupy a prominent role in the cultural politics of the emerging Christian Right.

# Chapter 2 | DAYS OF RAGE

Mary Calderone was not alone in her misplaced optimism about the progress of sex education. In a 1966 article on such programs in the schools, *Look* magazine's senior editor reported, "Backwardness is succumbing as surely as snow to spring."[1] It was, however, to be a fickle spring. During 1968 and 1969, at least forty states were snarled in sex education controversies and approximately twenty considered or implemented legislation regulating sex education. In 1969, *Good Housekeeping* ran an article that warned, "There will quite possibly be a knockdown, drag-out battle in your school district this fall over sex education."[2] When the attacks started, the Sex Information and Education Council of the United States (SIECUS) and many others were perplexed. Calderone said, "So we called the American Civil Liberties Union and said, 'What's going on, do you know? Because this is real character assassination.' And they put us onto a group called the Institute for American Democracy, the IAD, in Washington, [D.C.,] which began explaining the facts of life to us: that we were being attacked by two ultraconservative groups, the John Birch Society and people like them or who were in sympathy with them, and the fundamentalist religious groups."[3] Sex education was one of a range of single-issue battles fought by this emerging political coalition in the late sixties. These battles mark an early moment when the nascent Christian Right recognized the mobilizing power of sexuality.

Coming as they did at the sexual revolution's height of visibility, the sixties battles over sex education made tangible the competing tendencies in the sexual culture. However media-hyped the sexual revolution might have been, the term captured the reality of deep and significant changes in America's sexual culture. Youthful exuberance may have provided the impetus for a climate in which "there was a search for fresh language, there was an epidemic of cant, there was universal love, there was the right to say 'fuck' on the movie screen. For every face of authority, there was someone to slap it."[4] It is no surprise that the battles against sex education were inflamed by such youth rebellions. One sex education opponent, for example, carried the *Life* magazine featuring the Woodstock cover story when she did her talks. And perhaps even more threatening to the face of authority was that these cultural transformations were brought about not only by radical groups in bohemian enclaves but also by mainstream Americans throughout the country.[5] Still, there were equally deep and abiding pockets of resistance to the cultural changes of the sixties, resulting in tensions that would later be dubbed a moral divide or a culture war. If the sexual revolution challenged an entrenched emotional climate of shame, the strategies of the sex education opposition showed both the persistence and the significance of sexual fear and shame, not only for the regulation of sexuality, but also for political mobilization. Sexual politics helped launch the American right wing out of dormancy into a prominence from which they reconfigured American politics.

TEACHING SEX IN A REVOLUTION

SIECUS espoused the ideal of sexual liberalism, which celebrated sexuality and pleasure as long as they were controlled within marriage or stable heterosexual relationships. By the decade's end, this ideal had collapsed. The increasing commercialization of sex, greater media explicitness, and diverse shifts in attitudes and behavior all marked the transition from the midcentury's sexual liberalism to a more sexualized society.[6] Public sexual speech—characters saying "fuck" in movies—was, of course, a hallmark of the late sixties. Young people had seemingly boundless opportunities for such expression. Song lyrics continued their evolution toward more explicitness; for example, the Beatles moved from "I Want to Hold Your Hand" to "Why Don't We Do It in the Road?" Although radio stations typically censored Jefferson Airplane's lyrics "up against the wall, mother-fucker" on the song "We Can Be Together," the record nonetheless became a late sixties anthem. The Broadway play *Hair* featured nudity and songs about masturbation and cunnilingus, while a full depiction of intercourse prompted at least part of the controversy over the Swedish film *I Am Curious (Yellow)*, which was released from customs seizure by a landmark court decision in 1967. A spate of films featured homosexuality, such as *The Fox*, *The Killing of Sister George*, and a number of independents, prompting *Women's Wear Daily* to proclaim, "Movies Are Gayer Than Ever."[7] It may have afforded sex education opponents satisfaction to shut down sixties sex education programs, but as the Christian Crusade's Reverend Billy James Hargis later conceded, "I don't think we won that fight on immoral sex."[8] Widespread transformation in the sexual culture had already far outpaced the efforts of school sex education.

Although students may well have learned more on the schoolyard than in the classroom, school sex education expanded through the sixties. Emboldened (or terrified) by the times—the summer of love, the counterculture, the Woodstock nation—many communities initiated programs or amplified those already being implemented.[9] Educators were bolstered by a series of resolutions in support of sex education from professional organizations like the American Medical Association, the National Education Association, and the American Association of School Administrators. Federal funding through grants from the U.S. Office of Education helped further encourage efforts to teach about sexuality in the public schools. Busy SIECUS activists comprised one wing of a broader effort to fight sexual ignorance. They worked through the decade to help educators bring accurate information and a pluralistic approach to sexual values into the classroom.

As interest in sex education heightened through the sixties, SIECUS received hundreds of requests for help from schools nationwide. Not infrequently the response was a visit by Calderone or Esther Schulz, who became SIECUS's first education director. Schulz insisted on a show of community support, even if she herself drummed it up, before visiting. She remembered: "I maneuvered some way that I was invited. . . . I would get a community that would back me in planning what we were going to do, who we were going to tap, what organizations, what groups that you would tap to help set up the program. It might be an embroidery club or it might be a farmers group."[10] Towns that successfully engaged with the need for sex education were sometimes transformed. One community leader described the town's experience in 1966: "What has been going on in our community resembles a sort of mass therapy process. Those of us involved have found it necessary to reexamine and reevaluate our thinking not only with regard to 'What do I believe?' but also 'Why?'"[11] But sex educators did not count on such commitment. Even when a community indicated overwhelming support for a school program—for example, the 92 percent of Anaheim, California, adults who expressed a wish for sex education[12]—educators like Sally Williams organized information workshops for parents in order to keep their support.

Students' responses to school sex education programs were frequently positive. One town newspaper interviewed a range of students, all of whom expressed strong support for sex education, saying, "You have taken this out of the gutter."[13] In Anaheim, Williams remembered students as overwhelmingly appreciative: "Oh, their response was grateful, really. We got many, many letters from students thanking us. And when I visited in the classroom, you know, I'm supervising the teachers, and some teachers would introduce me as the one who had helped get the program started, and the whole class would turn around—I'd be sitting in the back—and mouth 'Thank you.'"[14] Some students were uncomfortable and reportedly asked their parents to get them out of the class.[15] But most Anaheim students remained in the sex education classes, if participation is any evidence of enthusiasm.

The sexual revolution aside, students in the late sixties were unlikely to hear radical messages in their sex education classes. By the decade's end, a number of organizations had circulated guidelines for comprehensive K–12 programs.[16] The earliest grades stressed the simplest instruction about privacy, hygiene, and respect for the body. These lessons might include a comparison among plant, animal, and human reproduction. In Cedarburg, Wisconsin, kindergarten classes, for example, children watched chicks hatch from eggs in an incubator.[17] The most advanced students in some senior high schools confronted issues of dating, marriage, and of course the thorny discussion of premarital intercourse. Along the way, some schools took up questions about masturbation, birth control, and homosexuality. Many others avoided these topics, however. In some fashion, all curriculum guidelines stressed the interaction of "home, school, church, and community all working cooperatively."[18] And although they were in line with SIECUS's position of avoiding punitive judgmentalism, many educators recognized the importance of teaching morals and values to students, not just providing information. Some educators acknowledged and attempted to negotiate the complex role of the public schools, as illustrated in this statement from an Illinois school district:

> Illinois youth are growing up in a democratic pluralistic society wherein many traditional ways and standards are being challenged. In sexual matters they are being confronted—in news media, magazines, advertising, movies, plays, TV, radio, and books—with "situation ethics" and an emerging, but not yet widely accepted, standard of premarital sexual permissiveness with affection. They need to be sex-educated so they can meet and adjust to current conditions by making intelligent choices and sound decisions—based upon progressive acceptance of moral responsibility for their own sexual conduct as it affects themselves and others—when faced with alternative standards and patterns of behavior.[19]

In short, sex educators tried to teach values in a diverse and rapidly changing world. Necessarily, they could not present an absolutist moral system.

Even the innovative programs of the era presented moderate messages. For example, journalist Mary Breasted chided the pervasive family focus of the Anaheim program for its "basically conformist philosophy."[20] After quoting the goals of the Anaheim curriculum, with such sentiments as preparing students to establish "a family with strong bonds of affection, loyalty, and cooperation" and "a family whose members are happy and enjoy living together," Breasted concluded:

> In short the . . . curriculum had been designed to prepare the Anaheim students for a family life that was like none you or I had ever seen. Oh, we had seen it, but only in the pages of our own elementary school health textbooks or in the glossy color pages of the *Ladies Home Journal* or *House and Garden*. It was a family without pettiness or passion or jealousies or any of the real anguish that has kept our divorce rate up so high that we might as well stop marrying each other to save ourselves the legal fees.[21]

Such a moderate program was the rule rather than the exception.

In communities like Anaheim, with widespread community support and student backing in a climate of sexual transformation, the growth potential for sex education must have seemed boundless. Indeed, if social change progressed seamlessly, sex education would likely only have grown in pedagogical sophistication and cultural influence. Instead, the Anaheim program was soon dismantled to a "birds and bees"[22] level, and the entire Cedarburg program was suspended, with the mother who provided the chicks protesting, "If I'd known what the school was up to they never would have got their hands on my eggs."[23] By the decade's end, communities across the nation were disrupted by controversies. One article observed, "Put a finger almost anywhere on a map and chances are it will land on a town where the radio talk shows and letters to the editor are stoking the controversy over sex education in the schools."[24] Williams hypothesized that the opposition purposefully waited until 1968: "I felt that the reason why they left us alone in the beginning was so that we got a large support group and demonstrated what a worthwhile program it was. And then they attacked us and destroyed it. So I think they were letting us build our support, and that gave them a bigger group to destroy."[25] But there was no such conspiracy. The opposition simply appeared in its moment, as much a part of the times as SIECUS was.

BUILDING A MOVEMENT

In January 1964, only four months before the founding of SIECUS, Barry Goldwater declared his candidacy for the United States presidency. There was, of course, no connection between the two events, yet they bespoke the tensions of the decade, as each represented the coalescing of a movement committed to widespread but very different cultural transformation. Goldwater's failed presidential campaign resonates in the collective imagination of conservatives with the same vibrancy Woodstock has for counterculturists. Indeed, his campaign catalyzed a political alliance of social conservatives, intellectual right-wingers, and evangelical Christians. Noted Goldwater organizer and Equal Rights Amendment foe Phyllis Schlafly recently observed, "Nineteen sixty-four was the year when grassroots conservative Republicans took control of the Republican Party, and they've had it, more or less, ever since. . . . I doubt if there's ever been anybody else who lost an election who had as big an impact as Barry Goldwater did."[26] The Goldwater effort showed millions of Americans that their disaffection with liberal social changes was shared. Significantly, it suggested the potential for political power among a grassroots coalition of conservatives. Goldwater's mailing list was used by conservative fund-raiser Richard Viguerie to launch just such a coalition. By 1968, a conservative alliance of Americans from diverse backgrounds dominated the Republican Party.[27] In many ways, 1968 was a watershed year. Sociologist Allen Hunter argues that at the beginning of the year "it seemed as though 'history' was on the side of liberal progress; at the end of 1968 that 'history' came to be associated with conservatism, with retrenchment."[28] The liberal consensus had given way.

It was not just sex education. A conservative ethos nurtured the proliferation of single-issue oppositional groups in the United States in the sixties. These backlash movements, deplored by John F. Kennedy in the early part of the decade as "crusades of suspicion," attacked everything from pornography to rock music to fluoridation of the water.[29] The opposition's attacks on sex education were most significant and have enormous importance for several reasons beyond the immediate impact on the field. First, these attacks signal the growing political visibility and viability of the right wing by the end of the sixties. Second, they helped foster the alliance among disparate conservative elements, from national secular right-wing groups like the John Birch Society to fundamentalist organizations like the Christian Crusade, to conservative Republicans, and finally to a fearful grassroots constituency. Third, the single-issue groups of the late sixties helped launch the more consolidated movement that by the mid-seventies would be known as the New Right. And finally, the sixties sex education battles proved to the emerging Right the power of sexual politics and sexual speech in provoking volatile local battles to further their goals.

The unsettled political climate of the sixties supported both the sexual liberalism represented by SIECUS and a coalescing right-wing oppositional movement represented by Old Right groups such as Billy James Hargis's Christian Crusade. In the same moment in which Students for a Democratic Society and the Black Panthers were organizing a defiant left wing on America's campuses, conservative and Christian evangelical groups like Young Americans for Freedom and Campus Crusade for Christ were flourishing. It would turn out that the right-wing politics of morality would have enormous appeal for many who had been disquieted by the instabilities of transition to a more sexualized society. In fact, the progressive social changes of the decade had nurtured a powerful coalition of conservatives and evangelical Christians that would unite in what 1966 gubernatorial candidate Ronald Reagan called a "moral crusade."[30] Although it caught many political commentators by surprise, this political efflorescence of evangelicals was not especially sudden or unexpected. Evangelicals had been largely insular since the humiliating Scopes "monkey trial" in 1925, favoring spiritual affairs over social activism. Yet sociologist Sara Diamond accurately notes that evangelicals in the first half of the twentieth century were "prepolitical" not apolitical.[31] The organizational infrastructure they built during these decades, in the form of radio and television broadcast networks and other ministries, would prove vital to their increasing visibility when, by the late seventies, the Christian Right had become a tangible political and cultural presence.[32]

The social and political changes of the sixties prompted this reinvigorated political mobilization among nominally secular conservatives and evangelical and fundamentalist Christians. They were outraged that the Supreme Court banned religious speech in public schools—including Bible reading and school prayer—while its other rulings relaxed prohibitions on literary speech formerly deemed obscene. The civil rights movement was an ongoing source of consternation to conservatives and right-wing groups, and the 1964 passage of the Civil Rights Act was met with public condemnation by many right-wing leaders and spurred an influx of members to their groups.[33] Lingering fears of a lurking "red menace" haunted the nation. Meanwhile, social anxieties had prompted widespread conversion to Christianity, defying sociologists' predictions that religion's influence would wane in a modern, scientific world.[34] Groups as diverse as "burned-out hippies to disillusioned liberals to ordinary seekers" flocked to fundamentalist churches.[35] The meteoric rise of evangelicalism, fundamentalism, and Pentecostalism offset declines in mainstream Protestant churches.

Fears of a sexual revolution were in the air. When Ronald Reagan condemned "sexual orgies and behaviors so vile I cannot describe them," he deployed sex as a metaphor to mobilize broad, inchoate cultural anxieties.[36] Sex education seemingly made these fears real. By the end of the decade, Mary Calderone and other SIECUS activists who toured the country talking openly about masturbation, birth control, and premarital intercourse had become targets. Sex education itself was a symbol for cultural decline. The right-wing leadership may not themselves have cared passionately about the teaching of sex in the public schools, but they discovered a small grassroots populace to whom such questions mattered deeply. The late sixties sex education controversies were short-lived, but they demonstrated a useful and critical strategy: that constituencies could be mobilized by strategic discourse which fostered the stigmatization of various social groups and sexual activities. In a few years, sexual issues would be at the center of the New Right's cultural agenda.

Once they started, there was a predictability to the outbreak of community sex education controversies. In the towns where conflict arose, programs were already well established or getting under way. Often parents had been informed and had had access to materials and the opportunity to comment on curricula. Typically one parent, or a small group, formed the epicenter of conflict and were quickly joined by other disgruntled residents. Although it is difficult to quantify precisely, by most accounts the sex education opposition remained a minority in nearly all places. Occasionally one or more of these parents were connected to national right-wing organizations but often they were unaffiliated. At some point, however, national right-wing groups influenced most community opposition, whether by sending speakers or disseminating anti–sex education literature. Despite the small numbers, opponents wielded enormous power to challenge school systems, disrupt communities, and even dismantle sex education programs. Sometimes the debates were simply part of everyday business. For example, a headline of one small-town newspaper flatly announced, "Roof Leaks, Sex Courses Are Taken up by Board."[37]

But in other places the sex education conflicts aroused passions that bordered on violence. Some school administrators reported death threats.[38] Schulz of SIECUS recalled "being spit on and having pickets walk outside the door while you were speaking to the community."[39] Calderone had a palpable fear of assassination: "Sometimes I would go to some central United States town and wonder if I was going to be shot at. Because there was violence in the air. When finally everybody was gone and you could release yourself from your audience and you and a few companions would go out to the parking lot, it would be almost empty. You'd wonder if you were going to be attacked at that time. Because a lot of people would think they were doing a martyr's job by killing this kind of woman who threatened them."[40] Fear became a significant emotional component of these early culture wars, as controversies fanned like prairie fire across the nation from Nashville and Baton Rouge to Chicago, Oklahoma City, and Anaheim.

Two national groups led the charge against sex education in the late sixties: Reverend Billy James Hargis's Christian Crusade followed by the John Birch Society. Other right-wing groups like the Liberty Lobby jumped into the anti–sex education fray, along with innumerable front groups for the Right with names like SOS (Sanity on Sex) or MOMS (Mothers Organized for Moral Stability). (Even in the late seventies the far right, white supremacist Christian Defense League recirculated all the sex education attacks in their lengthy recruitment broadside, "Sex Education: The Assault on Christian Morals.") The Birchers and the Christian Crusaders took the lead and were formidable because of their prominence and their collaboration. Their leaders endorsed each other, sold and reprinted the other's literature, and served as each other's advisers.[41] Their alliance signified a new willingness among certain right-wing fundamentalist leaders like Hargis to abandon separatism and forge political ties with others.

Founded in 1958, the nominally secular John Birch Society was known for broad, anti-communist conspiracy theories. In the post-McCarthy sixties, the Society incited controversy even among conservatives for its zealotry in mounting accusations that prominent public figures (Dwight Eisenhower among them) were communist agents or dupes. Although Birchers may have acquired a reputation for extremism, they had the potential to exercise influence in the Republican Party.[42] One membership study showed a well-educated, upper-middle-class, conservative Christian, Republican constituency.[43] Clearly it was a group that would have no trouble finding common cause with organizations like the Christian Crusade, and after about six months it followed the Crusade into the sex education battles. It was the proliferation of Christian evangelical and fundamentalist groups, however, that was the hot news in right-wing politics. The rapid social change of the sixties provided ample fodder for leaders at the pulpit to fan apocalyptic fears of Satanic Communism's threat to a Christian United States. They could, as historian Richard Hofstadter points out, unite the fundamentalism of the cross with the fundamentalism of the flag.[44] Probably no right-wing preacher excelled at this more than Reverend Billy James Hargis.

Hargis's meteoric career spanned his early obscurity at Ozark Bible College in Bentonville, Arkansas, to national notoriety in the sixties to political invisibility by the end of the seventies. His break came as chairman of the Bible Balloon Project, an enterprise that floated thousands of Bible excerpts into Iron Curtain countries on balloons launched from the West. He founded the Christian Crusade in 1948, claiming it to be part of God's plan to save America.[45] Eventually, Hargis's anti-communist diatribe became so forceful that Senator Joseph McCarthy cited his work as helpful for the McCarthy investigations.[46] Like many on the Right, Hargis had a proclivity to see the red menace in everything from rock music and sex education to civil rights. Whether or not he was a racist was the subject of some debate,[47] and Hargis himself insisted that he knew it was "wrong to deprive the Negroes of their constitutional rights."[48] However, he did write for explicitly anti-Semitic publications, continually excoriated civil rights leaders, and publicly condemned interracial marriage. Unlike some right-wing leaders who publicly repudiated or apologized for their earlier racist statements, Hargis continued to support a platform inimical to full civil rights.

Eloquent and charismatic, Hargis fashioned his Christian Crusade into one of the right wing's most powerful organizations by the early sixties. He was the focus of public attention, not all of it positive. His supporters saw him as an indefatigable crusader for the nation's protection. One associate noted, "The job of Billy James Hargis is to yell, 'Fire, fire, fire' till America awakens and realizes that there really is great danger to our way of life."[49] Hargis's detractors, who were legion, painted him variously as a zealot inspiring "orgies of hatred and fanaticism"[50] or a "doomsday merchant" profiting from Cold War cultural paranoia.[51] They pilloried his heavy frame, describing him as "rotund," "Oklahoma Fats," and "elephant sized."[52] *Hustler* editor Larry Flynt, of the magazine that courted SIECUS for a sex education column, called Hargis (among other similarly colorful epithets) a "lecherous bag of pus."[53] Nonetheless, the dynamic Hargis built an enormously powerful Christian anti-communist empire of radio ministries, publications, and training centers.

The Christian Crusade tapped a grass roots eager for information and support. In the early sixties, the organization's office processed two thousand letters a day, and Hargis's show was heard on two hundred and fifty radio stations and viewed on nine TV stations.[54] It published a weekly magazine, a tabloid *Weekly Crusader*, and sold taped sermons and separate Christian sex education records for boys and girls. The Crusade published countless small and inexpensive educational booklets, many of them written by Hargis himself. These included titles such as *Satanism—Diabolical Religion of Darkness*, *The Black Panthers Are Not Black—They Are Red*, and *Should We Surrender to Castro or Smash Him?* All of his publications were vehemently anti-communist, a tone that infused the anti–sex education critiques.

If they were not the engine of protest, the John Birch Society and the Christian Crusade were undeniably the rudder steering grassroots opposition to sex education. National publications disseminated sex education critiques—like *Is the School House the Proper Place to Teach Raw Sex?*—which were virtually reproduced in their entirety by local groups. Major figures such as Hargis and his associate Gordon Drake toured the country with their gospel of scathing sex education attacks. Their newsletter advertised "Would you like to have Dr. Gordon Drake, Christian Crusade's Director of Education, to speak in your community in opposition to unmoral sex education and 'sensitivity training' in your schools and in the churches of your area?"[55] Some of the local opposition groups were largely spearheaded by the Right or evangelicals, while others were explicit front groups, such as MOTOREDE (Movement to Restore Decency, an affiliate of the John Birch Society). Local churches acted as platforms for right-wing speakers and messages. With their resources and growing political acumen, these national groups helped bring together a diverse public.

Often local activists were evangelicals, deeply conservative, or actively associated with the Right. These were the "suburban warriors" described by historian Lisa McGirr—cohorts of middle-class women and men who helped effect the conservative revival in the late sixties through their fight against issues which to them represented domestic corruption.[56] A John Birch Society coordinator noted, "You'll find a member of the society active in every state where there's opposition to sex education," but an estimated 80 to 90 percent of MOTOREDE members were not Birchers.[57] Still, these opponents adopted the anti-communist and similar far right rhetoric. Other opponents tried to downplay it for strategic reasons. One activist in Wichita said, "We haven't even injected communism into it. I was afraid it would hurt us, that this would give people the chance to brand us as a bunch of far-out extremists," although he asserted that sex education is "either a Communist-inspired program or one inspired by those who believe in 'one world.'"[58] Whatever other personal interpretations or political strategies they might deploy, this cohort for the most part adopted the right-wing critiques of sex education.

Conservative Christian evangelicals added a strong religious critique to the movement. One parent said, "The creation of God is never mentioned in the instruction and kids think they are just another form of animal. Then they start regarding Mom as an old sow and Dad as an old boar. You establish an animal farm of people with this kind of teaching."[59] Evangelicals and fundamentalists were particularly stung by the Supreme Court decisions that had banned prayer and Bible reading from public schools. They insisted that sex education had to include religious moral teachings, which was now rendered impossible. Gordon Drake complained that sex education should be eliminated since "it cannot be taught within a Christian framework" because "God and the Bible have been kicked out of the schools."[60] In response, sex education teachers explained that although they could not teach Christian morality, they did in fact "teach within a moral standard of right and wrong, and if the students talk to their parents, or have anything to do with the church, our instruction can be supplemented."[61] But that was not enough for conservative religious critics who demanded that schools "inject Biblical morality."[62] Many conservative Catholics shared this view that, as one father put it, "Sex to us is religion [and] cannot be taught without reference to 'mortal sin' and 'venial sin.'"[63]

Two other overlapping sets of concerns prompted parents to join the anti–sex education movement. First, there was the argument that children were too young for sex information and would be harmed by any exposure to it. This notion was loosely extrapolated from Freud's discussion of a latency period in children aged six to eleven in whom sexual interest is sublimated. Manhattan analyst Rhoda Lorand became a national critic of sex education by arousing this fear. Lorand was a favored expert of the right wing, who quoted her frequently in their critiques. In one broadside published by the American Education Lobby, she warned, "Displaying a Kotex pad to a coeducational class of any grade is an appalling invasion of girls' privacy and can only seriously embarrass everyone. The graphics of the penis spurting semen and the head-on view of the vagina enlarged for screen viewing will unquestionably excite and frighten many, if not all, youngsters."[64] Parents were susceptible to these anxieties, like one New York writer and wife of a psychiatrist who was shocked that her eleven-year-old son had been told to look up "eunuch" for class. She complained, "At the age of 11, many boys are undergoing castration anxiety with the onset of puberty. It's exactly the wrong time to be forcing them to think about eunuchs."[65] Psychoanalytic language served a legitimating function for sex education opponents because it helped them avoid being branded as religious extremists.

Finally, numerous anti–sex education activists were simply motivated by the conviction that sexuality should be veiled. Whether they couched such notions in dignity, mystery, tradition, or plain modesty, these critics valued sexual reticence, not the openness SIECUS advocated. Discussion, they feared, could lead to promiscuity, confusion, or outright damage. There was certainly no need for it. One father of four justified this position by declaring, "My wife and I have never discussed sex in seventeen years of marriage."[66] Similarly, opposition leader Eleanor Howe described her indignation when she visited her sons' Anaheim sex education classroom: "There were so many things written on the blackboard. Here I was, I was in the service. I was married to a serviceman, and I didn't know what some of those things meant on the blackboard. And the kids all knew. But [the department head] Mr. Dirth told me what '69' meant, and I said, 'Isn't that strange? I ended up with four children. I was in the Air Force during the war, married to a Marine. And I lived all these years of my life not knowing what that meant.' You know, I couldn't understand it."[67] Not only did Howe believe her sons had no need of sex information, but she also felt exposure to it robbed them of something crucial: "And they took away from my children the mystery, the wonderful experience of my wedding night."[68] According to this view, sex education is a violation.

SIECUS and other analysts attributed the anti–sex education movement to the organized right wing and some deluded parents. Although there was some truth to this assessment, the movement could not have coalesced and spread so rapidly if it had been confined to the right wing. And the involvement of national right-wing groups like the Christian Crusade and the John Birch Society was complex, supplying vital resources to the sex education opposition but bringing a taint of "extremism" that allowed some to deride or simply dismiss their claims. The significance of the late sixties anti–sex education movement is the way the Right used sex education debates to mobilize a broader constituency. Although many of these people might disagree with right-wing ideology, they appropriated its ways of thinking and talking to express their own anxieties about sexuality and social change. National right-wing groups in local sex education battles exercised a powerful influence in shaping strategies of resistance. The Right's ways of talking became the vernacular of sex education opposition.

## TALKING BACK

The discursive practices of the emerging Christian Right, like those of all social movements, were intended to define the social world, create a volatile emotional climate, and mobilize people to action. Key strategies of sixties sex education opponents included anti-communist rhetoric, the dissemination of depravity narratives, sexual scapegoating, and a practice of strategic distortion. They drew on languages and images of danger and shame available in the broader sexual culture and made them specific to debates over sex education. These were more than expressions of fear and anxiety, although they certainly were that. They were rhetorics designed to outrage and thereby mobilize a diverse constituency. Anti–sex education discourses pushed back the border of sexual decency to exclude from acceptability the teachers, parents, and other advocates of open sexual discussion with young people. The grassroots resonance with anti–sex education rhetoric demonstrated to an emerging movement the enormous power in its strategic use of sexual speech.

This style of Christian Right sexual politics would not have been so effective without the long cultural history in the United States of political groups using sex as a mechanism for intimidation, blackmail, and shame. The purity crusades of the Ku Klux Klan in the early twentieth century are a good example of a far right group attempting to achieve its political goals through manipulating fears of sexuality.[69] The Klan's lynchings of black men for alleged, usually fabricated sexual crimes against white women show how race and sex intersected in strategies of intimidation. More institutionalized and mainstream through the sixties and into the seventies were the tactics of sexual blackmail employed by FBI director J.

Edgar Hoover. Capitalizing on the paranoia, moralism, and homophobia of the Cold War era, Hoover kept extensive files on the sexual lives of countless Americans in order to intimidate them for his own political purposes.[70] In addition, in the late fifties, Congress had given the U.S. Postal Service broad powers to enforce obscenity laws, leading to sweeping raids and stings. Lives were ruined, such as that of Smith College professor Newton Arvin, who was arrested in his home in 1960 for the possession of erotic pictures received through the mail.[71] The politics of sexual speech that would emerge out of the late sixties sex education battles drew on already familiar features of sexual persecution in American culture.

Yet however ordinary were their strategies of sexual intimidation, organized sex education opponents widened the scope of those who could be shamed and discredited on account of sex. In an understated recollection, early SIECUS board member John Gagnon mused about the group's activists, "I don't think anybody in that group really had any sense of the trouble they were going to get into."[72] This is not surprising. Largely they were men and women of social and economic privilege whose sexual lives were at least publicly discrete. However, as cultural theorist Michael Warner notes, despite the contemporary public visibility of sexuality, "Anyone who is associated with actual sex can be spectacularly demonized."[73] Still, the attacks on Calderone and other early SIECUS activists went even beyond this tendency to stigmatize based on sexual identity or sexual acts to include those who publicly spoke about sex. Like Joycelyn Elders almost thirty years later, and Margaret Sanger several decades before, SIECUS associates advocated open discussion with young people about sexuality, leaving them vulnerable to scapegoating for political purposes.

One way in which this happened was that opponents smeared them as communists. The anti-communist rhetoric laced through anti–sex education documents today reads as strident, hyperbolic, or even quaint. Yet it was consistent with the late sixties lingering cultural concern about the red menace. Although fierce McCarthyite paranoia was waning by this time, the fear of communism persisted through the country's preoccupation with the Cold War, the Cuban government of Fidel Castro, and the expansionism of Nikita Krushchev. An accusation of "communist" served as code for a diffuse set of overlapping transgressions. In particular, sixties sex education opponents tended to fuse sexual perversion and secular humanism when they railed against communists. In the late sixties and early seventies, innumerable anti–sex education tracts appeared, like *The SIECUS Circle: A Humanist Revolution*, *The Child Seducers*, *Is the Schoolhouse the Place to Teach Raw Sex?*, and *SIECUS: Corruptor of Youth.*

Sectors of the opposition "borrowed" freely from each other and many anti–sex education documents read like carbons of each other, typos included. They shared the anti-communist, conspiratorial tone of naming sex education, in particular SIECUS, a threat both to innocent children and to morality in American life. For example, conservative Christian author Claire Chambers in *The SIECUS Circle* charged that "sex education is just one of the many deadly weapons in the armory of the Communist-Humanist complex."[74] And *Pavlov's Children (They May Be Yours)*, the film and accompanying pamphlet that opponents used to link sex education to communism, warned that sex education was part of a one-world conspiracy to "reduce morality of all to the standard of the most immoral." The end result—that "people will no longer unite behind a shared outlook in religious, ethnic or racial groups"—appealed to midcentury nationalistic and racist sentiments.[75] Sex educators became much more menacing when linked to a communist plot.

Sex education opponents connected with national groups like the Christian Crusade or the John Birch Society were the most seriously and explicitly anti-communist in their challenges. In one of the most influential Christian Crusade booklets, *Is the School House the Proper Place to Teach Raw Sex?*, written by education director Gordon Drake, Billy James Hargis claims to have amended the title to read "'little red school house,' put a picture of a red country church on the cover, and sold one million copies."[76] A scant forty pages, *School House* railed against the "rawness" of sex education, "the SIECUS SEXPOT," and the "revolutionary gospel" of Mary Calderone.[77] Published in September 1968, the booklet did not single-handedly launch the late sixties conflicts over sex education. Similar critiques had already run in the right-wing *Herald of Freedom* and had been aired on the floor of the U.S. Congress by Representative John Rarick of Louisiana.[78] But *School House* was the most widely circulated critique in the sixties debates and hinted darkly at a communist agenda, warning that if "the new morality is affirmed, our children will become easy targets for Marxism and other amoral, nihilistic philosophies—as well as V.D.!"[79] At the heart of this anxiety was the notion that communists infiltrated societies by first weakening the moral fiber and then the military preparedness of the citizenry. It was thought that sex education, combined with rock music, pornography, and sensitivity training, would arouse carnal desires in children who would then devote themselves to the mindless pursuit of sex. The United States would thus be left vulnerable to takeover.

Conspiracy theories were the heart of right-wing anti-communism. Critics of sex education spilled a great deal of ink drawing labyrinthine connections to prove their allegations. SIECUS drew the most fire, especially because of board member Isadore Rubin. Like many citizens in the fifties, Rubin had been called for questioning about communist affiliations by the House Un-American Activities Committee (HUAAC) and had refused to testify. (He was doubly implicated in critics' eyes because he published *Sexology*, a sex information magazine that sported suggestive covers. Respected by experts, *Sexology* was such a target for critics that it was dubbed the *Das Kapital* of sex education.[80]) But no SIECUS associate escaped the "fellow traveler" taint. In a critique that was entered into the Congressional Record, Calderone was described as an "ultra-liberal one-worlder," a code for communist.[81] Her uncle, the poet Carl Sandburg, was cited as having a long history of communist affiliations. SIECUS cofounder William Genné had a file in HUAAC, which to critics suggested communist-front activity. *The SIECUS Circle* exhaustively listed everyone ever cited on a family life education bibliography and drew purported connections to communist ties in a section entitled "SIECUS's Core of Subversives." In addition to the usual suspects, other examples of alleged "communist-fronters" included Erich Fromm (suspect because of his membership in the ACLU and his critiques of capitalism) and Beacon Press (which publishes "a swarm of Communist-front authors" including John Dewey).[82]

Allegations such as these were widely quoted in both national and grass-roots oppositional literature. They were spread from town to town by local anti–sex education groups, especially MOTOREDE. MOTOREDE leaders were Birchers wedded to anti-communism and skilled at garnering publicity. A Utica, New York, newspaper headline was typical: "Sex Courses Tied to Red Plot by Area Decency Group Chief." The article continued: "Joseph Smithling of Syracuse, a member of the Movement to Restore Decency, told an Oneida County Patriotic Society meeting that the national sex education movement is a part of the 'International Communist conspiracy.' He said local teachers are being fooled by a Communist plot to take over this country by getting American children 'interested in sex, drawing them away from religion and making them superficial and less rugged.'"[83] But even some Birchers displayed a more moderate position, with one MOTOREDE leader in Hawaii noting, "I don't think sex education is part of a Communist plot to weaken the morals of this country. However, I believe that many sex education programs bear the stamp of SIECUS . . . and some SIECUS officers are either Communists or second-rate fellow travelers."[84] These allegations operated to raise suspicions about SIECUS in particular and increase anxieties about sex education in general.

But hard-line anti-communist convictions were not necessary for anti-communist rhetoric to be effective. Indeed, some of the most effective grassroots leaders claim never to have believed in the ideas of a communist plot. For example, opposition leader Eleanor Howe of Anaheim said that she used to argue to the local John Birch Society leaders that sex education was not a conspiracy: "The John Birch Society always made everything so mysterious that everything was underhanded and, for me, everything was out in the public, out in the open. Anybody could get the materials that I had. Anybody. And [sex education] wasn't a conspiracy, it was a program, and I'm thoroughly convinced it was a program to change the values of our society."[85] Howe's denial comes despite her having toured in the sixties showing the blatantly anti-communist film *Pavlov's Children*.[86] Retrospective memory is problematic and, especially in light of the dismantling of the Soviet Union, many activists may now be unwilling to admit having held such beliefs. Still, historian Lisa McGirr points out that by the late sixties, Orange County, California, had been dubbed America's "nut country," in part as a result of the apocalyptic and conspiracist rhetoric of its many right-wing groups.[87] It is not entirely unreasonable that even some grassroots conservatives themselves might have been uneasy with or skeptical of such rhetoric.

Howe's disavowal of her own anti-communism, if true, is instructive on several levels. First, it reminds us that social movements are fractured and do not depend on activists' complete adherence to achieve success. Claims can be effective even if the audience for them (or the claimsmaker herself!) does not believe them. Second, it suggests that anti-communist rhetoric could be broadly read by sex education opponents as a metaphor for other fears. Anti-communism became a symbol of intrusion by a menacing Other, intent on social subversion. Many characters could fill that role, including secular humanists, liberals, and anyone deemed a sexual deviant. And indeed, sex education opponents freely substituted these menaces in their challenges. This suggests that movement activists can be adept at transmuting symbolic systems in order to meet their own needs. The role of anti-communist rhetoric was powerful yet unpredictable. Taken literally, it galvanized some opponents but also opened the movement to ridicule from a late sixties constituency weary and wary of McCarthyism. Read more broadly, however, this rhetoric resonated for a range of opponents who feared the disruption of their cherished way of life.

In addition to anti-communist rhetoric, the sixties sex education conflicts marked the elaboration of the strategy I call the depravity narrative. These are tales about sex education that rely on distortion, innuendo, hyperbole, or outright fabrication. They draw their power from four sources. First, depravity narratives wield enough specific details to sound accurate, a move literary theorist Roland Barthes has described as the "reality effect."[88] Second, like so many other operations of sexual speech deployed by sex education critics, they depend on a compelling condensation of sexual threat, fear, and shame. They succeed because they appeal to a cultural logic that someone, somewhere might have done such a thing. Third, they exist in multiples. Sex education opponents routinely have a litany of such tales whose effect is synergistic. Finally, depravity narratives depend on a lack of information about the practices they describe, in this case about the truly limited nature of sex education in the United States.

Depravity narratives were designed to shock. Like urban legends, they spread rapidly and were seemingly legitimated by newspaper stories; narrators reported them with the certitude of knowing a friend of a friend to whom this had happened. Depravity narratives derived extra potency from the element of sexual perversion. Like anti-communist rhetoric, they were broadly expressive of deeper cultural anxieties, in this case about childhood sexuality. Their proliferation in the sex education debates marked an important early phase of the Christian Right's political deployment of provocative speech to arouse powerful emotions of fear and anger in local citizens.

Of the many depravity narratives circulating in the late sixties, two were especially prominent. The first simply recounted that a sex education teacher had had intercourse in front of the class as a pedagogical strategy. When asked thirty years later why he opposed the Anaheim sex education program so vehemently, activist James Townsend said, "It got so wild that one teacher even went so far as to have intercourse in front of her class."[89] In a variation of this narrative, male students raped a sex education teacher after watching a film in class. A version from 1969 held that seventeen males participated in the attack; when it reappeared in a broadside of the far right Christian Defense League in 1979, the number had increased to twenty male students, one of whom allegedly said, "Didn't she spend the whole year telling us how to do it, when to do it, and how much fun it would be?"[90] A second widely circulated depravity narrative alleged that a sex education teacher got carried away and disrobed in front of her class. Narratives placed the incident in numerous cities, including New York; Wichita Falls, Texas; Minneapolis, Minnesota; and Flint and Lansing, Michigan, prompting one weary health administrator to quip, "It's as though that teacher were on a burlesque circuit."[91] Other tales circulated to the effect that children were being encouraged to fondle each other, sexual intercourse would be taught in kindergarten, schools would install coed bathrooms with no partitions between stalls, and youth were being told about bestiality with donkeys and sheep.

Racial anxieties amplified some depravity narratives. Sex education opponents could portray programs as even more threatening if they seemingly promoted interracial sex. In one Christian Crusade publication from 1969, Gordon Drake claimed that "many" white teenage girls were interested in interracial sex in order to "atone for white guilt." He also condemned SIECUS for the organization's criticism of racism, and he speculated that SIECUS would soon be producing slides for young children which depicted a black father "on *top of* [a white] mother engaged in intercourse."[92] Interestingly, these explicit appeals to race-based fears were not routinely featured in the otherwise highly provocative and conspiratorial attacks on sex education by national right-wing groups, including Drake's most influential document, *Is the School House the Place to Teach Raw Sex?* This is noteworthy since so many of the late sixties anti–sex education documents are virtual reproductions of one another.

However, it is likely that many of the social changes through the sixties led some right-wing groups like the Christian Crusade to restrict such blatant appeals to racial bias out of the recognition that they might backfire.

And indeed, widespread fears of race-mixing were diminishing by the late sixties. In 1967, when the U.S. Supreme Court declared anti-miscegenation laws to be unconstitutional, only sixteen states still had such laws on their books, compared with twenty-nine in 1959.[93] Whites' attitudes were changing as well. Between 1958 and 1968, whites' approval of interracial marriage jumped from 4 percent to 20 percent, and as historian Renee Romano notes, its outspoken critics "were on the defensive."[94] Clearly, the Christian Crusade could count on a receptive audience among many whites for Drake's complaint that "apparently SIECUS-sex educators are planning to use their courses to educate children not to discriminate sexually because of race, or national origin."[95] But a very visible civil rights movement had helped render such explicit racist appeals culturally unacceptable and therefore strategically risky for a social movement.

There was no such public disapproval to deter the Right from its broad use of sexually stigmatizing depravity narratives, however. These narratives fueled intense battles. They provoked an immediate emotional reaction and were notoriously difficult to refute. The polarization prompted by depravity narratives usually precluded real debate about these questions. As one Nashville paper headlined, "Smears, Ignorance Cloud Issue of Sex Education."[96] Anaheim's Sally Williams encountered "horrid stories attributed to the Anaheim program" all over the country. She recalled that people felt "if there's so much smoke, there must be a little fire somewhere. And every time they accused us of doing things . . . it's very hard to get your point across. If you didn't do something, they would say you just denied it. How can you defend something that you didn't do? Well, I never found a way to do it."[97] In a 1970 interview, Mary Calderone responded to these depravity narratives:

One of our board members tracked it down and found that, in a health class at a Flint, Michigan school, a teacher demonstrated how different ways of dressing expressed different personalities, mores and manners. She modeled a number of dresses to illustrate these points and changed behind a screen. She was never without her slip. And bear in mind that this was an all-girl class. So you can see, these simple facts have been grossly distorted. A number of other untrue stories have been making the rounds; for example, it's alleged that in some schools, kids are herded together in closets so that they can feel each other, and that kindergarten children are taught to model genital organs out of clay. These tales are utter nonsense and are never substantiated by name, place or date. I look upon them as blatant insults to the integrity and intelligence of the teachers in our nation's schools.[98]

Largely, though, SIECUS did not have the resources to track and refute the countless depravity narratives of the late sixties sex education controversies.[99]

The popular media, however, took up the challenge as many newspapers and magazines launched their own piercing investigations of the opponents' allegations. For example, *Parade Magazine* followed two narratives, including the widely circulated story about a twelve-year-old boy who tried to experiment on his four-year-old sister after he learned about sexual intercourse: "'Intelligence Report' tracked this story down, learned that it originated with a Fundamentalist Protestant minister who heard it from a parishioner, who heard it from another woman who was not particularly noted for her emotional stability."[100] And when California Representative James Utt sent out a newsletter attacking SIECUS, one newspaper devoted full coverage to it. In a scathing critique, the article began:

> Rep. James B. Utt said Tuesday that sex education and rock 'n' roll music were part of a Communist conspiracy to destroy America. The California Republican also contended Communists had infiltrated all levels of the clergy in an effort to destroy moral standards as one step in a worldwide conspiracy. Statements and charges in the 1,200-word newsletter also involved the Beatles, the American Legion, psychiatrists, hypnotism, homosexuality, free love, sex life in Scandinavia and Pavlov, the Russian psychologist.[101]

The article then concluded: "Virtually none of the charges and statements was supported by evidence."[102] The piece exposed so many lies and distortions that it effectively humiliated the newsletter's author, Robert Geier, who defended himself at the end of the article with, "I'm not writing a thesis . . . to get a degree. If there is some jumping around or not tying together, I don't see how I can be responsible for that."[103] However embarrassing to the opposition, such exposés did little to derail the critics' momentum. The same tales surfaced in town after town, stirring fear and anger among local residents. They were a powerful tool of the opposition, regardless of whether parents took them literally.

Truth was irrelevant. If an incident did not happen, well then, it could and probably would in some town or another. James Townsend, the outspoken Anaheim opponent, acknowledged this complex power of belief systems as he discussed the tales of teachers stripping and engaging in public intercourse: "If it didn't happen, it certainly was out as happening and was being run around the country, talked about on radio and TV. So, happened or didn't happen, in the minds of the people, it happened."[104] And even more important was the emotional climate of danger and shame that was reinforced by the repetition of depravity narratives, even if an audience was skeptical. The tales exploited popular anxieties about the destructive power of unleashed sexuality. Their constant repetition, even amid some disbelief, reveals the anxious pleasures that were involved in speaking out against sex education.

Depravity narratives were the scaffolding for another tactic of Christian Right sex education opponents: creating a climate of blame in relation to individual sex educators. Critics portrayed sex educators, especially the most visible leaders, as sexually troubled, out of control, or perverted. Hate mail flooded SIECUS: "Sex-seducers & Sex-Maniacs" and "Mary STINKEN Calderone, Mistress of the Devil; Misfit Prostitute of Hell."[105] Although some of this material was clearly extremist, even the *60 Minutes* title for its interview with Calderone, "Dirty Old Woman," played on this sentiment. One parent on a news broadcast at the height of the Anaheim battles demanded that "in order to protect the children . . . all people with any affiliations to this program be investigated concerning their private and public lives and be given tests by a psychiatrist to see if they are considered sexually normal. These results then should be made public."[106] Along with depravity narratives, these accusations helped foster a climate of sexual suspicion in which sex educators might well be molesters for whom the classroom was the perfect vehicle for predation. Years later, Calderone said that the attacks had inflicted "lasting damage" on her since, as she was apparently considered too dangerous to be around children, she stopped being invited to speak to youth groups.[107]

The final strategy of sex education opponents was one of systematic distortion. The innuendo deployed in anti-communist rhetoric and the hyperbole of depravity narratives certainly figure as tactics of distortion.

However, this strategy warrants additional attention because of a broader range of practices such as decontextualization, omission, shock value, and "cut and paste" methods. Not uncommonly, for example, opponents claimed that sex education materials were pornographic, and they would read these aloud during school board meetings. Undaunted by imposed three-minute time limits, opposition leader Eleanor Howe of Anaheim told me how they would line up at the microphone and simply hand off the material to the person behind them like a baton in a relay race.[108] Often, however, the materials in question were not used with students but were in fact teacher resources, library books, or in some cases even doctored documents. One leaflet, for example, spliced a photograph of Michelangelo's *David* into a brochure supposedly from a San Diego program for five- to eight-year-old children.[109] These events were highly effective media stunts, garnering headlines like "Teachers Using Pornographic Sex Material, Woman Claims"[110] and "Parent Reads Textbooks, Causes Gasps and Giggles at Sex Education Hearing."[111] In such cases, the media helped foster the volatile emotional climate.

Sex education advocates were especially vulnerable to tactics of distortion. They were the speakers, the advocates for openness and explicit sexual speech. Calderone later said, "I didn't mind saying penis and vulva in public . . . but I wasn't doing it to shock but to make it easier for people to say the words themselves."[112] So it was not difficult with activists like Calderone for opponents to simply lift a few sentences out of context and make her sound like the dirty old lady which they had accused her of being. In *Is the School House the Place to Teach Raw Sex?*, the Christian Crusade's Gordon Drake did just that, with such a widely disseminated selective quotation that it is worth reproducing here as an example of such tactics. Drake claimed that Calderone had said, "What is sex for? It's for fun . . . for wonderful sensations. Sex is not something you turn off like a faucet. . . . We need new values to establish when and how we should have sexual experiences."[113] This misleading selective passage was widely reprinted. In fact, however, these words had been lifted from the text of a talk Calderone had given at Blair Academy for boys:

What is sex for? It's for fun, that I know, for wonderful sensations. It's also for reproduction, sedation, reward, punishment. It's a status symbol, a commercial come-on, proof of independence, a form of emotional blackmail. Many of these are negative ways of using sex. What we are trying to feel our way toward are the positive ways. Sex is not something to be feared or degraded or kicked around or used. Sex is not something you turn off like a faucet. If you do, it's unhealthy. We are sexual beings, legitimately so, at every age. Don't think that sex stops at the age of fifty. It doesn't.[114]

The full quotation, of course, conveys quite a different message and tone. Once again, this distortion underscores the vulnerability of sex educators to strategies which would discredit them. SIECUS did little to defend itself.

Even in the face of unsuccessful initiatives, strategists on the Right have been deft at transforming failures into creative efforts to recruit and mobilize supporters.[115] In this case, the question of success or failure in the sixties sex education wars is impossible to answer. Clearly there were tangible consequences in the short term: teachers lost their jobs; towns were polarized; neighbor fought neighbor; and sex education programs were dismantled. Quantification is difficult, but by the end of this period controversies had divided communities in close to forty states. In some cases, there was a chilling effect. For example, one teacher in a small Kansas town who had been forced to resign over the sex education attacks was quoted at the time as saying, "I was ready and willing to bring some responsible leadership to this movement [the family-life program] but now I'll not get involved in it in any way in my next position."[116] Another sex educator told me she received dire warnings when she started her job: "So they told me when I was hired that I couldn't teach about contraception, I couldn't teach about abortion. I couldn't teach—well, they didn't even mention homosexuality, forget that. This was 1970; it wasn't even mentioned. And I couldn't use any materials from this communist organization named SIECUS."[117] No matter that she had not even heard of SIECUS at the time.

In later reflections, activists on both sides of the sex education controversies expressed a sense of long-term failure. For example, in 1987, Calderone said, "It doesn't seem to me we've made any progress at all in the [past] ten years. Any. On the contrary, I think it's degenerated, because our children are more exposed, not having any training in thinking, intellectualizing about one's sexual aspects."[118] Calderone's pessimism was mirrored by her critics but, not surprisingly, from a different point of view. Eleanor Howe is proud of shutting down the Anaheim program and said:

I've been vindicated. I made the statement at a school-board meeting that if they continued with this type of sex instruction—I never called it education—that they were going to find it necessary to distribute condoms and other birth-control devices in our junior-high schools, and everybody laughed. They just thought that was the funniest thing. And yet that's precisely what they're doing now. . . . That's how far this whole thing has gone toward changing the values of an entire society. That's what I foresaw, and now all I can say is, "I told you so some twenty-some years ago."[119]

Likewise, Billy James Hargis later admitted his sense of defeat at stopping what he sees as the immoral sexuality of contemporary culture.[120] Both sides felt disheartened, regardless of whether programs were dismantled.

When asked what she thought triggered the controversies, SIECUS educator Esther Schulz said, "Oh, the whole idea that you didn't say 'sex' out loud."[121] In fact, not only did the Right fail to stop sex education, the controversies themselves proliferated public sexual speech. This happened in two ways. First, the conflicts made sexuality visible. At least in the short run, the sex education movement had been slowed but not stopped. The conclusion of a 1969 review article in the *Washington Post* was summarized in the headline "Despite Opposition, Sex Education Spreads in Schools."[122] In survey research published in the mid-seventies, political scientists James Hottois and Neal Milner concluded that most of the sixties sex education conflicts resulted in the programs' continuation or expansion.[123] Despite limitations in their sample, theirs is the only empirical study of those controversies. Their conclusion is not far from Calderone's later assertion that the controversies "made the name SIECUS famous. They really helped us more than they hindered us."[124] Both nationally and locally, sex education and therefore sexual topics suddenly occupied media attention in a way they had never before done. Students openly discussed the conflicts in their schools. Sex was everywhere spoken.

Second, the late sixties sex education controversies helped launch Christian evangelicals and fundamentalists into the realm of sexual politics. Throughout the course of the 1968 and 1969 sex education conflicts, those who wanted to silence talk about sex became the most ardent sexual speakers. Like censors through history, anti—sex education activists found themselves speaking that which they sought to render unspeakable. In attempts to prompt feelings of disgust and outrage, opponents dominated school board meetings with lengthy readings of sex education materials which they called pornographic. They produced countless documents—brochures, leaflets, books, slide shows—recirculating this alleged pornography. Groups like the Christian Crusade developed their own sex education materials. Front groups and spin-off groups "sprouted like mushrooms after a rain," according to the *New York Times*.[125] This helped effect a profound change both in the emerging Christian Right and in the future course of sex education debates. The late sixties sex education controversies demonstrated the political opportunities inherent in mobilizing around sexuality. This strategy would take hold more fully in the mid-seventies, as conservative Catholics, evangelicals, and fundamentalists came together to form the "pro-family" movement. The sixties sex education conflicts foreshadowed the prominence sexuality would come to hold in America's reconfigured political landscape.

# Chapter 3 | BORN-AGAIN SEXUAL POLITICS

In the late seventies, the Christian Right burst onto the political landscape. Of the scores of both single-issue groups and expansive national organizations, none was more influential than Jerry Falwell's Moral Majority. In 1980, Falwell repeatedly told a story about how he had been at the White House and asked the president, "Sir, why do you have homosexuals on your senior staff in the White House?"[1] Jimmy Carter allegedly responded that he had had to hire some homosexuals to prove he would represent *everyone*. When the *New York Times* and other major news media revealed that the exchange had never happened, Falwell claimed he had been recounting a "parable" or "allegory." Hearing this, another minister dubbed Falwell's explanation "a new name for a lie."[2] Was it an allegory or a lie? Scholars of political movements, and even some prominent leaders of the Christian Right itself, have claimed that the movement routinely distorts the truth and even fabricates many of its claims.[3] However, in her study of Falwell, anthropologist Susan Harding argues that it is misguided to read narratives such as the Carter story literally, outside of the context of fundamentalist speech communities. Falwell's speech is not secular, Harding argues, and his followers read him figuratively, not literally.[4] In a sense, both interpretations are crucial to understanding how the national rhetorics of sex education opposition evolved in the aftermath of the late sixties conflicts. Still, the disagreement over whether Falwell told a lie is emblematic of the polarizations that would arise from the Christian Right's fusion of religion and politics.

Christian Right activists have been more culturally powerful in sex education debates than have sex education advocates. To understand their ways of talking about sex education, we must examine several interrelated factors. Historical and political context shape a social movement's speech. Conservative Christian activists in the late sixties, allied with groups like the John Birch Society, had spoken out against sex education at a transitional moment in the American right wing. The Old Right was waning. Soon, however, they found themselves part of a reinvigorated national movement. It was a movement for which matters of sexuality and the family would figure prominently in building a sophisticated infrastructure of advocacy, research, and legal organizations. Moreover, the Christian Right's mass base is Protestant evangelicals and fundamentalists. Fundamentalists constitute a "community of discourse"[5] which interactively produces "truth" and religious and social identities through particular rhetorics, symbols, and ways of talking. Like all social movement activists, fundamentalists used language and images to foster an emotional climate that would capture the attention of diverse and often indifferent audiences, convince them that a problem exists, and mobilize them to action. Their ways of talking became political speech; traditional right-wing and fundamentalist strategies inflected the rhetorical style of sex education opponents. At a time of broad transformations in civic life and rapid changes in the sexual culture, their oppositional ways of speaking found a national audience and helped turn the late sixties controversies over sex education into widespread, unremitting opposition in later decades.

## PRO-FAMILY POLITICS

In the late sixties, Mary Calderone and other SIECUS advocates had encountered passionate opponents of sex education. By the mid-seventies, these episodic moral protests had evolved into a cohesive political movement.[6] Billy James Hargis was in many ways a transitional figure from an older right wing to a refurbished seventies New Right and its submovement, the Christian Right. The New Right was a face-lift for an Old Right in need of a fresh image and some distance from its explicit racism and the conspiracist thinking of organizations such as the John Birch Society.

The New Right coalition of corporate sponsors, cohorts of Republicans, and a grassroots, largely religious base backed familiar right-wing projects such as aggressively anti-communist foreign policy, increased military spending, and an economic agenda of corporate tax cuts and expansive capitalism. Like the Old Right, the New Right pushed for the dismantling of social welfare programs and government regulation. However, it downplayed the anti-communism of yore to foreground social issues. The "red menace" was displaced by a campaign against godless secular humanism. This emphasis allowed it not only to attract kindred born-again spirits, but also to draw more widespread support from those who might be indifferent to right-wing foreign policy and conspiracy theories but were worried about social chaos and moral decline. This emphasis on social issues, particularly sexuality, marked the coherence of a strategy that had already begun to emerge. The sex education controversies of 1968 and 1969 had been a profound lesson in the opportunities for mass political mobilization available through organizing around sex.

As schools developed and revitalized sex education programs during the seventies, so too the Christian Right was gaining power. Honed by the Goldwater campaign and strengthened by decades of institution building, evangelicals and other conservatives displayed remarkable organizational acuity. By the decade's end, they not only had spawned numerous groups—such as the Religious Roundtable, the Christian Voice, and the widely discussed Moral Majority—but also had developed sophisticated networks for political mobilization. Throughout the seventies, the Christian Right would more successfully forge ties among those with whom it might otherwise disagree theologically. This strategy, called cobelligerency, allied former antipathetic groups.[7] In historically unprecedented coalitions, conservative Catholics, conservative Jews, along with Christian evangelicals, fundamentalists, Pentecostals, and even some Muslim allies abrogated denominational loyalties to fight for "traditional values"—a move which united opponents of sex education. Several studies between 1976 and 1981 showed that, compared with other religious individuals, evangelicals were the most politically involved.[8] And by 1988, regular church-attending evangelicals constituted a larger voting bloc than mainline Protestants.[9]

The late seventies marked the clear articulation of pro-family politics, a development that would prove vital to the success of the New Right and the Christian Right. Activists condensed opposition to a series of social issues, including abortion, the Equal Rights Amendment, pornography, sex education, and homosexuality, under a "pro-family" rubric. The family represents the "seedbed of virtue" for neoconservatives,[10] while for evangelicals, pro-family politics expressed a concept of gender relations in which a male-headed family structure replicates God's authority over the churches, as expressed in Ephesians 5:22: "Wives, submit to your husbands as to the Lord. For the husband is the head of the wife as Christ is the head of the church." In fact, the "traditional family" that is so celebrated by conservatives and fundamentalists is less than historically accurate. It is, for one thing, a nostalgic and idealized late nineteenth-century middle-class family in which men and women operated in "separate spheres."[11] And as theologian Rosemary Ruether argues, the Bible, including the New Testament, articulates no single model of the family and, at times, is even anti-family.[12] Nevertheless, the pro-family moniker proved to be politically astute, since it helped swell the ranks of New Right groups. It was rhetorically powerful in that it linked opposition to a range of social justice issues and couched them as a defense of the American family against the incursions of feminism, gay rights, and sex education.

Two public events helped launch the pro-family movement: the 1977 International Women's Year (IWY) Conference and the 1980 White House Conference on Families. Their significance is largely symbolic, since neither event broke new public policy ground. They were, however, moments of galvanizing rage for a range of conservatives who viewed each conference as government legitimation of what they considered destructive social trends. The broad constituencies mobilized by the Christian Right demonstrated the widespread political appeal of social, and particularly sexual, issues. These rancorous debates over a social vision for America forecast the divisive culture wars that would unfold in the eighties and nineties.

The IWY Conference, held in Houston in November 1977, showed that the path to women's equality was strewn with obstacles. The national conference was the capstone event in the United States of the United Nations International Women's Decade, which had begun in 1975. Congress had appropriated $5 million for the conference to develop a National Plan of Action to identify and eliminate "barriers that prevent women from participating fully and equally in all aspects of national life."[13] The plan that eventually passed, which had largely been crafted beforehand at regional conferences, was a sweeping endorsement of goals compatible with feminism, such as the extension of Social Security benefits to housewives, funding for rape prevention and battered women's shelters, federally funded child care, the passage of the Equal Rights Amendment (ERA), and an end to discrimination against lesbians.[14] While some of these resolutions were not controversial, the endorsement of the ERA, abortion rights, and lesbian rights triggered vehement criticism. Internal battles over endorsement of the platform helped consolidate local right-wing networks in particular states, and ultimately Christian opponents organized a national counter-rally. Over ten thousand people attended the gathering, most bused in from church groups (including a vast Mormon contingent) as well as anti-abortion and StopERA organizations.[15] Some journalists reported a discernible John Birch Society and Ku Klux Klan presence.[16] In her analysis of IWY, sociologist Alice Rossi showed that the anti-plan delegates left the conference more unified in vision and strategy than ever.[17] As national activist Jo Ann Gasper told me, "The extremely liberal women's movement had been chugging along pretty much unchallenged, and conservative women who are primarily concerned with hearth and kin, family and their home and their local community had no grandiose idea about remaking the world in a feminist kind of mind-set. The International Women's Year movement and the state meetings gave conservative women, for the first time, an opportunity to see in the flesh what the liberal feminist movement meant."[18] This crystallization of an oppositional ideology in Houston marks IWY as a "cohering moment" of the national pro-family movement[19] and led to the establishment of many right-wing local networks.

The egalitarian vision of the International Women's Year Conference provoked the emerging pro-family movement. Conservatives saw key features of IWY goals—specifically the endorsement of abortion rights, lesbian rights, and the widespread sentiment against rigid gender roles—as antithetical to the survival of what they deemed traditional morality and family values. Phyllis Schlafly, then of StopERA, captured these fears in her charge that there was "the use of tax funds to promote ERA, lesbian privileges, government-funded abortions, witchcraft, Marxism, obscene performances, and Marxist literature."[20] This acute sense of danger was amplified by Robert Shelton, Imperial Wizard of the United Klans of America, who reportedly announced that the KKK would be present at

IWY, asserting that "our men will be there to protect our women from all the militant lesbians."[21] Although perhaps cartoonish, this rhetoric of risk concerning homosexuality at IWY foreshadowed later debates over the White House Conference on Families.

Called by President Jimmy Carter in 1978 as a national forum on family policy, the White House Conference on Families was an obvious target for the emerging pro-family movement. Planning broke down over irreconcilable differences among disparate constituencies regarding the meaning of "family." When an announcement of the conference changed the title from "family" to "families," right-wing activists seasoned by IWY were alerted to what they saw as code for "gay rights." They were poised to strike. Schlafly told a *New York Times* reporter that the rules were "rigged" against them at IWY but "now we know what to look for, and we're prepared."[22] Prepared they were indeed. They fought over the definition of family, constituted a considerable presence at the conference, and ultimately organized a counterconference of over three hundred pro-family groups called the American Family Forum. By the end of the White House Conference on Families, the pro-family movement had shown its muscle.

Anti-homosexuality was the nucleus of opposition to an expansive definition of family. This was political appeal to religious conviction, since the movement was an emerging coalition of evangelicals, fundamentalists, and conservative Catholics. As the *New York Times* conference coverage concluded about them, "The 'pro-family' forces . . . describe themselves as 'grass roots,' and as religious."[23] And so the conservative activists pushed a definition that stressed "a family consists of persons who are related by blood, marriage, or adoption."[24] Single mothers were barely tolerable, as were children raised by grandparents but not homosexuals. Beverly LaHaye of Concerned Women for America said, "Early in 1980, we saw that homosexuals were driving in, because they wanted to be part of the whole definition of the family. And we objected to that."[25] Although the pro-family movement did not prevail at the White House Conference on Families, that failure pales next to its blossoming political and organizational strength. The explosive events of IWY and the White House Conference on Families demonstrated to the New Right the potential political power of pro-family politics. And sexual issues would form the nucleus of these politics. Sex education, abortion, pornography, gay rights, AIDS, feminism, sexually explicit art, and popular culture all eventually became targets.

The movement grew exponentially over the decades. Like other social movements, the pro-family movement exaggerates its strength.[26] Still, its infrastructural expansion on the national, state, and local levels was enormous. In 1997, the Christian Values in Action Coalition produced a compendium of 1,450 organizations solely dedicated to promoting family, marriage, and home schooling.[27] This was *not* the entire Christian Right—a hefty companion encyclopedia listed 7,400 organizations with varied goals[28]—it is merely a subsection of groups "to help individuals put into practice family building and marriage enrichment principles."[29] These were specialized groups spanning a range of issues: for example, Teen-Aid, which produces abstinence-only sex education curricula; Liberty Counsel, which provides anti-abortion legal services; Morality in Media; and the anti-gay Oregon Citizens Alliance. Opposition to comprehensive sex education became a central goal of large national advocacy organizations such as Focus on the Family and Concerned Women for America and legal centers like the Rutherford Institute. By the end of the nineties, the pro-family movement was constituted by large numbers of interconnected, multilevel organizations with myriad initiatives from electoral politics to cultural reform.

## GOING LOCAL

From its emergence in the mid-seventies through the end of the twentieth century, national pro-family organizations came to figure prominently in local debates over sex education. Some sociologists have dismissed the significance of national, or "tertiary," associations, arguing that mass-membership organizations have little impact on the political cultures and social capital of communities.[30] However, broad changes in American civil society through the last half of the twentieth century heightened the potential for the pro-family national infrastructure to exercise wide influence. Local community boundaries eroded from the nationalizing effect of the federal government, the market economy, and mass media like radio and television. As Beth Bailey put it in her book on the sixties sexual revolution, "The increasing power and presence of national institutions and national culture upset 'traditional' ways—be it Jim Crow or sexual mores— and created openings for contestation and change."[31] In addition, changes in civic affiliation over the past several decades transformed the ways in which people connected to their neighbors, communities, and a broader political process.[32] The sixties through the nineties was characterized by the proliferation of what sociologist Theda Skocpol describes as "relatively centralized and professionally led organizations focused on policy lobbying and public education."[33] The power of national organizations like Concerned Women for America and the earlier Moral Majority grew as a result of the civic shift away from popularly rooted membership associations toward national advocacy groups. This shift in American associational patterns strengthened the nationalizing influence on ways of thinking and talking in local sex education debates. As it turned out, not only did national institutions help create the conditions for social change but conservative organizations would also exert pressure for the reimposition of "traditional ways."

The pro-family movement's local impact was also enhanced by astute organization building. For example, right-wing investors funded the types of infrastructural elements that build a movement, such as research centers and think tanks, rather than advocacy and social service programs that progressive foundations tended to fund.[34] And in her study of both left- and right-wing sixties activists, Rebecca Klatch found that as they reached adulthood, Students for a Democratic Society (SDS) and other leftist activists settled into nonprofit organizations, education, and social services, while Young Americans for Freedom and other activists on the right gained power in the political world as consultants and advisers.[35] Conservative sixties activists helped initiate the cultural swing to the right in the eighties, which in turn launched them to political prominence. The end result of all this was an expansive national right-wing infrastructure powered by trained activists with more capability than progressives to shape political debates.

The Christian Right grew to outweigh progressives in its advocacy infrastructure related to sexuality and the family. The Center for Reproductive Law and Politics noted that, throughout the nineties, the number of anti-abortion legal groups alone had risen from two—Americans United for Life and the National Right to Life Committee—to over eighteen such organizations so that anti-abortion legal groups outnumbered pro-choice organizations by almost ten to one.[36] The numbers are even more disproportionate for sex education. There are over two dozen large national organizations that oppose comprehensive sex education, such as the Eagle

Forum, Focus on the Family, and Concerned Women for America (see the Appendix for a list). SIECUS, on the other hand, is the only single-issue, pro-comprehensive sex education national organization, although other groups have intermittently dedicated part of their policy work to monitoring sex education.[37] Opponents of comprehensive sex education, moreover, have far greater financial resources available to them. For example, one Christian Right national organization, Focus on the Family, has an annual budget of over $110 million and broadcasts a daily radio show on fifteen hundred stations in North America.[38] In 1999, SIECUS's budget was not quite $2 million.

Unlike progressive groups, which tended to maintain large, professionally staffed offices in New York or Washington, D.C., the right wing's national organizations went local.[39] By 1995, for example, the Christian Coalition had established seventeen hundred chapters in voting districts throughout the United States. Concerned Women for America, which is opposed to comprehensive sex education and gay rights, is organized on the local level in Prayer Action Chapters led by Prayer Action Captains.[40] The national parent organization often coordinates efforts at the state and local levels.[41] On the state level, the Right established myriad think tanks designed to advance public policy and train activists.[42] Linked to the Republican Party, these state-level think tanks formed a web of influence linking national organizations and local politics.

Indeed, a commitment to seeking local public office became one distinguishing feature of the Christian Right. In 1980, *Newsweek* quoted a local Florida minister who observed, "We're running for everything from dogcatcher to senator."[43] By the early nineties, Ralph Reed, then director of the Christian Coalition, noted that conservative Christians were more interested in community positions, such as school boards and city councils, than in national politics.[44] School boards were a particular focus for Christians. In 1985, Robert L. Simonds of Citizens for Excellence in Education first released his well-known text *How to Elect Christians to Public Office.*[45] Revised in 1996, this guide exhorts Christians to seek political office in order to save the nation from "atheistic secular humanists."[46] Simonds's thesis—that "government and true Christianity are inseparable"[47]—is the hallmark of dominion theology, a philosophy calling for the establishment of a theocracy in the United States.[48] Although not many Christian Right activists advocated the establishment of an Old Testament—

based theocracy, there was growing interest among fundamentalists in a "softer" form of dominionism characterized by seeking public office to shape policy and law.[49]

Organizations like the Christian Coalition actively sought to bring this about. They held hundreds of training seminars across the country on how to win local offices, specifically school board seats.[50] During a hot 1993 city-wide school board election, Brooklyn's Christian Coalition chapter provided IRS lawyers to advise pastors on how to advocate for Christian candidates while maintaining tax-exempt status: "He can't say, 'Our Susie is running for school board and you should vote for her.' [B]ut he can say, 'Our Susie is running for school board, let's all pray for her!'"[51] The Christian Coalition widely distributed voter guides, some forty million nationwide in 1993, which endorsed Christian candidates. During highly contested 1993 statewide elections, in which sex education was a central issue in many towns, a local Christian Coalition chapter in Massachusetts distributed nearly four hundred thousand such guides. In a letter to local pastors, the Coalition coordinator declared that "'separation of church and state' is a bogus phrase. Our country was founded on Biblical principles and we need to turn back to God and His precepts."[52] He offered to come to local churches to distribute materials. In community debates, then, when comprehensive sexuality educators advocated for open sexual discussion with young people, pro-family activists had the organizational structures and material resources to show up and talk back.

SEX, LIES, AND NATIONAL RHETORICS

The pro-family movement became a formidable opponent. Cultural conservatives were galvanized by the high visibility and the many political gains won by feminism and the lesbian/gay movement. The women's and gay movements had, since the sixties, effected widespread changes in social policies such as anti-discrimination laws, more inclusive family initiatives, and efforts to end sexual violence and ensure reproductive rights. Although they were slow and uneven, cultural assumptions about the role of women and the possibility of equality for gay people tangibly shifted. The pro-family movement concretely addressed fear and confusion among some Americans arising from these tumultuous social changes involving the structure of families, relationships between women and men at home and in the workplace, reproductive issues, teenage sexual activity, and social acceptance of lesbians and gay men. It pointed to teenage pregnancy, sexually transmitted diseases, sexual openness in the media, and other changes of the increasingly sexualized society of the seventies and eighties as evidence of moral decline. Feminism and gay liberation, it charged, along with organizations like SIECUS and Planned Parenthood, fostered a dangerous climate of immorality.

Sex education in the public schools symbolized an increasingly profligate sexual culture, and dismantling it became a high priority for many national organizations. Because public opinion has generally favored sex education since the sixties, the pro-family movement had to change minds. Failing that, it had to discredit sex education sufficiently to discomfit potential supporters. It would do so by what I have called oppositional speech strategies. These national rhetorics sought to establish common meanings about sex education and to set an emotional tone in community sex education debates across the nation. Many of these strategies had been used during the late sixties controversies. They were ways of talking that were rooted in the movement's history.

"Words are . . . bullets" in the culture wars that divide America, according to James Dobson, founder of the evangelical group Focus on the Family.[53] His metaphor captures the sense by which, in opposing sex education, national organizations would use language as a weapon. As we shall see throughout the rest of this book, these oppositional strategies would include the repetition of evocative sexual language (calling a health education text "pornography"); establishing sex educators as targets for blame (they have been called everything from Communists to dirty old women to pedophiles); the invention of depravity narratives (circulating fictive tales to scare parents and discredit sex educators); the claim that sex education speech is performative (that talking about sex enacts sex); and the secularization of religious arguments (using medical claims that may be misleading or inaccurate to advance religious morality). These ways of talking were shaped by the rhetorical styles of the right wing and its evangelical and fundamentalist constituents.

Right-wing movements in the United States have a long tradition of crusading against groups or ideas which they consider alien and dangerous.[54] Many scholars have pointed out the right-wing style of paranoia, fears of conspiracy, and a tendency toward demonizing its enemies.[55] In earlier times, this has taken the form of nativist movements during waves of nineteenth-century immigration, the anti-Catholicism of the Ku Klux Klan, and the virulent anti-communism of the McCarthy era. By the seventies, as traditional anti-alien rhetoric lost its symbolic power, the Right turned to different adversaries and ideologies. As the Old Right morphed into the New Right, notes political researcher Chip Berlet, "the dynamic of demonization, scapegoating, and conspiracism remained largely intact."[56] In the early eighties, political scientist Rosalind Petchesky argued that feminists and homosexuals had displaced Communists as the scapegoats of the New Right.[57] Seen as promoting sexual deviance and immorality, sex educators also fell among the ranks of the enemy. As we saw in the sixties, and as we shall see later in Chapter 5, opposition to sex education would not uncommonly take the form of attacks on individual sex educators.

Such forceful anti–sex education rhetoric is consistent with evangelical and fundamentalist communities of discourse. Fundamentalism, in particular, is characterized by an absolute morality in which right and wrong are seen as literally written into the Scriptures. This tradition fosters particular ways of thinking, feeling, and talking. An unwavering belief in an absolute truth can lead to what sociologist Nancy Ammerman describes as rhetorics of purity, totality, and certainty.[58] Fiery ways of speaking can be stoked even further by righteous and passionate anger about transgression against God's way. Christian Right leader Jerry Falwell once defined a fundamentalist as "an evangelical who was mad about something."[59] When they politicized their morality and coalesced as part of the pro-family movement, fundamentalists brought along these strong feelings and rhetorics.

The amalgam of right-wing and fundamentalist styles translated into specific tendencies in pro-family politics. For one, a fixed worldview allowed for no compromise in political battles over issues for which they believe God has issued direct commandments. Moreover, some members of the national Christian Right leadership asserted that the Scriptures allow them, since they are on the side of righteousness, to mislead their opposition by withholding information, allowing others to arrive at false impressions and employing what they call "mental reservation"—a process by which they make a statement while "holding back some of our true feelings, some concealment of our true design."[60] Christian Right activists

William Marshner and Enrique Rueda of the powerful Free Congress Research and Education Foundation explained how, for Christians, manipulation of the truth is not inevitably immoral in political contests: "Scripture teaches us that mental reservation is sometimes acceptable. It can be a morally acceptable means to achieve important ends."[61] This was, perhaps, a modified version of Falwell's "allegory." Finally, politics seem to require of them strong, even provocative language. In an article entitled "Why I Use 'Fighting Words,'" evangelical leader James Dobson defended as necessary his metaphors of violence and war since Christian Right activists see themselves as engaged in an age-old struggle between righteousness and darkness, God and Satan.[62] Falwell urged his followers to "speak harsh language" because change doesn't happen "if you don't make people mad."[63] Many of them followed his advice and his example. And while sex education opponents were not all fundamentalists or evangelicals, these ways of talking became idiomatic.

National rhetorics of sex education opposition emerged. Leaders of national organizations chose highly evocative sexual language to discredit sex education as little more than pornography. The Moral Majority, for example, was adept at appealing to the complicated culture of sexual anxiety and excitement. This was especially the case in direct mail, which is, as one consultant put it, "a medium of passion."[64] In the first sentence of one Moral Majority anti–sex education fund-raising letter, Falwell told readers, "You are going to be shocked when you open the sealed envelope I'm sending you today."[65] The enclosed envelope, which contained excerpts from one health textbook, was emblazoned with the enticing warning "ADULTS ONLY! SEXUALLY EXPLICIT MATERIAL."[66] Another early eighties fund-raising letter illustrated their heavy reliance on sexual issues. After the front page questioned "Is Our Grand Old Flag Going down the Drain?" the letter answered, "YES! . . . Just look at what's happening here in America." And, in what follows, *all* of the five examples appealed to presumed sexual fears about gay teachers and pornography.[67] Falwell claimed that every month the Moral Majority newspaper went to six hundred thousand readers; "That's a stack 2½ miles high . . . or 10 times higher than the Empire State Building."[68] This was almost certainly an exaggeration, and yet Falwell's message was so effectively disseminated that his words reached nearly everyone in the country who kept up with the news in the eighties.[69] National rhetorics went local.

These rhetorics used emotionally resonant language to create an unsettled collective mood. One sex education critic explained that explicit sexual language was necessary to provoke aversive feelings:

> The revolting nature of the acts I have just described, illustrate the predicament that writers like myself face when trying to explain to the uninitiated the perverse nature of sex education and the putrefactive character and morals of [sex educators]. If one tells the truth, then one must accept the risk, that truth intended to inform, may corrupt or tarnish the person so informed. If one holds back and simply refers to the perversity in non-offending terms, then the reader is unlikely to be moved to action because his sense of outrage has not been triggered.[70]

Sex education critics used sexual words and images to arouse anxieties, even taking them out of context or, as was sometimes the case, even when they were not part of the sex education program in question. For example, Christian Coalition founder Pat Robertson said about Planned Parenthood, "It is teaching kids to fornicate, teaching people to have adultery, teaching people to get involved in every kind of bestiality, homosexuality, lesbianism—everything that the Bible condemns."[71] Debra Haffner described how she repeatedly faced inflammatory allegations when she was president of SIECUS: "I was on CNN with this guy who's the deputy director of the American Life Lobby and he said, 'Debra's organization promotes necrophilia, bestiality, coprophilia.' I looked at him and I said, 'You know you're making this up. I can't even respond. Let me tell you what we talk about.' And I said to him later, 'You know, the only people I know who use those words are you guys when I debate you on television.'"[72] The point, however, was to use words that could provoke images and fears of perversion, especially as they might relate to children.

Throughout the last decades of the twentieth century, national Christian Right organizations refined various anti–sex education speech genres. Some of them were familiar from the sixties; for example, new versions of the depravity narrative were continually reinvented. Others evolved from debates in other social movements, such as feminism, about the consequences of speech, as we shall see in Chapter 6 regarding the allegation that sex education is child abuse. All of these genres featured the repetition of sexually stigmatizing terms, following Falwell's and Dobson's charge to use harsh language. The AIDS epidemic prompted new vocabularies of opposition. Increasingly, sex education opponents couched their arguments in medical rather than religious or moral terms. They were designed to appeal to the broadest possible audience of not simply religious conservatives but anyone who might have—or be persuaded to have—misgivings about sex education. Even more so than in the sixties conflicts, as a result of the impressive coalescence and expansion of the pro-family movement, the national vernacular opposing sex education diffused to local communities.

Sexuality education, then, had proven to be an effective bridge issue from the Old Right to the New Right for rhetorical as well as mobilization purposes. Sexually stigmatizing rhetoric came to operate in many of the same ways as the overtly racist appeals used by some in the Old Right. Both the Old Right and the New Right had understood the political capital to be gained as a result of white anger toward the civil rights movement and growing black equality. The energy behind George Wallace's 1968 and 1972 presidential campaigns had demonstrated the continuing power of racial anxieties in American political life. However, explicitly racist claims lost social and political acceptability, becoming a strategic liability as racism in mainstream discourse became more encoded. On the other hand, the Right found that public arguments about sexuality could perform significant rhetorical work. For one, they could serve as a code for race; a way to implicitly tap racial fears. Welfare, teen pregnancy, public funding of abortion, and rock and later rap music were all issues that melded race and sexuality. Petchesky argues that part of the Right's power has been this ability to fuse diverse fears: "The 'freedom' that white parents want is clearly the 'freedom' to keep their children away from black children; their fears of 'racial mix' are in no small part bound up with sexual-racial stereotypes and the fear of their children's sexuality."[73] Moreover, many of the features of racist appeals that the Right had found so effective could readily be employed in rhetoric about sex: the construction of differences and hierarchies; linking difference to disease and contagion; and the use of scientific language to legitimize claims.[74] In the late sixties conflicts, sex education had turned out to be an issue in which demonization of sexual differences for political purposes proved to be acceptable. The right had found that drawing sexual boundaries and creating enemies through provocative sexual speech promised political rewards.

National pro-family organizations speak against comprehensive sex education with a consistent voice. Given their size and resources, they are powerful members of religious conservatives' community of discourse. Movement leaders, however, do not always speak for the grass roots. There are important distinctions between prescriptive discourse and how ordinary evangelicals and fundamentalists navigate their faith, daily lives, and politics.[75] Conservative Protestants differ among themselves as to whether the Scriptures serve as the absolute authority on all matters of daily life, including politics. There is a significant commitment among many to a literal interpretation of the Bible. One evangelical minister insisted that there was a scriptural mandate for his opposition to teaching about gay families in the New York schools: "This is Leviticus Chapter 18.22: 'Thou shall not lie with mankind as with womankind. It is an abomination.' See, this is not interpretation. This is clear. It is not—'Oh, but the Bible, they interpret the Bible wrong.' What is there to interpret? It's clear, it's fact."[76] Others, however, may not be so literal and disagree about whether the Bible is the actual or the inspired word of God. Susan Harding claims that Bible-believing Christians exercise complicated interpretive practices which she calls "'flexible absolutism,' a rhetorical capacity and will to frame new and internally diverse cultural positions as 'eternal absolutes.'"[77] Indeed, these different interpretive strategies shape varying evangelical approaches to what is perhaps at the heart of the pro-family movement—the male-headed family. Some strictly adhere to this hierarchical model, sometimes because it confers structure on an otherwise failing marriage. A small minority of couples interpret the Scripture as supporting *mutual* submission, while many other evangelicals work out situational compromises with the notions of submission and accountability.[78] Such internal diversity among religious conservatives about the nature of God's word and how it should be lived is an important factor in their political participation.

Politically, conservative Protestants may sometimes belie popular stereotypes. They are not inevitably foot soldiers of the Christian Right. Although they tend to be more influenced by the movement than Americans in general, over two-thirds of them say that they are not supporters of the Religious Right.[79] Individuals themselves and even particular churches may demonstrate more flexible moral boundaries and cultural accommodation than would be expected from their sectarian traditions. Sociologist Christian Smith argues that evangelicals are not out of step with mainstream Americans in their views about issues such as whether teachers should lead prayers in public schools or whether women should stay in the home.[80] However, Smith found that evangelicals expressed contradictory sentiments: for example, that same-sex marriages should be outlawed but that laws should not regulate sexual lives, or that Americans should follow Christian morals but they should also be free to pursue any lifestyle, including non-Christian ones.[81] Moreover, three-quarters of evangelicals said that morals should be based on absolute, unchanging standards, and a majority of fundamentalists believe that Christian morality should be the law of the land, even though not all Americans are Christians. The rhetoric of the national pro-family movement, therefore, does have a potentially receptive audience.

In particular, the sexual rhetorics of the national Christian Right can receive a sympathetic hearing among grassroots religious conservatives. Even researchers who argue that evangelicals are increasingly heterodox and tolerant note that such open-mindedness diminishes with regard to sexual morality. For example, Smith's evangelical and fundamentalist respondents are consistently much more negative toward homosexuality and abortion than are other Americans.[82] And in her study of contemporary families, Judith Stacey found that sexuality was the most inflexible dimension of evangelical gender ideology. She notes, "Even most biblical feminists find it difficult to overcome scriptural and personal antipathy to homosexuality and abortion, and the popular evangelical literature is almost uniformly reactionary on these issues."[83] Stacey adds that it is in the area of sexuality in which the Christian Right has scored its most significant political and ideological victory. There can be a congenial fit, often, between national rhetorics opposing sex education and the conservative sexual morality of local conservative Protestant residents.

For many reasons, then, national ways of speaking against sex education strengthened and spread. The pro-family movement lent coherence and infrastructural power to the oppositional voices that spoke out in the late sixties. Scores of national research, advocacy, and legal organizations prioritized efforts to dismantle sex education in the public schools. Their impact on local debates was enhanced by changes in civic life that fostered a national culture. Their ways of thinking and talking about sex education appealed not only to many religious conservatives. Parents could be frightened by allegations about their own school programs, and those anxious about changes in the sexual culture might easily respond to the secularized arguments crafted by Christian Right national organizations. Meanwhile, in the seventies, the movement expanded beyond oppositional speech. No longer simply agents of resistance to modernity, Christian evangelicals stepped into the sexualized society as participants. As sexual experts in their own right, they developed their own sex education programs and expanded their movement.

# Chapter 4 | THE NEW SEXUAL REVOLUTION

Like Hollywood, the Christian Right found that sex sells. Evangelicals Tim and Beverly LaHaye are a case in point. Tim was an original board member of the Moral Majority and later established the American Coalition for Traditional Values, and among his countless books is a strong indictment of secular humanism, *The Battle for the Mind*.[1] Beverly is the founder of Concerned Women for America, a large national organization dedicated to furthering goals of the pro-family movement such as opposition to feminism and gay rights. Together they have authored books and led seminars for conservative Christians on a range of family issues. But many of these accomplishments were yet to come when, in their 1976 book *The Act of Marriage: The Beauty of Sexual Love*, they advised that God made the clitoris for women's pleasure and urged their readers to put Jesus at the center of their sex lives.[2] The LaHayes claimed that they were reluctant to write their conservative Christian sex manual—afraid that it would be inappropriate in its frankness and concerned that it would be misinterpreted.[3] Instead, the book went on to sell two and a half million copies, and the LaHayes's prominence as a power couple only grew. As it turned out, their sex counseling was evidence of a profound sea change: the sexualization of Christian evangelicalism.

Evangelicals, and by extension the Christian Right, entered a new phase in sexual politics. Instead of a movement only opposed to the sexual culture, conservative evangelicals and fundamentalists also developed a proactive movement for sexual change. In the sixties sex education battles these groups had spoken against sex with the angry voices of censors. By the mid-seventies, however, many of them had found a different voice that celebrated sexuality. They began to speak about sex not simply to oppose social change, but also as therapists, educators, even sexual confidants. And they built their own alternative sexuality industry. Their timing was flawless. The seventies was a watershed moment, capped by a 1976 *Newsweek* cover story heralding "The Year of the Evangelical" and citing a Gallup poll numbering them at fifty million Americans.[4] Evangelicals and other religious conservatives began to position themselves as sex experts precisely as they became powerful political actors. As we shall see, this development is not without tension within the Christian Right itself. But the burgeoning of Christian Right sex-related organizations, research institutes, and networks of committed grassroots activists devoted to sexual issues would radically reshape sex education while expanding the movement's political power.

## SEX, "TRUTHS," AND EVANGELICALS

Evangelicals' first steps into sexual counseling were understandably defensive. Those early writers were, after all, countering a long-standing association of Christianity with sexual prohibition and denial. Tim and Beverly LaHaye tried to finesse Christianity's responsibility for anti-sex moralizing, instead blaming "pagan philosophy" during the "Dark Ages," but finally they admitted that "confused church leaders of the past" might have contributed to the notion that sex is evil.[5] In fact, the Christian sexual tradition is complex. Christian dogma tenaciously advanced the idea that original sin has a toxic effect on all of humanity, including human sexuality.[6] Historically influential Christians such as Augustine and the Apostle Paul had denounced the sin of lust, yet Christianity has not been uninvolved in the widespread changes in sexual culture over the past century. The work of many of the nineteenth-century sexologists who had helped effect the medicalization of sex was inflected by their religious backgrounds.[7] Similarly, the various social purity crusades against prostitution and venereal disease bore an evangelical stamp. All contributed to an increasingly public sexual discourse. Religion scholar Peter Gardella argues for Protestantism's central role in dispelling sexual guilt and advancing an ethic of marital sexual pleasure in America.[8] And, as we saw in Chapter 2, mainstream denominations had been addressing questions of sexuality and religion intensively since the early sixties.

Still, evangelicals are renowned for their repudiation of sins of the flesh. So it was nothing short of revolutionary when, in 1973, an evangelical house-wife penned a bestseller advising her sisters-in-faith to greet their husbands at the door clad in erotic costumes and ready for sex.[9] And while Marabel Morgan's "total woman" may have been on the far edge of the evangelical sexual frontier, she was still on the map. By the mid-seventies, evangelicals had generated a boomlet in sex advice material. In line with the mainstream commercialization of sexuality, scores of sex manuals appeared with titles like *Sex for Christians* and *God, Sex, and You*.[10] Christians could be coun-seled on sexual problems in a wide range of programs—such as the Family Life Seminars, Total Woman workshops, or Fascinating Womanhood—or they could listen to advice cassettes at home. This proliferation of sexual self-help prompted one pundit to conclude that "the sexual revolution has pen-etrated even the self-enclosed world of right-wing fundamentalism."[11] And, with major qualifications, this assessment had some truth to it. By the early seventies, Christian evangelicalism had undergone distinct shifts in sexual ideology away from a singularly restrictive tradition.

Evangelicals began to celebrate sex, but only divinely approved sex. Evangelicals believe that there are absolute truths for sexual morality, know-able through the Bible. Despite their own growing participation in a pub-lic sexual arena, they are critics of a "sex-saturated culture where not much is really sacred."[12] For example, strictures against masturbation had markedly relaxed since the end of the nineteenth century, in part through the efforts of modern sexologists. Even liberal religions accepted the prac-tice, thereby aligning themselves more with a SIECUS-style ethic than that of evangelicalism. Pastor Howard Moody, in an article on sexual pleasure in *Christianity and Crisis*, sounded not unlike SIECUS founder Mary Calderone when he avowed, "Masturbation is not a disease of the human sexual condition. It is a means of pleasuring endowed in the very nature of our bodily creation by a good and loving God."[13] Calderone and SIECUS had frequently maintained that masturbation was a positive means of sexual pleasure.[14] In contrast, the LaHayes warned in 1976 that "we do not feel it is an acceptable practice for Christians."[15] Rather, evangelicals should resist the sexual temptations of a secular age. God, they assert, "never intended the cheap, perverted, publicly displayed sex we see today."[16] Christians are called to self-denial for the sake of God's kingdom, despite living in a modern age of indulgence. Therefore, they are staunch opponents of any expression of sexuality that is not marital, potentially procreative, and devoted to the preservation of the nuclear family.[17]

The scriptures are the center of Christian sex manuals in the way that their secular counterparts revolve around the texts of sexologists Alfred Kinsey and Masters and Johnson. Evangelical sex advisers look to the Lord for guidance in all matters. In their sex manual, the LaHayes discuss the need to discern the wishes of their very personally involved God. After having been approached by a Christian publishing house to write a religious sexual self-help book, they decided to pray about it:

> At first Bev was reluctant to get heavily involved with the endeavor until the Lord gave her a specific sign. Within the next two months she counseled at least ten frigid wives. The success these women soon achieved in their love lives convinced her that God required her active participation in the project. As we began to read current literature on the subject, convinced that God meant lovemaking to be mutually enjoyed by both partners, we prayed that He would lead us to make this work fully biblical and highly practical.[18]

God-centeredness and the claim that "religion is good for sex and that sex is good for religion" pervade evangelical manuals.[19]

Although confined by their reading of scriptures to marital intercourse, Christian sex counselors nonetheless brought exceedingly good news to contemporary evangelicals. Sexual pleasure was part of God's plan; "God designed our sex organs for our enjoyment."[20] The evangelical God is a personal God and, they argued, He so wants us to have good sex that He has been known to directly intervene to help hapless Christians. In *The Act of Marriage*, the LaHayes tell of a recently saved married couple, in which the wife could not achieve orgasm. They were advised by their minister to pray about it. That night they went to a party where they happened past a couple just as that husband threw his arm around his wife and exclaimed, "Hasn't our relationship been beautiful since we discovered clitoral stimulation?"[21] Thus the first couple was led "out of the wilderness of orgasmic malfunction" in this sexual parable which reassures readers that no dysfunction is too complicated or trivial for divine healing.[22]

Many evangelicals who have taken up sex counseling argue that confining sex to heterosexual marriages is not just morally correct but also affords a better sexual experience. And the rich pleasures of marital sex promised by Marabel Morgan, the LaHayes, and other contemporary evangelical sex advisers are reserved for the devout. Using a range of secular and religious surveys, these sex manuals claim that Christians have better sex than non-Christians.[23] If this turns out not to be the case for some couples, there are shelves of self-help books such as Morgan's titillating strategies in *Total Woman* for spicing up Christian marriages. Morgan, a self-described "little bumpkin from Ohio,"[24] became internationally famous as a result of her Total Woman seminars and her spate of books advising women how to save their marriages. She combined a more risqué, secular style—always be ready for sex, make love under the dining room table, wear a range of sexy costumes—with scriptural messages about the purity of marital sexual pleasure. Her inspiration for writing *Total Woman* was both her own failing marriage and her biblical conviction. She said:

> It definitely was from reading the Bible. There were a number of portions, like Song of Solomon. I read that and I probably blushed. I thought, "Good heavens! This is amazing." And I remember there was a verse in Hebrews that said something like, I can't remember it exactly, but the idea that the wedding or the marriage bed is undefiled, that God created it and we're to enjoy it, that the main purpose isn't really procreation but enjoyment and recreation within the parameters of marriage. And that's really all I needed. I mean, I bought it, hook, line, and sinker.[25]

Morgan's books and the Total Woman seminars continue to enjoy phenomenal popularity, a success she attributes to there being "a lot of bumpkins out there just like me. And I don't mean that in a derogatory way."[26] Total Woman seminars are conducted in far-flung locales such as Japan and Australia. Bearing their message of biblical sex, Morgan, the LaHayes, and scores of other evangelical sex advisers staked out their ground in the until then largely secular realm of sex experts.

The sexualization of evangelicalism has not come without controversy, however, and it has generated some internal tension in the Christian Right. Although their message is much more restrictive, there are still similarities to the secular fields of sexology and comprehensive sex education. Evangelical advisers have become defenders of the goodness and pleasures of marital sex, and they experience themselves as pioneers speaking out against a destructive tradition of sexual silence. In a comment reminiscent of Calderone, Morgan said, "Back in 1973, people spelled 'sex' in a sentence when they spoke about it. I've had people say, 'Well, you know, S-E-X.'"[27] Like their secular counterparts, these evangelical sex experts have discovered an audience eager to speak openly about sexuality and pleasure. Again, sounding uncannily like Calderone describing SIECUS's early years, Morgan speaks of the "tens of thousands of letters" she had received in response to her books and seminars:

> It was just incredible to me. I mean, the hurting people in the world. They would say, "Dear Marabel, I would like to tell you a little bit about my situation and maybe you can give me some advice." And then they would write five or six pages about their lives. And, of course, I wasn't a psychiatrist but I would write back and give them as much hope and practical advice as I could. And then finally I couldn't handle [it], we were receiving bags of mail. And so I hired some of my girlfriends. One time we had a little warehouse made available to us. So on Tuesdays and Thursdays ten of us would go over to the warehouse and work for about four or five hours and answer letters. And we had to answer them right away because if you didn't, in two weeks here they come again with another bag of letters. . . . But there were many that I wrote to and said, "Please call me." I mean, their stories broke my heart. So I was having conversations with people all day long all over the country. And I became friends with a lot of those people. People flew into Miami just to meet for an hour. It was amazing to me.[28]

Evangelical sex advisers had found their market.

Controversy was inevitable. Some criticism came, not surprisingly, from sexual liberals. Morgan's advice for women to submit to their husbands like they submit to the Lord coincided with a reinvigorated feminist movement which disdained this kind of advice. For evangelical women like Morgan and LaHaye, the family replicates the church, with the husband at the head in the Christ-like position and the women assuming the role of the obedient flock. And so, while evangelicals excoriated feminist ideas about gender and sexuality, feminists fired back at writers like Morgan. Magazine headlines denounced "The Books That Teach Wives to Be Submissive."[29] Feminist critic Barbara Ehrenreich likened fundamentalist imagery of women's submissiveness to classic sadomasochism.[30] In an interesting turn, however, Calderone, who was still president of SIECUS, defended Morgan out of "a feeling of camaraderie" that they both shared the goal of "the real liberation of women."[31] Calderone, as I've detailed in earlier chapters, had had her own qualms about feminism. And forever the crusader, she believed, no doubt rightly, that "Marabel Morgan's book and classes would probably reach a group of women who would not be reached in any other way—certainly not by anything SIECUS had to say."[32] Calderone rejected as false the assumption "that there is only one 'right' way to interpret these facts or to incorporate sexuality into one's life." By her criticism of liberal and feminist critics, whom she thought unfairly dismissed Morgan as "sexist," Calderone displayed striking generosity toward a conservative evangelical despite the personal attacks on her by some in the Christian Right.

The new evangelical sex advisers also encountered criticism from other Christians. Some were offended by what they saw as an unseemly emphasis on sex. For instance, liberal religious scholar Martin Marty, who wrote critical reviews of Morgan's books in the religious journal *Christian Century*, joked about "fundies in their undies" and quipped that Morgan's later book *Total Joy* displayed a "costume fetish [that] would dazzle Krafft-Ebing."[33] Pastor Tim LaHaye said that his colleagues advised him against writing his sex manual: "Way back then it was not popular for ministers to speak about sex. But I was led of God to write against the tide. . . . One of my dear friends, we laugh about it now, he said, 'Tim, you're going to ruin your reputation.'"[34] There was danger in speaking openly about sexuality, and indeed LaHaye did incur some criticism for being too liberal by refusing to outright condemn birth control for married couples.[35] But ultimately he did not ruin his reputation. That he and his wife Beverly remain prominent Christian Right leaders speaks not only to the cultural legitimacy that sex counseling acquired among evangelicals and fundamentalists. It also reveals how central the Christian Right sexuality industry was becoming to the movement's political goals.

Fundamentalism in the United States is characterized by separatist institution-building.[36] The establishment of a conservative Christian sexuality industry was consonant with this tradition. Fundamentalists and evangelicals are also committed to winning souls to the salvation found in Jesus Christ. Add to this mix the powerful entrance of conservative Christians into the political arena in the mid-seventies and it was not surprising that they became intent not on simply injecting morality or even religious considerations into the sexual culture. Rather, they were determined to broadly establish sexual mores that were congruent with their interpretation of biblical standards. They began efforts to implement public policy regarding teenage sexuality. The new Christian Right sex experts set about to regulate teen sexuality so that young people would wait until after marriage to enjoy the divine sexual gifts of the sort Marabel Morgan had promised. In their efforts to reshape the sexual culture according to their own values, the conservatives and evangelicals declared "Abstinence: The New Sexual Revolution."[37] By the early years of the Reagan administration, they had orchestrated the passage of the Adolescent Family Life Act (AFLA), Title XX of the Public Health Service Act, to achieve this goal.

## BUILDING A MOVEMENT THROUGH CHASTITY

The New Right and the Christian Right vaulted to surprising political influence in the eighties. Although pundits argued about the extent of their impact on Ronald Reagan's election in 1980,[38] the visibility of groups like the Moral Majority was unprecedented. Along with Reagan's election, Republicans also seized control of the Senate for the first time in twenty-six years. The New Right organized heavily around sexual issues— for example, teenage pregnancy, sexual explicitness in the media, and opposition to feminism and gay rights. In addition, two other important sex-related issues during the mid-seventies to the mid-eighties helped set the context for AFLA: abortion and AIDS. Both of these issues, along with AFLA, reveal the tensions in the changing sexual and political cultures.

Opposition to abortion was perhaps the most powerful unifying issue for a range of secular conservatives and religious groups on the Right. Even before the passage of *Roe v. Wade*, which legalized abortion in 1973, the Catholic Church had been organizing right-to-life committees.[39] Protestant evangelicals and fundamentalists on the Christian Right would join them by the mid-seventies. Important to women's sexual autonomy, abortion is therefore a vital target for right-wing efforts to control sexuality, reproductive rights, and the family. Shortly after the passage of *Roe*, a series of legislative initiatives eroded women's access to abortion. By 1977, Medicaid funding for abortion was restricted, thereby cutting off access for poor women. States began to pass parental consent provisions, requiring teenagers to go to court unless they could secure permission from one or both parents. A range of other unsuccessful efforts, such as the move to pass a constitutional amendment prohibiting abortion and state attempts to require waiting periods even for married women, contributed to the erosion of state and cultural legitimacy for abortion rights. (In 1979, Planned Parenthood Federation of America founded its Department of Education. Given its association with two profoundly controversial efforts—abortion and sex education—Planned Parenthood sexuality educators became a much maligned cohort.) AFLA, designed to prohibit discussion of abortion services in its programs with young women, emerged in this anti-abortion climate.

Like anti-abortion initiatives, the AIDS epidemic provided a platform for the right wing to enact policies and influence attitudes about sexuality. AIDS also made more visible the contentious question of what sexual topics should be taught to young people. Familiar Old and New Right leaders voiced their customary opposition to sex education of any kind. Phyllis Schlafly, for example, said she would rather see her children infected with sexually transmitted diseases than for them to know about condoms.[40] But AIDS marked an important dividing line in the Christian Right's approach to sex education. After Surgeon General C. Everett Koop's controversial 1986 AIDS report calling for detailed sex education including information on heterosexuality and homosexuality starting "at the lowest grade possible,"[41] the health crisis made it less viable for conservatives to call for the dismantling of school sex education programs. Even Koop, the erstwhile ally of conservatives before refusing to use his office to aggressively oppose abortion, grudgingly said about his AIDS report, "You can't talk of the dangers of snake poisoning and not mention snakes."[42] Yet the Christian Right blamed mainstream sex education organizations like Planned Parenthood and SIECUS for fostering sexual immorality, and so they constructed a distinct alternative to comprehensive sex education—one that would talk of snakes. With the Adolescent Family Life Act, conservatives launched a national project to establish chastity among youth. In the process, and with federal support, they built a vast national network of new organizations and research institutions dealing with sexuality.

AFLA was the prized child of Reagan's first term, the "highwater mark of the right-wing conservatives who were elected to the Senate in 1980."[43] Passed without debate as part of the massive Omnibus Budget Reconciliation Act of 1981, the Adolescent Family Life Demonstration Projects earmarked federal funding for prevention, care, and research related to adolescent pregnancy. Congress, however, had already funded several such programs since the early sixties: Title X of the Public Health Act and Titles V, XIX, and XX of the Social Security Act, which funded public contraceptive programs.[44] Organizations that discussed birth control and abortion, like Planned Parenthood, received such funding. Significantly, AFLA supporters cast it as an alternative to these programs. AFLA was their conspicuous attempt to shift the discourse on the prevention of teenage pregnancy away from contraception and instead to "chastity" or "morality." But Janet Benshoof, then a lead attorney for the ACLU (which eventually filed suit against AFLA), saw its passage as a trade-off so that conservatives would not slash Title X along with the other social programs being gutted at that time: "It was passed as a benign gift to the right wing, saying 'You give us our two-hundred million dollar a year Title X program and we'll give you your little ten-million dollar AFLA program.' It was 'You let us have this and we'll let you have this unconstitutional thing.'"[45] This deal would have far-reaching consequences for everyone involved.

AFLA, from its inception, sought to further the Christian Right's cultural and political goals. Cosponsored by Senators Orrin Hatch, a Republican from Utah, and the newly elected one-term Senator Jeremiah Denton, a Republican from Alabama, it was widely acknowledged to be Denton's pet project. Like many other Reagan conservatives, Denton had campaigned on a pro–traditional family, "traditional values" platform. A Roman Catholic, he also had strong ties to the emerging New Right. He was widely backed by the Moral Majority and adopted many of its positions once he was elected.[46] He had been a consultant for the Christian Broadcasting Network and founded the Coalition for Decency, a nonprofit pro–traditional family organization.[47] Denton inspired widespread media attention after his election, since he was a colorful, and some thought heroic, figure. After his release from a seven-year confinement in North Vietnamese prison camps, he had stepped to the microphones in 1973 at Clark Air Force base and said "God bless America."[48] As a politician, he opposed "secular humanism,"[49] called the family "the most critically endangered species in America,"[50] championed "self-discipline,"[51] and felt called upon to reassure the citizenry after his election that he "never seriously proposed the death penalty for adultery."[52] Although he was not totally uncritical of the Christian Right (he challenged the Moral Majority on its racism),[53] Denton was the quintessential representative of the movement's social values. His election was celebrated as making concrete a new alliance between Catholics and evangelicals. As New Right strategist Paul Weyrich observed, "My proudest moment was when an article appeared that said right there—jumped out of the page—that Catholics in areas like Dubuque, Iowa, had helped elect the evangelical [Charles] Grassley, and evangelicals in places like Mobile helped elect the Catholic [Jeremiah] Denton. And I looked at that article, and I stared at it, and I said, 'By golly, it really has happened.'"[54] The Christian Right could unite disparate cohorts and flex its political muscle.

AFLA was evidence of a culture clash between those like SIECUS and Planned Parenthood, who supported a pluralist sexual value system and those like Christian evangelicals, who demanded adherence to biblical sexual morality. Depending on your standpoint, AFLA was a blessing or a debacle. Religious conservatives and fundamentalists felt that they were finally getting long-deserved recognition. A witness at the reauthorization hearings enthused, "We feel that the Government, by funding grants such as ours, has taken a positive step to support and serve another section of the population—a section that chooses to reserve itself sexually until marriage."[55] From the Christian Right's point of view, AFLA interrupted what they saw as an unfair federal privileging of comprehensive sex education with its pluralist values. Jo Ann Gasper, who eventually succeeded antiabortion movement leader Marjory Mecklenberg at the Office of Adolescent Pregnancy Programs (OAPP), said:

> One of the things that I wanted to do was get some money out of the established grantee network, if you will. In other words, Title XX came out of Title VI, and so when I got there, most of the people who were getting money were still the old Title VI grantees. And I realized that for the Title

XX program to work the way the Title XX program is supposed to work, it has got to get outside to people who have new and different ideas on how to deal with this issue and how to promote abstinence. So we very simply wrote up the policies and procedures that would give them a fair playing ground so that they could compete. And then when they competed and were fundable, we funded them.[56]

AFLA, from this perspective, was an equalizer.

But critics saw AFLA as a powerful example of the state providing structural support and therefore legitimation for a specific set of religious sexual values, in this case, largely evangelical and Catholic. As Benshoof noted, "Evangelical Protestants got a foothold in getting federal funding for the first time under the AFLA program."[57] Furthermore, critics claimed that government agencies, under the control of Religious Right directors, engaged in corrupt and deceptive practices to further their own moral and political goals. Attorney Benshoof claimed that the ACLU's lawsuit against AFLA revealed the inner workings of the Reagan administration: "The right wing completely took over this branch of [Health and Human Services] and used the AFLA program as the vehicle for right-wing funding. The discovery in the case on AFLA showed just horrible, horrible abuses of government power and violations of the constitution and sleaziness and corruption. So it turned out to be this huge kettle of corrupt fish that we uncovered that made the violation of church and state look like white toast."[58]

Several features, which critics would later decry as unconstitutional, distinguished AFLA. The law was rigidly anti-abortion. AFLA—which imposed speech restrictions on grantees about abortion, encouraged adoption, and mandated parental consent for teenage girls' involvement in funded programs *unless* the parents supported abortion—was part of the post-*Roe* proliferation of legislation eroding abortion rights.[59] AFLA disallowed funding for groups that offered any abortion-related services. Grantees could only refer teenagers to other clinics for abortion counseling if both parents gave permission. AFLA was designed not simply to prevent young people from having sex (the original language stated that one purpose was "to promote self-discipline and chastity," which led to its nickname, "the chastity act"[60]). It also expressly encouraged pregnant teens to carry the fetus to term and give the child up for adoption. This stipulation, then, meant that only those religious groups that were anti-abortion would qualify for funding. Indeed, of the eight church-affiliated groups first funded, six were Catholic, one was Mormon, and one was the Lutheran Church–Missouri Synod.[61] All are strongly anti-abortion.

Significantly, AFLA mandated that to qualify for funding, programs involve religious groups. The ACLU would later charge that not only did it violate the constitutional requirement for separation of church and state, but its implementation also resulted in discrimination among religions. One of the ACLU plaintiffs was a minister who, as Benshoof put it, "taught sex education twenty miles away from a [AFLA funded] Catholic sex education session. So here you have directly a minister of a Protestant denomination teaching sex education without state support and another religious leader teaching sex education with state support."[62] By promoting the social programs of anti-abortion religions like Catholicism and evangelical Protestantism, AFLA helped foster the growing political collaboration among these churches.

Although animated by an anti-abortion agenda, AFLA also funded "prevention" of adolescent premarital sex. Therefore it exercised a profound effect on sex education in the United States. AFLA is evidence of, and also helped fully effect, a transformation in conservative discourse on sex education between the sixties and the eighties. First, there was a shift from outright opposition of sex education to support for alternative programs. As Jeremiah Denton had remarked at a hearing, "I personally am a supporter of family life and sex education. . . . I have found, however, that the best sex education includes the parents and relies upon the cooperation of teachers, social workers, the medical community, and representatives of community and religious organizations with parents to develop the curriculum."[63] These alternative programs were to be congruent with evangelical sex/gender values. Still, this was a radical departure from Billy James Hargis's condemnation of all sex education as a godless, communist plot.

Second, AFLA proponents embraced the cultural move toward sexual openness. Some grantees sounded remarkably like the comprehensive sex educators. Catholic Family Services of Texas, for example, employed the classroom technique popularized by Sally Williams of Anaheim and Esther Schulz of SIECUS in which students wrote anonymous questions on cards for the teacher to answer. Sister Mary William Sullivan told a congressional committee that students wondered "What is oral sex?" and

"Where do babies come from?"[64] She noted, "Our presentations cover information, attitudes, and frank discussions of 'myths,'" and she concluded that "having the opportunity for open discussion with significant adults and with their peers takes some of the 'behind the barn' mystic [*sic*] out of the truly beautiful and natural power that is theirs."[65] Again, this was a far cry from the sixties, when opposition leader Eleanor Howe had deplored the fact that her sons were being taught about oral sex and had complained that her children were being robbed of the mystery of sexuality.

In principle, then, these sentiments were not dissimilar to the SIECUS philosophy of openness, which stressed parental, community, even spiritual involvement in teaching sexual values. In certain respects, AFLA helped cement the foundation of school sex education for young people. It did not eclipse all the opposition; certain far-right organizations continue to condemn all sex education programs. But AFLA helped secure the transformation of community sex education debates away from conflicts over *whether* sex education would be taught in public schools. Rather, post-AFLA debates are defined by conflicts over *which* curriculum will be offered to students. They are conflicts over what will be spoken about sex. This is a crucial tactical shift. Although, as we shall see in succeeding chapters, these contemporary debates entail a range of strategies reminiscent of the sixties—for example, the depravity narrative—the boundaries of the current conflicts are less starkly defined and therefore more confusing to parents unfamiliar with sex education programs. In fact, camouflage was vital to the implementation of AFLA throughout the eighties as grantees became adept at concealing conservative religious doctrine in seemingly secular programs.

Comparatively, then, AFLA was a small program with a big impact. Never fully funded, it was a demonstration project for which Congress authorized $30 million for 1982 but appropriated $10.9 million. This sum was only slightly increased over the next two years.[66] By its reauthorization in 1984, there were fifty-nine demonstration projects, of which sixteen were for prevention programs, thirty for care programs, and thirteen for combined prevention and care.[67] Nevertheless, AFLA amplified the conservative religious pro-sex movement. It provided federal funding to a religious cohort already engaged in sex education and counseling and was a resource for the establishment of new programs for young people. But the explicit alliance of church and state that AFLA represented would not go unchallenged. In 1983, the Reproductive Freedom Project of the American Civil Liberties Union filed suit against the Department of Health and Human Services.

The lawsuit was massive in scope. Filed in federal district court in Washington, D.C., a U.S. district judge in 1987 found AFLA facially unconstitutional, since it advanced religion and resulted in the entanglement of church and state. The case was eventually heard by the Supreme Court, which in 1988 overturned the district court but remanded the case for investigation as to whether the ways in which it was administered rendered AFLA unconstitutional. Ultimately, the incoming Clinton administration settled the case in 1993. During this decade of work on the lawsuit, ACLU lawyers garnered documentary evidence of AFLA's implementation from over twenty grantees across the country.[68] The civil action (*Chan Kendrick et al. v. Margaret Heckler, Secretary of Department of Health and Human Services*) was filed on behalf of three United Methodist ministers, a Unitarian Universalist minister, the American Jewish Congress, and several taxpayers. Known as *Kendrick v. Heckler*, the lawsuit sought to enjoin AFLA because it violated the Establishment Clause of the First Amendment. The suit stated, "The Adolescent Family Life Act is a unique piece of federal legislation in that it funds the teaching of traditionally religiously based values which are susceptible to the infusion of religious dogma: the values of premarital chastity and of continuing pregnancies over abortion."[69]

Indeed "unique," AFLA reflected the efforts of the Christian Right, newly empowered in the Reagan administration, to enact its own social programs. Although Reagan broke his promise to ministers that evangelicals would comprise appointees in his administration proportionate to their numbers in the population, he nonetheless filled a number of prominent and lesser posts with religious conservatives. For example, James Watt, a member of the Assemblies of God, was appointed Secretary of the Interior; Robert Billings, the Moral Majority's executive director, was named to a top post in the Department of Education; and anti-abortion activist C. Everett Koop was appointed to the Department of Health and Human Services (HHS) and later appointed Surgeon General.[70] These appointees, and newly elected religious conservatives such as Jeremiah Denton, formed the nucleus of efforts to implement projects including constitutional amendments to ban abortion or allow school prayer. They lost many of their efforts during Reagan's first term. AFLA, however, was their stunning success.

It was not as though AFLA inadvertently spawned some problematically religious programs. The law was designed by Denton and implemented by Reagan appointee Mecklenburg at the OAPP to purposefully entwine conservative religious doctrine into the care of teenage pregnancy and the prevention of adolescent sexual activity. Jo Ann Gasper remembers when the secretary of the HHS asked her to replace Mecklenburg, "Mrs. Heckler asked me to take over the office, and the mandate I was given was clean up the management of it and be pro-life."[71] The selection of grantees was central to this mission. Mecklenburg (who was later forced out of office for an alleged affair with a staff member[72]) oversaw the selection of external reviewers of the 405 applications for AFLA funding. She disregarded the recommendations of her professional staff and instead chose reviewers from religions with anti-abortion platforms. The reviewers were crucial since, as then ACLU attorney Nan Hunter put it, "If you bring in Sister Mary Katherine Louise Flanagan, not to indulge in stereotypes, or if you bring in somebody from Planned Parenthood, you're going to have very different outcomes. One of the first things the Reaganites did was get rid of many of these people who had been review panelists for the last ten years."[73] In the final list of seventy-two reviewers, nineteen were employees of religious groups, eight were employed by Catholic Charities, and ten others had significant religious backgrounds.[74] Their comments on the grant proposals reflected these backgrounds. One Baltimore reviewer wrote, "There is missing a decided pro-life commitment in this proposal. . . . Lacking is the kind of counseling that you get in Catholic Social Service, for example."[75]

Politics, specifically religious politics, drove the selection of grantees. For example, despite high scores from the HHS staff, the University of Arkansas was denied AFLA funding because of pressure from anti-abortion activists that their materials were "Godless."[76] In addition, two members of Mecklenburg's staff testified that she utilized a "hit list" of organizations compiled by New Right activist Richard Viguerie in the journal the *Conservative Digest*. Organizations on this list, such as the Urban Institute and the American Bar Association, were not recommended for AFLA funding even though they received very high scores on their proposals.[77] While Mecklenburg's successor Gasper had no specific knowledge of the hit list, she pointed out that it would have been "a dumb thing to do" because, in fact, Mecklenburg could have achieved her goals without such a list: "You have to follow the law. Now, I will also tell you that, given the constraints of the law, you can still jolly well fund whoever you want to."[78] AFLA, therefore, was implemented in a fashion to ensure that the programs that received funding would be well equipped to develop religiously oriented sex education programs. And, in fact, they did so.

### The Pre-Kendrick Era

The *Kendrick v. Heckler* lawsuit represented a distinct shift in AFLA implementation. The pre-*Kendrick* era was characterized by the unrestrained development of religiously oriented sexuality and pregnancy programs. The OAPP had given grantees no guidelines on restricting religious content. During this time, then, programs used federal funding to develop explicitly religious sex education curricula. St. Margaret's Hospital in Dorchester, Massachusetts, is a prominent example of AFLA-funded religious programming. A nonprofit Catholic facility, St. Margaret's operated a home for single pregnant women and offered a sex education and natural family planning program that relied solely on a version of the rhythm method. The hospital received AFLA grants starting in 1982 for both care and prevention services.

Catholic doctrine infused St. Margaret's general operation, as the hospital did not offer sterilizations, abortions, or any contraception except natural family planning. The mission statement proclaimed the hospital was committed to providing care that was consistent with the guidelines of the Committee on Doctrine of the National Council of Catholic Bishops and the Archdiocese of Boston. It read in part, "St. Margaret's Hospital for Women accepts the basic principles of Christian social living. It recognizes the dependence of man upon God, his Creator."[79] It is not surprising, then, that St. Margaret's AFLA-funded program propounded a good deal of Catholic doctrine. The early care and prevention services were almost entirely religious. The grant application approved by the OAPP listed a nun as the AFLA program administrator. Staff were prohibited from mentioning abortion, even when teenagers asked for such information.[80] Most of the sex education classes offered by St. Margaret's were held in Catholic schools. These were all features that the ACLU later argued constituted excessive entanglement of government and religion.

St. Margaret's prevention curriculum, illustrative of many AFLA-funded programs, shows how this federal program helped transform the sex education debates. First, it was rife with Christian references. Students on the elementary level were taught religious beliefs: that God created them, that life begins at conception, and that they should aspire to "Christian values and goals."[81] Second, it explicitly promulgated Catholic doctrine. A middle school curriculum contained a statement by the Pope on "The Role of the Christian Family in the Modern World."[82] A section for high school students included "The Church's Teaching on Artificial Contraception."[83]

A later section entitled "The Church's Teachings on Abortion" stated that "no reason, medical, economic or social, can morally justify a deliberate and direct attack on the life of an innocent human being regardless of age, mental or physical condition, or social status" and went on further to quote from the Second Vatican Council.[84] Finally, the curriculum contained many medical inaccuracies designed to buttress anti-abortion and contraception instruction. A section on abortion techniques, for example, listed death first in the series of possible complications.[85] It did not differentiate between first- and second-trimester abortions and failed to note that early, legal abortion is safer than childbirth.[86]

These characteristics were not unique to St. Margaret's; rather, they were shared by many AFLA fundees. Catholic Charities in Virginia, which presented its sex education program only in Catholic schools in those early years, included a section on church teachings. The priest in charge announced to the parish that the sex education program would approach the issues "within the context of the church's framework of values."[87] Some programs used AFLA funding to instruct teenagers that natural family planning is the only acceptable contraception method.[88] Catholic Family Services of Amarillo, Texas, developed a curriculum replete with references to God, while St. Ann's in Hyattsville, Maryland, used Bible quotations to illustrate Catholic teachings on masturbation, homosexuality, and abortion.[89] Throughout the country, religious groups received federal grant money and developed sophisticated sex education programs that promulgated Catholic and conservative Christian beliefs.

### Kendrick and Beyond

The *Kendrick v. Heckler* lawsuit initiated the second era in AFLA programming. The suit occasioned depositions and investigations of programs around the country, putting Health and Human Services on notice of alleged Establishment Clause violations. This prompted the agency to issue guidelines—belatedly—prohibiting the use of AFLA funding to promulgate religion. In addition, the HHS contacted certain programs regarding violations. In April 1984, for example, Mecklenburg wrote to Sister Kathleen Natwin, the administrator of St. Margaret's Hospital:

> As you know, this Department is currently defending a legal challenge to Title XX of the Public Health Service Act, *Kendrick v. Heckler.* . . . As you are also aware, in the course of defending the lawsuit, we have had occasion to look particularly closely into St. Margaret's Title XX project. While we continue to be very impressed with the project as a whole, we now find that one aspect of the Family Life Education component of the project raises troublesome issues of potential Federal funding of religious activity."[90]

The letter goes on to detail many of the violations I have described above and suggests that Sister Natwin contact the HHS for help resolving them.

Once again, and as would be expected in a culture clash of this magnitude, perspectives differed concerning the sincerity and usefulness of efforts to resolve AFLA violations. AFLA fundees and supporters tended to view the ACLU criticisms as ideological and believed the lawsuit had led to undue scrutiny of their programs. One abstinence-only educator whose curriculum was vetted by the ACLU during the *Kendrick* case said,

> If someone is misusing federal funds, then yank it. I mean, they're not allowed to do that. I don't want my taxpayer's money to promote one type of faith or another, right? But if you're going into any setting, and you're teaching something that is well documented, and primary citations . . . and you don't use Christian references or resources, then I don't think there's a problem with that. But you know what? It's just too sticky. It really is, because when we had the grant, if we went into any church or any synagogue or anything, we had to cover any religious artifact with a cloth. Yeah, we had to go there and cover everything, pictures, a crucifix one time, a statue. We had to cover them just because it was so controversial.[91]

Another educator described what she saw as a chilling effect: "Principals will bring me in and say, 'This isn't religious is it?' Every principal that allows me in goes out on a limb, because they're afraid you're going to say 'God.' They're more afraid of me saying 'God' than if I'm up there and did a series of expletives, which is not what I do, but, you know, they're petrified. The ACLU will come in and that will be it."[92] Such scrutiny aggravated Christian Right activists, who by the nineties began to complain that they represent a persecuted religious minority.

At the same time, liberal critics saw AFLA's post-*Kendrick* era as initiating stealth tactics to conceal the religious character of the programs. The ACLU's Janet Benshoof claimed that staff had lied about their programs during depositions: "One nun in a deposition was denying that anything was religious, and when we asked her, 'Well, what's that around your neck?' she said, 'It's a "T."'" They denied that the Pope was Catholic. I mean, really, come on, a 'T'? That's how secular they were getting."[93] But whether the nun was actually wearing a "T" or a crucifix, AFLA personnel could not conceal the actual documents from their programs, the explicitly religious curricula. In response to the *Kendrick* lawsuit, many programs claimed they had developed measures to separate religious dogma from AFLA programming. In many cases, their efforts were tantamount to claiming that a crucifix was a "T."

The main outcome of the lawsuit against AFLA has been the "virtually secular" sex education program. Post-*Kendrick*, many programs crafted public school curricula devoid of explicit references to God. Generally, however, they still expressed Catholic or evangelical doctrine and routinely distorted medical information. For example, St. Margaret's Hospital submitted a public school curriculum for approval to the HHS in 1984 after *Kendrick* had been filed. The curriculum, which the OAPP approved, continued to list death first among possible abortion complications and asserted that there are no medical or psychological conditions for which an abortion might be indicated.[94] *Kendrick* called it "virtually identical to the Catholic curriculum."[95] The Committee on the Status of Women, a conservative, pro-life Illinois group which employed AFLA funds to develop the very popular curriculum *Sex Respect*, also revised the manual for public schools. While most religious references were expunged, the manual still included supplementary references with sentiments such as "Pray together, invite God on every date and enjoy His friendship."[96] One educator, who says "my goal is to promote chastity," insists that "the public schools are the mission fields" and "in the public schools never am I changing the message. I'm changing the way I deliver it. . . . Instead of saying [like] in the Catholic school, I'll say, 'Sexual intercourse belongs in marriage, what God intended it to be.' In a public school I'll say, 'Place sexual intercourse in marriage where it belongs.' In other words, I gave the same message, I just didn't say 'God.'"[97] The post-*Kendrick* era spawned many ostensibly secular curricula which became the nucleus of contemporary community sex education controversies.

From the late eighties into the nineties, AFLA-funded curricula proliferated. AFLA also funded evaluation programs, thereby launching religious-based organizations which published often questionable reviews of the curricula.[98] Though they camouflaged their specific Catholic or evangelical affiliation, all of these programs fulfilled the AFLA mission of being alternatives to comprehensive sexuality education. Generally called "abstinence-only" or "abstinence-only-until-marriage" curricula, they typically omit any discussion of topics including masturbation, homosexuality, abortion, and contraception. And while the evangelical orientation was not necessarily discernible to the average parent or citizen caught up in a community debate, their religious intent was well known by the Christian Right, which came to support many of the programs. For example, the evangelical organization founded by Beverly LaHaye, Concerned Women for America (CWA), endorsed the AFLA-funded Teen-Aid, Inc. Teen-Aid provides community support groups and specifically targets public schools. LeAnna Benn, Teen-Aid's director, wrote in a CWA newsletter:

> George Grant's book *Grand Illusions—The Legacy of Planned Parenthood*
> describes Planned Parenthood as a "disease" with the cure being the Word of
> God. It sounds like a wonderful idea and it surely is the solution to stop the
> pushers of birth control, purveyors of pornographic educational materials,
> and proselytizers of abortion on demand. Then how does one go about
> getting Godly principles disseminated in the public arena? . . . Teen-Aid,
> Inc. has written value-based materials for public schools making sure that
> the tenets of nearly all major world religions would not be offended.[99]

Benn's comment shows the continuing ire of conservatives against comprehensive sexuality educators. Her charges are familiar from sixties debates but they carry new weight. A dynamic and powerful alliance of newly politicized religious conservatives had taken up the sex education battles in a way that groups like Billy James Hargis's Christian Crusade simply did not. In addition, Benn reveals in this evangelical forum that she and her allies are interested not just in their own cohort but in spreading their values in the public domain. In reflecting on the *Kendrick* case, lawyer Nan Hunter commented, "The concern was that [AFLA] was a major development in funneling public funds to religious or conservative groups in the area of sexuality. Both we and the Right saw this as possibly a model, as perhaps something that would become institutionalized, would stay with us, and become very difficult to dislodge. And in fact, that's what happened."[100] That is, indeed, precisely what happened.

AFLA, which was created in the propitious seventies fusion of evangelical sexualization and Christian Right political power, prompted major institutionalization of evangelical sexual morality as public policy. AFLA allowed for the creation of new Christian Right sexual discourses in which conservative evangelical sexual morality is the only "normal" and "healthy" option. After *Kendrick*, the recognition of the need to conceal the promotion of explicit religious values led to secularizing strategies which have afforded these discourses on sexuality and young people enormous power on both the national and local levels. For example, major state support for the singular sexual morality of abstinence-only sex education came in the form of the welfare reform law of 1996. Spearheaded by a cohort of national pro-family, conservative organizations and research institutes—such as the Heritage Foundation, Concerned Women for America, the Christian Coalition, and the Eagle Forum[101]—Section 510(b), Title V of the Social Security Act created a new entitlement program for abstinence-only education. This provision, signed into law by Democratic President Bill Clinton, allocated $50 million annually over five years for sex education programs. However, a program would only be funded if it "teaches that a mutually faithful monogamous relationship in the context of marriage is the expected standard of human sexual activity."[102] The law demonstrated the power of the Christian Right at the end of the century to legislate its own particular sexual value system.

AFLA also generated an abstinence-only sex education industry. Commercially oriented, this industry has allowed for unprecedented grassroots organizational expansion. At the end of the nineties, there were over twenty major abstinence-only curricula commercially available for public schools. Many of them were originally developed with AFLA funding as explicitly Christian programs and then the wording was secularized. There are countless other less prominent curricula produced by religious groups. And a small cottage industry of abstinence-only commercial artifacts has appeared. In addition to curricula such as "Sex: A Christian Perspective" and "Pure Talk/Sex: When, Where, & Why and What Is the Truth," one can buy a growing selection of items like Passion 4 Purity rings, True Love Waits pendants, Don't Be a Sucker lollipops, and Sexless in Seattle nightshirts. There are over thirty major educational organizations, including A is for Abstinence and the Just WAIT Project, which offer speakers' bureaus, videos, conferences, and other abstinence-only services. These networks, connected to national Christian Right organizations or simply supporting Christian Right goals, are able to influence national policy.

In the post-*Kendrick* era, the new abstinence-only proponents are careful to maintain their virtual boundary between the religious and the secular. For example, the national *Directory of Abstinence Resources* states, "This directory contains resources suitable for public school settings along with those resources that contain Christian content. Resources containing Christian content are noted as such. All other resources are suitable for public school settings."[103] "The Chastity Challenge," for example, is available in both secular and Christian versions. However, many of these materials for public schools, as the educators themselves are aware, still carry a spiritual message cloaked in secular language, prompting the SIECUS criticism that "religious bias influences the curricula and only one viewpoint on sexual behavior is discussed."[104]

Finally, this alternative sexuality industry allowed for a significant Christian Right organizational development—the establishment of local service groups in sexuality-related areas. Over the past decade, the numbers of pregnancy crisis centers, abstinence-only sex education providers, and ex-gay ministries have skyrocketed. These groups, often linked to national Christian Right organizations, extend the reach of legal and political groups. They constitute an organizational network of thousands of grassroots groups, linking millions of activists and sympathizers. And by allowing the Christian Right to offer alternative services—adoption rather than abortion, conversion to heterosexuality rather than support for gay rights, limited rather than comprehensive sex education curricula—they more fully position the Christian Right as an active player in the sexual culture.

The current level of proactive Christian Right engagement with sexuality issues is unprecedented. So far these developments have almost uniformly served to strengthen the movement. On the one hand, the sex-related infrastructure has given the Christian Right a much broader reach than ever. Moreover, the Christian Right's positive engagement with sexuality may assuage some of the antipathy provoked by the evangelical and fundamentalist reputation for extremism.[105] Rather than being only judgmental, some on the Christian Right currently encourage therapeutic talk about sex. As conservative Catholic chastity educator Molly Kelly said, "Is sexuality dirty? If it's dirty, nobody should be talking about it. If it's a gift from God, what are we afraid of?"[106] They are working hard to distinguish their own positive messages about sex from what they see as a broader culture of flagrantly immoral, crass sexual freedom.

On the other hand, open sexual speech may allow for trouble in the Christian Right. Tim and Beverly LaHaye voiced the problem of needing to be frank, since "evasiveness is not adequately instructive," but wanting not to replicate the "crude language" of secular books.[107] Religious conservatives have always faced the tricky negotiation of openly speaking about that which they condemn. A very early example is the author of the eighteenth-century anti-masturbation tract *Onania* who felt compelled to address critics who thought that to speak about masturbation, even to vilify it, would be to incite such action among those who would otherwise have been innocent of it.[108] The new evangelical sex advisers, however, were extolling sex, not inveighing against it. While it is important not to overstate the transformation, there is in fact a change in both scope and tone. As Marabel Morgan recalled about her work, "I was talking about sex, trying to make it light and funny and happy and exciting."[109] This is, for evangelicals, a new genre of sexual speech. And so the establishment of a proactive sexuality industry may generate in the Christian Right important structural and ideological contradictions.

Open and positive sexual speech from the Christian Right carries two risks for the movement: dividing its constituencies and putting its sexual message at odds with itself. First, there is still a vocal cohort opposed to sex education of any kind. For them, any open sexual discussion is unacceptable. The AFLA-funded abstinence-only curricula have alienated some in the Christian Right who are still vehemently opposed to any type of sex education. Several Catholic groups denounced the abstinence programs as "more coarse than chaste."[110] The ultra-conservative Catholic organization Human Life International, for example, criticized Molly Kelly's chastity programs for not upholding "Catholic or Christian morality, but [upholding] the criteria of the U.S. Office of Adolescent Pregnancy [Programs] in Washington."[111] The Catholic critics were annoyed that Kelly had failed to even discuss the Sixth and Ninth Commandments, and in a complaint that could have come from the ACLU but for opposite reasons, they charge, "She mentions God eight times in the book."[112] Clearly this is not often enough for Human Life International, while it is far too often for other groups.

When comparing Christian Right sex education programs with comprehensive sex education, conservative critic Melvin Anchell said, "Arsenic also is less injurious than cyanide, but neither should be given to students."[113] Randy Engle, also associated with Human Life International, excoriated AFLA-funded efforts to combine "sexual morality or prudence with explicit sexual information," including those of the wildly popular Coleen Mast of Sex Respect fame, calling them "sex education in Catholic drag."[114] Internal dissent is not uncommon in social movements, as such movements are not singular undertakings. And yet it is possible that such hyperbolic criticisms represent not so much simple disagreement as painful expressions of schismatic tendencies in the Christian Right. As Kelly said about Human Life International's criticism of her chastity programs, "They're basically opposed to talking about sex. Period. And I am not going to do what they do."[115] There is a strain between those committed to sexual silence and those who now advocate more open sexual discussion.

Second, there is an important tension between this new endorsement of sexual discussion and traditional Christian Right speech strategies that rely on sexual shame. Comprehensive sex educators have long poked fun at what they consider to be contradictory cultural messages: Sex is dirty; save it for someone you love. There is now a similar contradiction in the Christian Right's sexual discourse. Sex, on the one hand, is "pure as cottage cheese" and a divine gift.[116] The movement, on the other hand, depends on the power of sexual shame to scare, intimidate, and humiliate. Although both messages are ultimately political, the therapeutic approach is at odds with the regulatory tactics.

It remains to be seen whether the development of an alternative sexuality industry and the proliferation of positive sexual speech will prove to be "potentially subversive"[117] for the Christian Right. Currently they are negotiating any contradictions by emphasizing that sex is only blessed within marriage and comes with many divine restrictions. In the abstinence-only curricula, fear is used to mediate the positive messages about sex. But the paradoxes resulting from proactive sexual speech may produce unmanageable strains. AFLA was designed to restrict sexual speech and although it does that, it also spawned a vast sex-related network. Once the movement has introduced and sanctioned widespread talk about sexuality, such speech is out of its control. Although the speakers may resolutely "talk about sex and God in the same breath," as Marabel Morgan put it, they cannot control how the audiences will interpret and internalize those messages.[118] Speech is unpredictable; the word "is half someone else's."[119] Audiences who hear a message linking sex and God are quite capable of embracing sex while minimizing God. Morgan's workshops were met with such eagerness by conservative Christian women that she remembered thinking, "We were just holding a tiger by the tail."[120] Candid discussion of sex was emotionally pleasurable and financially lucrative. This opened the Christian Right to the same commercial and ideological influences as the mainstream sexualized society, potentially pushing some of its endeavors beyond the confines exerted by evangelical beliefs. Traditional evangelical dictates about sexuality might shift, along with the regulatory force of sexual guilt. Instabilities of speech and its interpretation are part of what allow for social change and, in this case, changes in the sexual culture. Still, it is impossible to predict the impact of these internal contradictions within the Christian Right's sexual culture or the direction of any potential changes. In the meantime, the Christian Right's sexual speech has so far proven to be an extraordinary resource for the movement. By the late eighties, local communities would feel the influence of the varied Christian Right rhetorical strategies in debates over sex education.

## Chapter 5 | VICTIMS, VILLAINS, . . .
## AND NEIGHBORS

It was crucial for communities in the post–Adolescent Family Life Act (AFLA) era to talk about sexuality education. Suddenly there was an important choice: Would young people in the public schools be taught a curriculum that included information about birth control and safer sex, or would they only be taught to abstain from all sexual activity until marriage? On the one hand, comprehensive programs—which stressed abstinence and generally included information on the so-called hot-button issues of contraception, abortion, masturbation, and homosexuality—were supported by a wide range of religious and public health agencies such as the American Medical Association, the American Academy of Pediatrics, and the United Church Board for Homeland Ministries.[1] On the other hand, abstinence-only curricula had as their "exclusive purpose teaching the social, psychological, and health gains to be realized by abstaining from sexual activity."[2] Abstinence-only curricula were supported by conservative, Christian evangelical, and Catholic organizations, such as the Eagle Forum, Concerned Women for America, Focus on the Family, and the National Association for Abstinence Education ("just say NAAE"). These programs were developed to promote the moral position that sexual behavior, especially sexual intercourse, is dangerous and wrong before marriage; they were sometimes dubbed "fear-based" curricula by detractors or "chastity education" by some supporters. The choice facing communities through the eighties and nineties was which curriculum to adopt in their public schools: comprehensive or abstinence-only.

The argument could not be solved empirically. The answer to the question "what works?" is exceedingly complicated and, as we shall see, was itself politicized.[3] Rather, each side had to mobilize arguments to convince a broader public of its merits. In efforts to be persuasive, villains and victims appeared in the rhetoric on both sides. Opponents of comprehensive sex education abandoned the outdated communist conspiracy theories from the late sixties, although suspicion that sex education was part of a broad secular humanist agenda persisted. Aided by the growth of their own research institutes, conservative and evangelical Christians developed a new sophistication at using the language of science and medicine for their moral protests. However, they continued to use evocative sexual language and themes of sexual danger as ways to discredit their opponents. For their part, advocates of comprehensive programs were not silent like Mary Calderone and her Sex Information and Education Council of the United States (SIECUS) associates had been in the sixties controversies. Rather, they launched initiatives to educate communities about the merits and shortcomings of different curricula. They also drew on the rhetorical opportunities available to them, which was to lodge charges of extremism against their foes. Sometimes they succeeded. But when community discussions turned into fights, they were vulnerable to sexual scapegoating. Speaking out in support of comprehensive programs and resisting the stigmatizing charges from their opponents proved exceedingly difficult.

MAKING UP CHILDREN

Everyone agreed that young people were either the potential or actual victims of sex. Both sides of the debate pointed to specific developments which lent new urgency to this old fear. The visibility of sexuality was unparalleled. Even more so than when SIECUS was founded in the early sixties, sexual references now suffused public life. A significant number of teenagers reported that they had learned about sexual issues from television and movies, an inevitable feature of late twentieth-century culture which nonetheless enraged critics of popular media.[4] The AIDS epidemic, which conjured a diffuse sense of sexual danger, raised the stakes for adolescent sexual expression. Regardless, in the late nineties, roughly half of all seventeen-year-olds had had sexual intercourse,[5] and gay youth support groups popped up in public schools across the nation. In theory, the asexual child remained a powerful icon. But the Romantic ideal as cultural practice proved to be far more unstable. Ambivalence and confusion about the sexuality of young people heightened tensions in sex education debates.

Two tragic figures in particular lurked in the national and the local arguments about sex education: the pregnant teenager and the suicidal gay youth. Both images can be considered examples of what philosopher Ian Hacking terms "making up people," by which technologies of counting and measurement create new social categories into which "people spontaneously . . . fit."[6] Labeling and counting do not prompt behavior in any straightforward way—pregnancy and diverse sexual behaviors have long been among the experiences of young people. However, by organizing and regulating social lives, statistical classifications give rise to new categories and types of people. These types then assume lives of their own and appear in debates among the various organizations which gave rise to them and sometimes capitalized on their political usefulness. Acknowledging the rhetorical power in appeals to protect innocent children, cultural theorist Henry Jenkins notes that "almost every major political battle of the twentieth century has been fought on the backs of our children."[7] Such was the case with the pregnant teenager and the suicidal gay youth, who, at least as archetypes, figured prominently in sex education debates.

The image of the pregnant teenager sprang from the mid-seventies invention of an "epidemic" of pregnancies among adolescents. The adolescent birth rate had reached its highest peak in the fifties and had declined by the late seventies, but the pregnant teen as a type was never simply a product of straightforward measurement. She was, rather, a construct that reflected social anxieties about sexuality and race, meanwhile advancing the interests of family planners and demographers. Planned Parenthood Federation of America and its research wing, the Alan Guttmacher Foundation, first planted the idea of such an epidemic.[8] A 1975 Guttmacher statistic of a "million pregnant teenagers" a year showed up in articles and brochures everywhere. That statistic was misleading; it included married nineteen-year-olds along with younger, unmarried girls.[9] Although other Guttmacher figures were similarly misleading, the "epidemic" took hold in the public and political imaginations. In fact, the nonmarital birth rate was increasing—among white women. Sociologist Constance Nathanson

argues that in a crucial mid-seventies shift, "deviant sexuality and reproduction" transformed from a problem of poor, black women into a danger for the white, middle-class high school girl.[10] The white pregnant teen
became publicly visible in the late seventies. Through the eighties and
nineties, although the rates of teen pregnancy fell, she was a frightening
specter in sex education debates.[11]

Similarly, the suicidal gay youth emerged from statistical classification.
A highly controversial chapter in the 1989 Health and Human Services report on youth suicide estimated that gay adolescents were three times more
likely than heterosexuals to attempt suicide.[12] Subsequent research supported that estimate.[13] As Hacking notes, novel possibilities for action
emerge from new forms of description.[14] While there is no evidence that
gay suicide itself became contagious, the category generated prolific public testimony from and about suicidal gay youth. The 1992 video *Gay Youth*
profiled the suicide of twenty-year-old Bobby Griffin, who had hurled himself from a highway bridge into an oncoming truck. In Massachusetts, suicidal gay youth regularly lobbied for educational reform, such as one young
woman who described at a hearing how she cut her wrist with her father's
hunting knife in five suicide attempts.[15] The suicidal gay youth became a
symbol of the need for educational reform. There was little accord, however, on what kind of reform.

Both sides of the sex education debates condemned teen pregnancy and
gay youth suicide. But they remained far apart on the solutions. Sex education advocates called for more comprehensive programs. They considered
more information about a broad range of sexual issues as the way to address
important problems. Planned Parenthood, for example, said, "Americans
know that keeping children ignorant about sex hurts them. When teens are
given honest information they make more responsible choices."[16] Opponents
of comprehensive programs blamed an increasingly corrupt sexual culture
in which SIECUS and Planned Parenthood were central players. They used
statistics on teen pregnancy as a way to attack sex educators themselves. For
example, Focus on the Family said, "SIECUS also supports non-marital sex
among adolescents despite the fact that teen girls experience 1 million pregnancies and 3 million cases of STDs each year."[17] (Some went further, such
as Concerned Women for America, when it claimed, "The impact of
SIECUS-style sex education on America's children, teenagers and young
adults has been catastrophic. SAT scores and academic achievement have

plummeted. Moreover, destructive behaviors among youth have increased dramatically."[18]) Opponents of comprehensive programs also claimed that gay youth suicide was the result of the "deathstyle" of homosexuality itself, not the result of social oppression.[19] One opponent of comprehensive programs that would teach tolerance of gay people said, "You cannot make a case for the fact that teen suicide is caused by the rejection of people because they practice homosexuality. Here again we have a situation where government is non-family-friendly, embracing a lifestyle that destroys people. Now how on earth is that going to stop the abuses that they claim they're trying to stop?"[20] Sometimes the actual youths themselves receded behind the political deployment of the categories (for example, gay youth mounted resistance to the emphasis on suicide[21]). Still, in sex education debates during the final decades of the twentieth century, the pregnant teenager and the suicidal gay youth symbolized the universe of sexual danger for young people. Moreover, they underscored the very real differences among constituents who lobbied either for comprehensive or abstinence-only programs as a way of minimizing sexual risk.

CONSTRUCTING RISK

Conservatives seized the offensive against comprehensive sex education programs. They followed two lines of action: They characterized programs as inappropriate by using strong language and stigmatizing terms, and they employed the language of scientific medicine to argue that comprehensive sex education was dangerous to young people. Public ignorance and unease about sex education fueled the success of their initiatives. As one sex education teacher put it, "There is a real misunderstanding wherein people think that sex education is intercourse education. The fact that, of the thirty days in class, we didn't talk about intercourse that much, people think, well how can you have thirty days of sex education if you don't have thirty days of talking about intercourse?"[22] Another educator concurs: "People are always trying to make it sound more explicit. The Right loves to use terminology about courses being 'a how-to.' But nobody teaches how to perform oral sex. That is not what goes on in sexuality education. I think that most people, if they really knew, would feel like, 'Oh, this is kind of boring.' You know, family roles, body image, parenting skills."[23] Still, some comprehensive programs give information about historically taboo topics such as masturbation, birth control, and homosexuality. This left them vulnerable to stigmatizing characterizations.

Opponents fought these programs with strong language. For example, critics of a first-grade teacher's guide in New York City that mentioned lesbian and gay families dubbed it "the sodomy curriculum," which conjured up images of six-year-olds learning about oral and anal sex. In other venues, opponents described curricular materials as pornographic. Through the eighties and nineties, "pornography" was a familiar stigmatizing term used by conservatives against a wide range of expression, from the women's health book *Our Bodies, Ourselves*, to music and art with sexual themes, to sexuality and AIDS education.[24] This was the type of language that could mobilize residents, if they heard that pornography was being taught to children in the local public schools. In one such case, in Massachusetts, a controversy began when one parent objected to the use of an American Library Association award–winning text, *The New Teenage Body Book*, as an adjunct book in the school's sex education program. The *Body Book* covers teenage dilemmas from acne to asthma to sexuality issues.[25] It openly discusses masturbation, oral sex, and homosexuality, on occasion using what the media called street slang. The sections on sexuality stirred controversy. A local group, the Concerned Citizens Task Force, formed to ban the book.

Opponents of the book charged that it was pornographic. The claim was galvanizing and quickly spread through the community. The pastor of a Congregational Church complained, "I'm against pornography for ninth graders—pure, unadulterated pornography."[26] Critics of the book launched a petition drive demanding the permanent removal of the book because, they alleged, it contained "obscene passages" that "endanger the community" and "inevitably" cause an "increase in sexual promiscuity" and other dangerous sexual consequences.[27] The school board president at the time claimed that petitioners stood outside of church saying, "They're teaching pornography at Silver Lake. Sign here," and that some who signed later regretted doing so.[28] There were eight hundred signatures on the petition, from a town of approximately fifteen thousand people.

Strong language grabs attention and provides a framework for evaluating a sex education program. Some parents agreed with the claim that the *Body Book* was pornographic, complaining that it said too much, too explicitly. One mother objected to sections of the book dealing with topics that, in her opinion, "are not meant to be discussed openly."[29] Another complained that the students focused only on the "juicy sections" about sex.[30] The claim that comprehensive sex education is pornographic can succeed because open discussions about topics like masturbation can be discomfiting. The school board president said, "When I first saw the book I thought, 'Oh my God!' but a friend said, 'That's what kids need to know.' And I thought, 'She's right.'"[31] Her first reaction, however, speaks to broad cultural anxieties about children and sexuality. In that town the claim that the public school was teaching pornography tapped widespread disagreements about whether children are best protected by sexual discussion or sexual silence. While some parents tried to shield their children from sexual knowledge, others recognized the difficulty of doing so, such as one mother who said, "It's astounding to me that so many of these parents think this book is the first time their kids have heard about oral sex."[32]

Although strong language does not inevitably persuade, it often incites community discord. This controversy "pitted friends against friends."[33] Moreover, residents discovered the difficulty of speaking out on behalf of the sex education book. Eventually, when the book's most vocal opponent told the school board president that the pictures were pornographic, she told him, "They're explicit. They're not pornographic."[34] She knew, however, that evocative language such as "pornography," "obscenity," and "promiscuity" coded support for the *Body Book* as comparable to support for unacceptable and immoral sexuality. The book's primary opponent called her "perverted" because of her defense of the text. She complained "I've been married twenty-nine years and I don't teach my kids to run out and do it whenever they can. I'm affronted by these implications. They make you feel dirty."[35] She noted, however, that the *Body Book* became "the hottest read book in the town."

Along with using strong language, opponents told frightening stories about comprehensive sex education. These were updates of the sixties depravity narrative. Generally, they featured children being humiliated or inappropriately exposed to sexual material. Regardless of whether these narratives were actually believed, either by the activists themselves or their audience, they could foster intense emotions in communities. Conservative educator William Kilpatrick recounts a number of such narratives in his book *Why Johnny Can't Tell Right from Wrong:* "Another [sex education] strategy is to require each boy in a class to say 'vagina' out loud while all the girls say 'penis.' In one eighth-grade class, a girl who was embarrassed to do this was made by the teacher to come to the front of the class and say it loudly ten times."[36] Another narrative was repeated in a local community debate—"At a suburban high school in Massachusetts, tenth-grade students are given a homework assignment to go home and masturbate"— but the speaker refused to name the town.[37] There is no documentation for any of these narratives, so there is no way to verify or refute them. The president of the teachers union in one town described campaign tactics in a school board election in which fears were generated about the health education curriculum: "It got them elected because they were handing out pamphlets at the supermarket saying, 'Do you want your third-grader to learn about condoms? We'll put a stop to this.'"[38] In this context, as in others, sexual fears are mobilized for political purposes.

Depravity narratives operated by diffusing rapidly across communities. The narrators claimed to know someone who knows someone to whom it happened. For example, Leslie Kantor, formerly of SIECUS, told of a Texas opponent who criticized the state's sex education guidelines by comparing them with SIECUS guidelines: "She said, 'And what the SIECUS guidelines say are that five-year-olds should learn how to masturbate, how to be homosexual, how to use contraception, and how to do abortions.' And she distributed this one-page handout which pulled the most controversial topics in the guidelines completely out of context. This distortion was all over the state. I wish I had had a little map of Texas that could light up, because I was talking to people from all over."[39] The sheer ubiquity of depravity narratives lent credence to them, making them more difficult to refute.

By the mid-nineties, opponents of comprehensive programs augmented their rhetorical strategies with the language of medical science. This shift took place amid an extended cultural argument over the role of religion in public discourse and institutions. "Integralists" challenged the exclusion of, and hostility toward, religion in the public arena—the "naked public square" against which theologian Richard John Neuhaus had warned in the early eighties.[40] They argued for the importance of religion in solving social problems like teen pregnancy. However, while some social movement theorists argued for the potency of moral and religious discourse in mobilizing citizens,[41] religion became a red flag in the sex education debates. Stung by the ACLU lawsuit against AFLA, organized critics of comprehensive sex education became highly vigilant about public disclosures of religious beliefs. Local candidates often secularized their messages so as to avoid religion, like Merrimack school board member Shelly Uscinski, who wrote a chapter for the Christian Coalition's Leadership Manual advising, "Don't wear your religion on your sleeve. You may be religious but you must stay focused on school issues. Talk their language—they don't understand yours."[42] Conservative evangelicals and Catholics repackaged sexual morality into a secular vernacular of health and disease. For example, one opponent of the *Children of the Rainbow* teaching guide in New York City said:

> You can read every single communication we sent to the Board of Education, and there were dozens of them, pages long. There isn't a single one in which we make either a religious argument against *Children of the Rainbow* or even a moralistic argument. . . . Mary Cummins, myself, and her school board and our allies never once attacked *Rainbow* on biblical grounds. . . . And in the end we hammered at it so persistently, and we gave it so much empirical data drawn from medical journals, demographic journals, and other research sources. . . . I won't say that there weren't people in New York City who weren't outraged on religious and moral grounds. There were. We were. But these are public schools.[43]

Although sex education opponents continued to argue with harsh language, they increasingly adopted a medical idiom of powerful data sound bites.

Proliferation of medical research on sexuality helped effect this strategy. Sexologists were joined by some feminist and gay organizations which conducted research related to sexuality. And the AIDS epidemic prompted an escalation of sex research not only among these cohorts but also by public health epidemiologists and educators around the country, most notably at the Centers for Disease Control and Prevention (CDC) in Atlanta. Of crucial importance, however, was the entrance of Christian Right activists into sexuality research. An important way to foster morality in contemporary American culture is through the establishment of expertise. Conservatives and evangelicals had accomplished this through becoming sexual experts. The burgeoning infrastructure of Christian Right research institutes, such as the Family Research Council and the Medical Institute for Sexual Health, generated a steady stream of studies and statistics that activists cited as support for their arguments. Regardless of their accuracy, scientific data were vital resources for social movements because of the lingering cultural authority of medicine.

Anthropologist Mary Douglas has said, "When 'risk' enters as a concept in political debate, it becomes a menacing thing, like a flood, an earthquake, or a thrown brick."[44] This was precisely the effect conservatives sought. They hoped to dissuade communities from adopting comprehensive programs. Their data sound bites were hyper-condensed narratives which drew on the power of medicine while simultaneously playing to sexual fears and danger. Employing statistics and medical language, conservatives made graphic claims that comprehensive sex education enhanced young peoples' sexual risks.

The condom became a target of criticism. Conservatives charged that there are tiny (five-micron) holes in condoms that sperm are too big to penetrate but through which the HIV virus can pass. They cited official sources such as medical journals and public health agencies as documenting this claim. A report called "Condom Roulette," published by the conservative Family Research Council, asserted: "Researchers studying surgical gloves made out of latex, the same material in condoms, found 'channels of 5 microns that penetrated the entire thickness of the glove.' The HIV virus measures between .1 and .3 microns."[45] The report footnoted a one-paragraph letter in the journal *Nature* from 1988 in which several researchers had examined latex gloves under electron microscopy and found microscopic channels.[46] The claim was misleading, however. As Kay Stone, a medical epidemiologist at the CDC, points out, "Gloves and condoms are different. Other studies have examined latex and nothing gets through. It's really not generalizable to condoms at all. . . . That article has been literally blown out of proportion."[47] Latex condoms are virtually impermeable mechanical barriers against sperm and viruses. Indeed, there is overwhelming evidence from a range of research and public health organizations, including the CDC, that attests to the efficacy of latex condoms.[48]

Nevertheless, conservative national organizations such as the Family Research Council, the Medical Institute for Sexual Health, and the evangelical group Focus on the Family distributed materials alleging that condoms are unsafe because they have holes. The claim was a resource for community activists who then used it to underscore the risk of sexuality and AIDS education. One man at a contentious town meeting described the size of alleged condom holes versus the size of the HIV virus: "It's like shooting BBs at a tennis net."[49] A local Massachusetts group's newsletter warned: "AIDS IS 100% PREVENTABLE!!!!! If you have sex JUST ONCE with an infected person, YOU CAN DIE EVEN IF YOU WEAR A CONDOM."[50] This same publication features a compelling graphic of a large circle, a much smaller circle, and a pinpoint. The large circle is labeled "Sperm—about 45 microns in size." The smaller circle is dubbed "Standard Latex Holes—(voids) 5 microns in size, or 9 times smaller than sperm." The pinpoint is labeled "AIDS Virus—0.1 microns in size, smaller by a factor of fifty than the standard hole (void) in latex rubber."[51] All of these figures are footnoted in the text to sources such as the CDC and the Food and Drug Administration.

The claim that condoms have holes operated as an indictment of comprehensive sex education. Such programs often (but not always—see Chapter 9) provided students with information about condoms and safer sex. But even though untrue, the allegation that condoms have holes opened up these programs to charges of irresponsibility at the least and, as we shall see in Chapter 6, complaints that such education was tantamount to murder. Critics warned that "passing out condoms to teenagers is like issuing them squirt-guns for a 4 alarm blaze. Condoms don't hack it."[52] Moreover, since conservatives objected to condoms because they seemingly sanctioned sexual activity, their claim about condom holes was a reminder that sex was dangerous. Their texts were stern warnings to young people. A conservative newsletter said, "If you don't want to get AIDS, you don't have to. It's simple. Don't have sex."[53] One popular text cautioned, "Sex: What you don't know can kill you."[54] In the sex education video *No Second Chance,* a young man asks the teacher what if he does not want to wait until marriage to have sex. She replies, "Well, I guess you'll just have to be prepared to die. And you'll probably take with you your spouse and one or more of your children."[55]

As an antidote to what they saw as the risky comprehensive sex education programs, opponents championed their own curricula. Using program evaluation data, conservatives claimed that abstinence-only programs were more effective. For example, a press release for the popular program Sex Respect claims the curriculum changed teenagers' behavior and lowered pregnancy rates. However, the Office of Adolescent Pregnancy Programs reviewed the results of the evaluation and concluded otherwise.

It reported, "The lower incidence of pregnancy among female students participating in the program compared to non-program students cannot be supported by the evaluation methodology. There is not sufficient evidence to support assertions of change in behavior or long-term change in behavior or long-term change in either attitudes or behavior."[56] Program evaluations under AFLA were fraught with methodological shortcomings. Many of the programs allocated only 3 percent of funding for evaluation, whereas 10 to 15 percent would have been more appropriate. A number of them do not have appropriate comparison groups, they have fairly small samples, they were conducted over a very brief course of time, and they lack behavior measures or follow-up data.[57] Comprehensive reviews of evaluations in both 1997 and 2001 concluded that nearly all of the evaluations of abstinence-only programs were so flawed as to be meaningless, thereby offering no evidence that the programs delay the onset of intercourse.[58] Despite these dilemmas, advocates of abstinence-only curricula made claims about their programs' effectiveness.

The San Marcos "miracle" is perhaps the most striking example. Promotion materials for an abstinence-only curriculum by Teen-Aid boasted that two years after the program was implemented in a San Marcos high school, the adolescent pregnancy rate fell from 20 percent to less than 3 percent. San Marcos was widely discussed in community battles across the country because, indeed, it did promise a magic bullet. Teen-Aid, controversial for allegations that income from the curriculum has been used to fund an anti-abortion crisis clinic,[59] is promoted not just by the Teen-Aid organization itself but also by national Christian evangelical groups like Concerned Women for America (CWA) and Focus on the Family. The San Marcos claims were widely touted by these groups as well. For example, a newsletter from CWA said, "During the 1983–1984 school year, 178 high school girls, (1 in 5) had become pregnant. Adoption of [*Sexuality, Commitment, and Family* by Teen-Aid, Inc.] resulted in a dramatic reduction of teen pregnancies to only 20 in the 1986–87 school year."[60] The claims about Teen-Aid swept across the country, showing up in local debates. One woman testified at a school board meeting in Melbourne, Florida, "Don't our children deserve the best? In San Marcos, California, school systems they had 147 pregnant teens and after two years of Teen-Aid being implemented that number of pregnant teens dropped to twenty. That is an 86 percent decrease."[61]

Unfortunately, the San Marcos "miracle" turned out to be the San Marcos "myth," and one reporter noted that the story has proven "as tenacious as a virus."[62] Although no statistics were kept on teen pregnancies, the birth rate of San Marcos mothers aged fourteen through seventeen more than doubled through the eighties, according to the county Department of Health Services.[63] In fact, in the 1986–87 year during which Teen-Aid claims only twenty pregnancies, fifty-six babies were born to school-age mothers in 1986 and forty-seven were born in 1987.[64] These figures are up from the thirty-three births in 1984, before the introduction of the Teen-Aid curriculum. The story itself, it turns out, arose from loosely configured numbers kept by a guidance counselor to whom pregnant girls sometimes confided. Feeling overworked by what she thought was the sheer volume of such counseling sessions, in 1984 she began to count the number of pregnant girls who came to her. She revealed the figures, 147 girls or one in five, at the end of the year to the superintendent, who disclosed them to the press. Two years later, the school district reported only twenty such pregnancies, thus launching the San Marcos miracle. But the guidance counselor was quoted as saying about the new figure, "I think the district office made it up."[65] In light of the Department of Health Services statistics, the huge drop was clearly deceptive. One San Marcos counselor said, "It's a myth. It was used to sell Teen-Aid and all that [Teen-Aid] was trying to do."[66] In another venue he emphasized, "That simply didn't happen. There were no statistics to support that. There never have been."[67] Still, conservative and evangelical groups continued to boast of Teen-Aid's success.

Advocates for comprehensive programs launched their own initiatives. SIECUS and Planned Parenthood began to monitor community conflicts. They compiled information kits to help their advocates respond to criticisms against comprehensive programs. Leslie Kantor of SIECUS coached them on the political process, such as "talking to people about what they need to do to rally supporters by their side, so that they do not end up the lone voice waving this piece of paper saying, 'Condoms work,' and have three hundred people coming in saying, 'No, there are five-micron holes in condoms. What are you talking about?' And nobody is going to believe you when you are the only person and you are waving a little piece of paper."[68] In addition to advising community residents, SIECUS targeted abstinence-only programs. Kantor undertook a comprehensive review of the most prominent abstinence-only curricula. (She later joked, "Probably on my deathbed I will say, 'Now that I have checked every footnote in Teen-Aid, I can rest in peace.'"[69]) At a disadvantage because their own programs were stigmatized, comprehensive program advocates fought back with the resources available to them. SIECUS sought to discredit abstinence-only curricula based on criticisms ranging from medical inaccuracy to the charge that the programs fostered race and gender bias as well as sexual fear among young people.

Independent academic critics joined SIECUS to claim that abstinence-only curricula conveyed a moral message through distortions and medical inaccuracies.[70] Such biases, they charged, were for the purpose of heightening a sense of danger and were usually difficult to track because they involved misrepresentations of reputable studies. In one example, Teen-Aid claims that gay male sexual activity results in condom breakage half the time. It turns out that the cited reference in the British medical journal *The Lancet* is not a study but rather a letter referring to the experiences of three female prostitutes during anal intercourse, not to gay male sex.[71] Comprehensive program advocates worried that even if teenagers had the skills to evaluate the studies, it would be extremely unlikely that they would catch such errors by researching the original references in curricula. In another case, an early version of the program Choosing the Best advised young people who might have intercourse to use Lysol on their genitals after condom use. Alerted to this advice by SIECUS, the company that manufactures Lysol brand products sent a cease and desist letter to Choosing the Best's publisher, warning that the disinfectant is only for use on hard surfaces not on human bodies.[72]

Critics of abstinence-only programs also challenged the representations of gender and race in the curricula. They charged that the curricula were rife with stereotypic illustrations. For example, girls are depicted as nurses while boys are doctors, or girls are the only ones represented as involved in parenting. Illustrations also predominantly depict white young people. Researchers Mariamne Whatley and Bonnie Trudell at the University of Wisconsin pointed out that in response to criticisms of racial bias, some curricula made only "weak" attempts at multiculturalism by simply making the white faces darker rather than fashioning more diverse facial characteristics.[73] In the texts themselves, depictions of girls' and boys' sexuality mirror the notions of gender set forth in Tim and Beverly LaHaye's Christian sex manual *The Art of Marriage*, in which men are portrayed as instinctually sexually aggressive while women are considered to be passive and more interested in mothering.[74] Most of the gatekeeping messages are targeted toward girls, who are depicted as more vulnerable to negative consequences such as loss of a good reputation. In keeping with the Christian Right's focus on white, middle-class children in the sex education debates, most of the texts are silent about race and ethnicity. However, some critics wondered whether warnings such as that in the Teen-Aid curriculum, which tells high school students that "different cultural backgrounds are also hurdles too high for some couples to negotiate," might themselves constitute coded efforts to discourage interracial relationships.[75]

Finally, critics of the abstinence-only curricula charged that they created a climate of sexual fear, guilt, and shame. Indeed, a Florida school board member said, "Let's scare the hoo-hoo out of [young people]. Show them the pictures of the last stages of AIDS,"[76] which is what the curriculum Free Teens does. Many curricula included the familiar claim that condoms have five-micron holes. Amplifying that fear, the curriculum Choosing the Best says, "When you use a condom, it is like playing Russian roulette. There is a greater risk of a condom failure than the bullet being in the chamber."[77] In other curricula, young people are told that premarital sex will inevitably result in a wide range of personal disasters. The parent-teacher guide Facing Reality lists forty-five such disasters in one sentence, ranging from pregnancy and disappointing one's parents to suffering sexual violence and even death.[78] It stresses, "Premarital sexual activity does not become a healthy choice or a moral choice simply because contraceptive technology is employed. Young persons will suffer and may even die if they choose it."[79] SIECUS pointed out that the curriculum derides those who engage in premarital sex by calling them "selfish," while the Sex Respect curriculum calls them "stupid."[80] At the turn of the twenty-first century, almost one in five students reported that their sex education teachers presented sex as "something to fear and avoid."[81]

Sometimes foes of abstinence-only programs succeeded, particularly in their criticisms of medical inaccuracies. A few communities filed lawsuits against abstinence-only curricula for medical inaccuracies. After a lawsuit in Caddo Parish, Louisiana, for example, the highly popular Sex Respect program could only be used after medically inaccurate sections had been deleted. Despite their efforts, however, it proved to be very difficult for comprehensive sex education advocates to counter the combination of stigmatizing language and medical sound bites that had been lodged against their own programs. Kantor, who monitored hundreds of community conflicts while at SIECUS, said, "What people did not understand is that perception was going to be the only reality. To the extent that the far right got their message out and bought an ad in the local paper and lobbied the school board, it did not matter what the facts were anymore. All that mattered was political pressure."[82] As we shall see in Chapter 9, with some notable exceptions like New Jersey, comprehensive programs across the country narrowed in content and scope throughout the nineties.

Teachers themselves reacted with fear. In her ethnography *Doing Sex Education*, researcher Bonnie Trudell describes how teachers try to protect themselves by "defensive teaching." Sex education instructors reduced the curriculum to a series of facts that students learn for the exam but rarely discuss in class in an attempt to avoid controversy.[83] Talk about sex became a menacing act to be disavowed. One teacher who had supported a controversial multicultural curriculum that included information about gay families insisted, "Nobody is talking about sex. Believe me, I don't want to talk about sex to kids."[84] One professor noted that teachers understood their vulnerability to scapegoating and became "driven not by theories of education but by the fear of attack."[85] Many became unwilling to teach sex education at all. After bitter conflicts in Newton, Massachusetts, the director of physical education at one high school said, "Teachers feel they're going to be put through something as strict as like before you adopt a child" because they must complete a document "with everything they have ever done, why they want to teach this course, what are their religious affiliations, are they heterosexual, homosexual." They must, she added, "be somewhat ready for a backlash."[86] In fact, few in Newton were ready; only 6 of 450 surveyed teachers were willing to teach the pilot curriculum. Teachers might well have feared that if accused, they would be, like anthropologist Gayle Rubin's observation about sex itself, "presumed guilty until proven innocent."[87] As we shall see, those fears were not groundless.


MAKING UP ENEMIES

Along with efforts to discredit each others' programs, advocates and opponents of comprehensive sex education perhaps inevitably fought each other. Opponents of comprehensive programs targeted SIECUS, Planned Parenthood, and sex educators themselves, whom they described as "the pornographers in the public school system."[88] In a speech during one local controversy, national right-wing activist Judith Riesman implied that sex educators tend to be pedophiles who enter the field to have access to young people.[89] Focus on the Family dubbed SIECUS "a wolf in sheep's clothing" and suggested that SIECUS leaders supported incest and pedophilia.[90] Lawsuits became a mechanism of intimidation. The American Family Association (AFA) Law Center circulated letters threatening to sue schools and teachers who taught information on condoms. The AFA of Georgia sent a letter to the state's Sex Education Review Committee members warning, "It is our belief that public school systems are potentially liable for products recommended and for information disseminated that affect the health and well being of students. We will offer legal counsel to students we feel have been harmed by products or information provided for health reasons."[91] An AIDS educator was sued in Massachusetts for allegedly traumatizing students by her presentation, and sexuality educators around the country were threatened with lawsuits for criticizing abstinence-only programs.[92]

Comprehensive sex educators complained of stigmatization by these opponents. They described distortions of their comments or in-class activities. One teacher said:

> One of the things that we were accused of is this orgasm game. And there's
> one other teacher and myself who teach this advanced human sexuality class,
> and we know we never, ever did an orgasm game. But I think what they
> were getting at—or trying to get at—is that we did use the word "orgasm"
> in class, and we did talk about pleasure and we did do activities that helped
> people look at the various kinds of pleasure, and I don't mean all sexual
> pleasure, but, you know, like eating a hot fudge sundae, all those kinds
> of pleasure things, and what was it that kept us from being able to talk
> more openly in the classrooms and in our lives about sexual pleasure, and
> why was sexual pleasure so restricted, and what was so bad about masturba-
> tion, and all these other kinds of things.[93]

A teacher in suburban Philadelphia told of being transferred after the circulation of narratives about statements she had allegedly made in her sex education class. The superintendent had read her a list of alleged incidents.

"It was vast distortions of things I had said," the teacher recounted, "the most memorable being that I had had my best orgasm ever sitting in the back yard reading a book; that I had told [this to] a class of twenty-five students of ninth-graders."[94] Another rumor, which she said "took on a life of its own," was that she had told her students that she and her husband used chocolate syrup as a lubricant.[95] Neither story is true, the teacher maintained, and she struggled to imagine how these tales might have arisen. The backyard orgasm story might have emerged from a discussion with students that there are other joys in life than sex. She said, "Kids are saying our parents don't want us to have fun, and I'm saying, 'That's not the only fun, that's a dangerous fun. There are other things you can do, you can go for a walk together, go roller skating, read a book.'" But ultimately, she concluded, "I don't know how we could have argued, how could you prove whether I said those things or not. The lies can't really be challenged. I don't yet know how we fight that kind of thing."[96] This teacher's sense of helplessness about such distortion recalls that of sixties educator Sally Williams of Anaheim, who, having been similarly transferred out of her sex education class, felt that she never found a way to fight the charges levied against her.

Advocates of comprehensive programs had fewer strategies available by which to challenge their opponents. Sexual stigmatization, which could be used so powerfully by their opponents, was not a possible option for their side. A similar rhetorical disparity was evident in abortion battles, which were occurring alongside sex education debates and among ideologically similar cohorts. Sociologist James Davison Hunter describes how anti-abortion organizations decried their opponents as "murderers," "pro-death activists," "intolerable evil," "death merchants," and "blood-sucking hyenas." Pro-choice activists responded by calling their adversaries "extremists," "zealots," or "bigots."[97] Sex education debates followed this pattern. Foes of comprehensive programs had available a much richer array of characterizations, such as pornographer and pedophile, leaving advocates with the somewhat monochromatic countercharge of extremism.

Still, their claim was not without cultural power. They charged that religious extremists were secretly insinuating themselves into local political debates, attempting to impose their own moralities. They deployed powerful buzzwords like "fundamentalists" and "censorship." This claim was reinforced on the national level. For example, in its advocacy kits, Planned

Parenthood Federation of America circulated the article "The Typical Censorship Scenario."[98] In embattled communities, such material became an explanatory device. One local sex education advocate said, "We have a very good piece about the opposition and their stages of development. We're in about the third stage, which is that they are harassing."[99] This narrative was sometimes reinforced by the media, such as in headlines that blared "Sex Ed Foes Tied to Christian Groups" and "National Right-Wing Ties Alleged as Fight Enters Voting Booth."[100] One conservative Christian sex education opponent told me that her group had been called "theological skin heads" and that a reporter had gone out of his way to take a photograph of her in front of a religious picture in order to, she claimed, "make me a Bible-thumping nut."[101] Suspicion ran high among local residents. When she was asked what happened in her town, one teacher said, "I hesitate to label people with names, but I guess I would call it a group of ultra-conservative, right-wing Republicans, because they're Republicans, all of whom profess to follow the beliefs of the Christian Coalition. They kind of snuck in,"[102] In another town, a prominent sex education foe seemed to come out of nowhere, fueling speculation that she was a paid agitator. One resident said, "We don't know who she is. We don't think she could be doing this unless she was being paid to do this."[103] They were not simply paranoid.

The claim that religious extremists were sneaking into communities was given weight by two broad factors: the emergence of stealth tactics among national organizations and the public's apprehension about Christian fundamentalism. Stealth, which dated to the 1992 campaign season, is a strategy of conservative Christians running in local elections without identifying themselves as such until after they have won. After a victory in San Diego, the Christian Coalition's Ralph Reed made his infamous statement to the *Los Angeles Times* that campaigning was like guerrilla warfare and "it's better to move quietly, with stealth, under cover of night."[104] Reed and other evangelical activists later denied using secrecy as a campaign strategy. But "stealth" became the perfect metaphor for anxieties about sinister presences sneaking into the community.

This anxiety was heightened by popular antipathy toward extremely conservative Christians. Over the past several decades, the United States has undergone a religious revival that has raised important questions about the relationship between conservative faith communities and politics.

Public rhetoric, which can be judgmental and caustic, is often the only exposure mainstream Americans have to conservative and evangelical Christians. Perhaps as a result, many Americans are suspicious of, and antagonistic toward fundamentalist and evangelical Christians. In one study, almost one-fifth of respondents were significantly hostile toward fundamentalists, expressing less regard for them than for illegal aliens.[105] To mainstream Americans, evangelicals and fundamentalists may seem rigid, intolerant, anti-intellectual, and threatening.[106] One liberal school board member complained, "Every time you object to something because it isn't reasonable or sound and it doesn't make sense, they accuse you of bashing their religion and bashing their Christianity. . . . They tell you that they want to be a participant at the table, but that is not what they want. They want to own the table. And they want to saw the legs off of your chair once they get there."[107] Such resentments, plus the fear of stealth activists, clouded local debates and aggravated a mood of suspicion. Sometimes these anxieties about national Christian Right and fundamentalist incursions into community affairs were warranted. In other cases, the narrative was oversimplified and sometimes simply wrong.

In local neighborhoods, national politics typically played out in oblique ways. National right-wing activists might visit and actively consult with local communities. Still, it was local residents, who might or might not have already been activists or religious conservatives, who imported the rhetoric of national Christian Right organizations. One attendee at a Christian Coalition training workshop claimed, "People think we're out to take over, but we're really just neighbors."[108] Some residents who became anti–comprehensive sex education activists were already religious conservatives who actively sought assistance from national and state Christian Right organizations. Local affiliates of Concerned Women for America, Focus on the Family, and the Christian Coalition, for example, could supply a ready squad of neighborhood activists on alert to join or generate sex education battles. Religious activists, particularly evangelicals, are much more politically engaged in demonstrating, boycotting, petitioning, and voting than the average resident.[109] Describing how she became involved in the sex education issue, one Massachusetts activist said, "God struck me with a lightning bolt."[110] National groups were able to establish and flourish by targeting citizens like this woman who then became concerned about sex education.

Although many local religious activists secularize their strategies, some do not. One New Hampshire resident who describes herself as a fundamentalist Christian was elected to the school board in a highly contentious climate. She was remarkably candid about how religion shaped her political work on the school board, noting, "I think we look for certain things in a candidate. We look for, 'Is he a Christian? Is the candidate a Christian?' If we push a Christian, it's not because we're trying to push a candidate that would be imposing Christianity on the world. That we would not. But more, the Christian, Judeo-Christian values would be more of what we would want that candidate to pursue."[111] Her perspective reveals how fundamentalists can view as necessary the imposition of their religious beliefs in the secular political arena, and her own votes on the school board consistently followed fundamentalist tenets. For example, this school board member voted to prohibit discussion of homosexuality in public school classrooms. When she was asked about those who might have different beliefs, she insisted, "There is no such thing. The word of God is for all, it's not just for those that believe."[112] This woman's position was consistent with the overwhelming majority of activists in conservative evangelical groups who believe that most political issues have one correct, Christian view.[113]

There were powerful incentives for local residents to seek out national groups. Camaraderie is one advantage, especially because sex education opponents are sometimes an unpopular minority. One local activist said, "It was nice just to be in the company of people who felt as I did."[114] Furthermore, opportunities for recognition and training in leadership skills were compelling rewards. Christian Right organizations are adept at training locals and fostering the "embourgeoisement" of activists, especially women.[115] Perhaps reflecting this emphasis, one school board member said she viewed the Christian Coalition as a political, not religious, organization. At the time of her school board campaign, she claimed that she was "just a mom" and a not-very-active Catholic: "I didn't really identify myself as a religious person at that time at all. I mean, if I made it to church once a month, I was doing really good. But I guess the more I put my views out there I realized that I really was lined up with religious conservatives in this country."[116] She came to embrace the Christian Coalition. "As time went on, I learned very quickly what it was and I found out it was more a political group than religious. Just people of faith who had gotten into politics is what it is."[117] Rumors about this school board member's involvement with the Christian Coalition were substantiated when she appeared as a speaker at a national meeting in Washington, D.C., was on television with Coalition director Ralph Reed, and publicly accepted paid membership. The Christian Coalition became a source of political support and also a platform for her national visibility. She summed up the controversies in her community by saying, "A lot of good things have come out of all of that for me personally."[118]

The power and expanse of conservative national organizations in the sex education debates derive from an uninformed public. Many people are not fluent in civic matters or expert in social problems. This can be true even for activists. National organizations offered locals essentially endless resources. Residents who might not have been very informed about sex education when they became activists did not have to reinvent the wheel of debate. For example, when one parent was elected to the school board, she immediately solicited information from right-wing groups such as Phyllis Schlafly's Eagle Forum: "The first thing I get on the board and I started looking for conservative avenues."[119] Her companion on the school board also described herself as uneducated about many topics after her election. Conservatives actively reached out to her. She described the controversy over a proposal to teach creationism in the public schools:

> A news reporter asked me, "Well, what do you think about this?" And I said, "Well, if they teach about evolution, why not teach creationism?" It was sort of a very naïve position to take. I said to one reporter, "The closest thing I've come to dinosaurs is the wallpaper in my son's bedroom." I knew very, very little about creation science. Next thing I knew, I was getting letters, videotapes, and audio tapes and all kinds of things in the mail from people all over the place trying to educate me on creation science.[120]

One school board member of a small Massachusetts town said about a sex education opponent, "One day he was talking, 'You're perverted,' and the next day he's talking like he has a Ph.D. or something. We thought, somebody's giving him words. And we were right. Eagle Forum jumped on him."[121] The words that Christian Right national organizations offer can become a common language for a select cohort.

Still, despite the many advantages national Christian Right organizations offered to local residents, there were drawbacks as well. The heavy influence of conservative Christian organizations and the fear of stealth activists could foster the automatic assumption that local sex education opponents were "fundamentalists." As one conservative candidate who lost her campaign for the school board said, "All I could say when I was asked, 'Are you another stealth candidate for the Christian Coalition?' the answer is 'No.' But that can also be, in this community concerning that question, the very answer that incriminates you. So that was a no-win." I asked whether her religious beliefs had shaped her opposition to sex education, and she complained, "People always do say, 'Well then, you must be the religious right.' But they never ask, 'Are you the unreligious left?'"[122] The charges of fundamentalism and extremism could be stigmatizing and irrefutable in their own ways.

The Christian Right's mobilizations against comprehensive sex education attracted a diverse constituency of Christian evangelicals and fundamentalists, conservative Catholics, along with some Muslims, and conservative Jews. Indeed, the movement's power is that it can draw even nominally religious individuals and further build its strength. This was the case in Newton, Massachusetts, a liberal, upper-middle-class, heavily Jewish city. Jewish sex education opponents found themselves discredited as fundamentalists by liberals in the community. Rabbis at an influential Newton temple had sent out a letter saying that the anti–sex education activists were a Christian fundamentalist group which was attempting to insert Christian doctrine into the schools. One Jewish sex education opponent said, "Then a letter came out from the ACLU denouncing us. . . . We were being linked to right-wing Christian groups. And it didn't matter that [another opposition activist] was a Jew. It didn't matter that I was a Jew. It didn't matter that there were other Jews. There were Roman Catholics. So what I felt was going on was an attempt to silence us by calling us the worst thing you could possibly be called in Newton, which was right-wing Christian fundamentalists. Like being called a Jew in Mississippi."[123] Newton sex education supporters were not unreasonable to suspect outside infiltration of Christian fundamentalists. Panelists on a very well-attended opposition forum had included well-known representatives associated with the evangelical organizations Concerned Women for America and the American Family Association and the ultra-conservative Catholic group Human Life International. The forum had been widely advertised on the local Christian radio station and in a Christian book-store, and fundamentalist churches outside of Newton had bused in their congregation members to attend. And tellingly, the preponderance of the opposition's literature was lifted directly from national evangelical orga-nizations like Focus on the Family and Concerned Women for America, with Christian Right themes braided throughout. The presence of national organizations, even if only in the form of their materials and rhetoric, can mask any internal diversity in local community debates, leaving sex edu-cation opponents open to charges of religious extremism.

The century that had opened with calls for sex education in the public schools ended beset by local battles over what and how much to say to young people about sexuality. By the late nineties, there were more than seven hundred controversies throughout the fifty states.[124] On the national level, Joycelyn Elders's firing in 1994 underscored conservatives' success at limiting the terms of public conversation. The lack of a popular uprising on her behalf, and Clinton's pronouncement "That's not what schools are for,"[125] highlighted the ongoing risk of speaking out in favor of sex edu-cation. National rhetorics exerted paradoxical local effects. The ways that communities talked about sexuality education were often flattened by the scripted arguments of national organizations, which in one sense resem-bled what novelist and critic Toni Morrison describes as dead languages—those that "cannot form or tolerate new ideas, shape other thoughts, tell another story, fill baffling silences."[126] At the same time, evocative rheto-ric aroused powerful emotions that disrupted and lingered in communi-ties nationwide. As Kantor of SIECUS put it, "These battles tend to just go on and on. They do not really go away even after the vote is done."[127] Opponents of comprehensive sex education had evolved from the religious and conspiracy rhetoric of the sixties to the idiom of scientific medicine in the nineties. As we shall see in the next chapter, they also adopted the language of other social critics as well, including those of feminists and critical race theorists.

# Chapter 6 | DOING IT WITH WORDS

On the *Phil Donahue Show* in 1979, SIECUS founder Mary Calderone posed a riddle to the somewhat abashed host: "It's a four-letter-word ending in K and it means intercourse, and it's the most important intercourse there is—TALK."[1] Belief in "intercourse" was one thing that distinguished SIECUS not only from its critics but also from prior generations of sex educators who had feared that open talk about sex might incite sexual behavior. Social hygienists who had issued the first call for sex education in the public schools in the twentieth century had hesitated about the propriety of intruding on Victorian dictates regarding sexual modesty and innocence, especially that of women, by giving them explicit information about sexuality. Maurice Bigelow, a leader in the late nineteenth-century war against venereal disease, suggested an obfuscating educational strategy by which "Sex knowledge . . . can often be conveyed without the slightest consciousness on [students'] part that what they are receiving is sex instruction."[2] SIECUS, of course, had played an important role in advocating that classrooms become sites for open discussion of sexual matters, breaking with the normative position that such discussion could have dire consequences. However, broad political debates which surfaced in the eighties about the nature and impact of speech gave rise to innovative claims by conservatives about the ways in which talk about sexuality was destructive.

Through the eighties and nineties, some political and legal theorists began to argue that speech is conduct which enacts violence and discrimination. This notion extended philosopher of language J. L. Austin's contention in *How to Do Things with Words* that certain speech acts have performative power. Austin suggested that, depending on the "total speech situation," some utterances result in later consequences, while others perform certain effects in the moment of saying them.[3] This claim was put to good use by conservative opponents of sex education, who charged that talk of sexuality in the classroom was performative. Two versions of this allegation about sex education prevailed. One said that speech about sex acts as an unhealthy stimulus to sexual thought and practice among students. This anxious warning—that sex education makes kids go out and have sex—was as old as sex education itself. In the eighties, a second allegation about sex education arose that speaking about sex *is* sex. According to this claim, sexual speech itself enacts an emotionally abusive type of sex. In public arguments, critics equated speech in the classroom with violent conduct. The shift in oppositional vocabularies from provocative terms like "promiscuity" to ones like "abuse" performed its own unsettling effects in the already unsettled space of the sex education culture wars.

## SEX TALK / SEX ACTS

Sex education opponents played on long-standing fears that sex talk triggers sex. Sexual speech, these critics contend, provokes and stimulates; it transforms the so-called natural modesty[4] of children into inflamed desires that may be outside the child's control and thus prompt sexual activity. For example, Judith Riesman, who is associated with several national right-wing groups such as Concerned Women for America, the American Family Association, and Human Life International, is noted for her allegation that contemporary sex education is built on Alfred Kinsey's research and that as a result schoolchildren are being taught "a theory of indiscriminate sexuality."[5] "The Kinsey Grand Scheme" sexualizes children, Riesman claims, so as to "promote widespread promiscuity to create a sexual anarchy."[6] With these claims circulating on the national level, it was not surprising to hear them condensed in local debates, as with one parent who complained "the 'know-how' of safer sex is an invitation to promiscuous sex."[7] Another claimed that "sex education as taught in the public schools is a contributing factor to teen sexual promiscuity."[8] Sex education evaluations which consistently show that instruction does not result in increased sexual behavior did not allay this rhetorical strategy.[9] (Sex education advocates who argue that those very speech acts *deter* young people from these actions also engaged in claims of performativity—or perhaps anti-performativity.)

A version of the accusation that sexual speech produces sexual behavior was the charge that sexual speech constructs sexual identities. The fears, of course, travel in one direction—that by talking about homosexuality, otherwise heterosexual youth will be seduced into it. For example, in reflecting back on his vehement opposition to the influential Anaheim, California, program in 1968, journalist Jim Townsend recently concluded, "There were more homosexuals made in that sex education classroom than would have ever been here today if they hadn't told them, 'If you haven't tried it, don't knock it; it's just an alternative lifestyle.' Well, they tried it, and they didn't knock it, and a lot of them became homosexuals as a direct result of being taught that in the classroom. That's a fact."[10] Silencing classroom discussion through speech codes was an obvious tactic for sex education opponents who believed that talking about homosexuality condones and therefore encourages its performance.

By the mid-eighties, opponents of comprehensive sex education escalated their claims about the performativity of sexual speech. They continued to argue that sex education caused young people to engage in sex, but they also rhetorically fused speech and action to allege that speaking about sexuality in the classroom is tantamount to "doing it." Sex education, they charged, *is* sexual abuse. The title of national right-wing leader Phyllis Schlafly's 1984 book *Child Abuse in the Classroom*, a broad critique of public education, exemplified the trend.[11] A more developed argument appeared in the widely disseminated sex education critiques by psychiatrist Melvin Anchell, who pronounced that "seduction is not limited to actual molestation. A child can be seduced, in psychoanalytic terms, by overexposure to sexual activities, including sex courses in the classroom."[12] Contemporary critics condemned all classroom programs in which, they alleged, a broad spectrum of words in a range of contexts rape, seduce, or molest in the moment of their utterance. One text announced that sex education is not education at all, but rather a "legalized form of child seduction and molestation."[13] Another was entitled *Raping Our Children: The Sex Education Scandal.*[14] An amplification of more traditional allegations that sexual speech causes later sexual activity, these claims introduced the threat of immediate harm. One activist in the well-known anti-gay video *The Gay Agenda in Public Education* claims: "As a counselor I'm very concerned about the fact that the focus on the sexual at a young age is a kind of mental and emotional molestation, because these children are not meant to think about sex at such age and even if they are, not ever to think of it in the context that it's being presented because it's a false context and it will cause them to dwell on thoughts that should not be. And it will do damage."[15] The new twist on performativity expressed by "molestation of the mind" intensified the danger motif inherent in much anti–sex education discourse.

The extent to which speech performs that which is spoken is a subject of considerable academic debate.[16] Literary critic Shoshana Felman poses the question, "To speak an act: can this be done?"[17] Is, for example, burning a cross on the lawn of an African American family a legally protected form of expressive conduct or a hate crime? How is it similar to, or different from, hurling a racist epithet at someone on the street? What is the nature of the harm effected by either? Pornography has been the subject of similar contention, as some feminists argue that pornography is not speech but a discriminatory act of terrorism.[18] Campus speech codes, civil laws against pornography, and restrictions on sexual speech in the workplace are all measures, albeit profoundly controversial ones, that have been proposed or implemented to redress or protect from harmful speech. These broader cultural developments inflected oppositional rhetoric that comprehensive sex education speech actually performs harmful sex.

## ANTI–SEX EDUCATION SPEECH AND CULTURAL POLITICS

The discursive strategies of political movements depend on a broad mix of sociohistorical conditions. Sociologist Ken Plummer, in his analysis of sexual stories, asserts that particular stories can only be told when the cultural circumstances are such that there is a ready audience. Otherwise such stories lie "dormant, awaiting their historical moment."[19] I would also argue, concerning what he calls "the tale and its time," that historical circumstances are productive of narratives, not simply receptive. Narratives do not simply preexist, awaiting their moment; rather, the cultural moment is the fabric out of which new narrative themes and textures are constructed. Historical eras give rise to speech genres with particular vocabularies and meanings.[20] In particular, the crucial strategic shift from claims, common in the sixties, that talking about sexuality causes kids to have sex, to the more recent allegations that sex education speech *is* sex, specifically sexual abuse, depended on two crucial historical developments: first, the rise of "our culture's master narrative of child molesting"[21] and second, the widespread circulation of political arguments that collapse speech and conduct as similarly assaultive. With respect to the claim of mental molestation, then, the times spawned the tale.

"Emotional molestation" could only emerge as a culturally powerful rhetoric of fear in a broader context of high anxiety about potential dangers to children. Despite its long history, physical and sexual abuse of children received episodic attention throughout the twentieth century.[22] Only since the late seventies has child abuse most recently been framed as a widespread social problem. Newly formed agencies and organizations, such as the National Center for Missing and Exploited Children, had ushered through a host of laws, as forty-seven states passed legislation concerning child abuse and neglect between 1963 and 1967. By the seventies and into the eighties, professionals such as physicians and social workers and otherwise antipathetic political cohorts such as feminists and New Right activists allied in nationwide campaigns to protect children against a variety of abuses and abusers. Kidnapping, murder, sexual molestation, ritual abuse, and even Halloween sadism were among the many alleged dangers that child advocates targeted. By the mid-eighties had come a massive cultural shift in attitudes in which the vulnerability of children, and their need for protection, had become "national social orthodoxy."[23] Cultural sensitivity to child endangerment had reached new heights.

Activists effected social and legislative initiatives to address some very real problems. However, these efforts had the ancillary effect of contributing to a cultural climate in which abuse seemed to lurk around every corner. For one, some activists inflated prevalence figures. Along with journalists and politicians, they deployed often wildly exaggerated or unsubstantiated statistical estimates of endangered children.[24] Such claims of large numbers of victims exacerbated anxieties about child safety. Moreover, the definition of sexual abuse became elastic enough to encompass not only the physical violation of a child, but also such diverse behaviors as taking nude pictures and talking about sexuality with a child. Parents, for example, were arrested for photographing their children in the bath.[25] In addition, the subject of child abuse pervaded the media. By the nineties, coverage of what one reporter decried as "the most unspeakable of crimes, childhood sexual abuse,"[26] was so prolific that cultural critic James Kincaid observed, "There's a whole lot of unspeakableness going on."[27] And so when comprehensive sex education opponents coined the term "emotional molestation," it conjured up a host of sinister associations in a national affective culture wherein sexual abuse had become a ubiquitous fright. Through these allegations, sex education took its place in the pantheon of abusive contexts.

Along with the rise in attention to child victimization, a series of legal and political discourses blurred the boundaries of speech and conduct. These were crafted largely by progressives, some of whom described themselves as legal realists,[28] as well as by certain feminists and critical race theorists. Their arguments named particular types of speech acts as discriminatory, even abusive, behavior. Some critical race theorists, for example, described an alarming rise in the incidence of "assaultive speech, [e.g.,] words that are used as weapons to ambush, terrorize, wound, humiliate, and degrade."[29] Some feminists made claims about the performativity of sexual speech, that words are conduct in pornography and sexual harassment. Legal scholar Catharine MacKinnon articulated the most direct fusion of sexual speech and conduct: "Talking about sex can be speech, but doing it through words can be sexual assault. Harassment that is not sexual does its harm through its content, undermining equality, especially in universities, where the mind is the terrain of the equality as well as the speech. Harassment that is sexual does its harm as an act of sexual abuse, like, and sometimes as, pornography."[30] The idea that words wound or abuse has been heavily debated and contested within both the feminist movement and among critical race theorists. Debates over legislating against pornography prompted the volatile feminist sex wars of the eighties.[31] Feminist critics of MacKinnon's position argued that collapsing the boundaries between sexual speech and conduct was conceptually flawed and that putting this theory into practice would undermine free expression and work against women's interests.[32] Nonetheless, the concept that words wound, subordinate, and abuse circulated widely. It was not a vast conceptual leap for sex education opponents to adopt these strategies for their own purposes to allege that sex education speech molests.

Vocabularies of abuse construct an indisputable immorality.[33] And opponents of comprehensive sex education needed to enhance the cultural power of anti–sex education discourse by the late eighties. A range of AIDS educators, from those in gay-run service organizations to mainstream groups like Planned Parenthood, had incrementally challenged cultural resistance to frank safer-sex education. The Centers for Disease Control and Prevention (CDC) had trained Planned Parenthood affiliates in HIV prevention, and those educators were suddenly more in demand (although one educator in Salt Lake City reported that she had been asked not to mention condoms or even sex in her AIDS education workshop in the city schools).[34] Fear of death sometimes trumped the fear—long kindled by sex education opponents—that talk about sex would prompt kids to have sex. With the tide of the sexual culture flowing against them, sex education opponents needed even more dramatic strategies. Rhetoric that sex education speech is abuse countered AIDS anxiety with the urgency of immediate threat from dangerous classroom programs.

The claim that sex education speech performs (molests, abuses, assaults) in the very act of speaking accomplishes significant rhetorical work. First, it constricts the already minimal cultural space afforded to sexual pleasure. In sixties anti–sex education claims of performativity, the alleged consequence of sexual speech was arousal. A prominent sixties opponent of the sex education program in Anaheim, California, claimed to have been mobilized by comments such as those from one boy who said, "I never go to that class without stopping at my locker and getting a big book, because when I come out of that class I have to put that book in front of me."[35] Indeed, the notion that sex education would incite sexual passions in young people was the fear underlying that era's conspiracy theories. So although youths' sexual desires were themselves considered dangerous by sex education opponents, there was still cultural acknowledgment of childhood sexuality. However, only sexual danger inheres in contemporary claims that sex education speech is an abusive, molesting act. Anti–sex education speech thus shrinks the discursive space for pleasure and expands the climate of sexual fear and shame.

Second, it broadens the category of assaultive speech to include a wide range of talk about sexuality. Classroom pedagogy, by tradition, simply does not include graphic descriptions of sex acts, especially in this era of defensive teaching. Therefore, the kinds of sex education speech that are putatively performative, that opponents believe enact the rape or molestation of the mind, are any mention of homosexuality that does not utterly condemn it and nearly all other sexual discussion including safer-sex instruction or any mention of issues like birth control, masturbation, or heterosexual intercourse outside of marriage. To claim that talking about sexuality in the classroom enacts abuse or rape is to infinitely extend the reach of claims about the performativity of speech so that simply talking about sex in the classroom is doing it.

Finally, the claim that sex education is abuse creates a vast new network of sex offenders. If indeed it is abuse or "mental molestation," then someone must be the molester. This is the largely unarticulated leap in opponents' argument that sex education speech performs abuse. The perpetrator of the alleged mental or emotional molestation of youth in the classroom is often unnamed, thereby increasing both the anxiety and the imaginative possibilities. Of course, since much of the targeted pedagogy is speech about homosexuality, the perpetrator is a familiar figure—the child-molesting homosexual. But the scope of accusation is much broader to include sex educators in general. Peter Scales, a former education director of the Planned Parenthood Federation of America, recalls being picketed and called "America's Child Abuser Number One."[36] National activist Judith Riesman electrified an audience in Massachusetts with her implication that many sexuality educators in the schools are child molesters who enter the field to prey on children. At a community forum, Riesman asked, "Are we supposed to say that there are no pedophiles or pederasts amongst our teaching profession and that suddenly they're immune? Pedophiles and pederasts only go into the priesthood?"[37] As explosive as her charge was at the time, it was only inserting the subject into the sentence that includes emotional molestation. Usually amorphous, the concept of emotional molestation accomplishes a broad amplification of the already elastic culture of child molesting. Like not knowing which child might suddenly turn on his classmates and riddle them with bullets on the playground, emotional molestation is a concept beset with seemingly random danger. Any teacher is a suspect.

The rhetoric of national organizations rapidly diffuses into the culture, becoming common knowledge. Through the nineties, the claim that sex education speech is sexual abuse echoed in local community debates. Invoking the sexual innocence of the Romantic child, one conservative school board member noted

> I said [to the health curriculum committee], 'My children were outside in the snow, sled riding.' And we're talking about nine-, ten-, eight-, eleven-, twelve-year-olds. All they did all day was slide up and down that hill, up and down that hill. Do you think for one minute they had the thought of sex on their minds, or condoms or spermicide? No, that's not in their world right now. And why should we be forcing it on them? Why should we put that burden on them? You know, I think that's wrong. I see it as child abuse, I really do.[38]

Dolores Ayling in New York accused educators of homicide for suggesting that there are "promising treatments" available for HIV: "No one is safe from this disease and to even suggest that they can engage in sex and be safe from a virus like this is in my estimation actually committing murder."[39] Extending the analogy, she continued, "Would you like your child to take a gun and put one bullet in and play Russian roulette and take the chance that he will not kill himself? Well, basically what's happening here is the same thing."[40] Concepts like mental and emotional molestation, sex education as child abuse, and HIV education as murder were vocabularies of endangerment available to community residents who began discussions about local sex education programs. Intended to shape collective feelings, they framed comprehensive sex education as potentially even lethal to young people.

Such rhetoric escalated the affective pitch of the culture wars. The concerns of early twentieth-century social hygienists, or of sixties sex education opponents, that sexual discussion would encourage young people to experiment sexually had been repeatedly addressed. Independent researchers have found no evidence for earlier onset of intercourse among students who take comprehensive sexuality education.[41] Although these studies largely had not stopped critics from making this claim, the charge that sex education *causes* subsequent sexual behavior has been empirically investigated. But the charge that sex education *is* sex reconfigured the grounds for debate. Whether talk about sexuality constitutes molestation or abuse was largely a matter of individual belief, not subject to empirical investigation. Furthermore, such a charge demanded an immediate response, an end to the abusive conduct. The claim that children are being molested by talk about sexuality in the classroom was intended to foster intolerance toward sex education.

Sexual speech is not sexual behavior—talk and action are not precisely the same. Collapsing the two is, as philosopher Judith Butler observes, "a bit of a mistake."[42] Equally mistaken would be to deny the importance of public talk about sexuality. Sexual speech *is* powerful, although it is impossible to specify or predict exactly in what ways for which individuals. Public sex talk can conjure up a range of sexual worlds and possibilities. Classroom discussion might either reassure or frighten; it could disgust or even arouse. Information on safer sex could be life-saving but, in some contexts, information might mislead. The consequences of speech and the uses of knowledge are always unpredictable. It is precisely this unpredictability, along with deep uncertainties about sexuality and young people, that fueled the rhetoric of sex education opponents. Among the questions that faced each community and public school system in the nineties was to what extent its sex education program would allow for open discussion and the provision of information on sexuality—and to what extent it would restrict those possibilities. The fusion of speech and conduct, the use of terms like "abuse," "murder," and even "promiscuity," constituted political strategies which helped establish a volatile emotional climate in those debates.

## Chapter 7 | THE PASSIONS OF CULTURE WARS

On the chilly May night in 1993 when the Newton, Massachusetts, school board planned to vote on a highly contested sex education program, anti–sex education activist Brian Camenker was number sixty-three on the list of citizens who had signed up to speak. After three hours of tense debate in an auditorium marked by a heavy police presence, Camenker, who had been instrumental in leading the fight against the program, got his turn. He stepped to the microphone, paused, collapsed to the floor, and was carried out. It was later announced that he had suffered an intense anxiety attack. Camenker's statement, which was read to the school board by someone else, announced, "My feelings on this issue are well-known. So is my disgust for the tactics being used to silence us. We won't stand for it in Newton, we won't stand for it in Massachusetts, and we won't stand for it in America."[1] Camenker's rhetoric reflected the embattled tone of the debates in Newton, which one father had described as a "civil war."[2] And yet his inability to speak his own refusal to be silenced was a poignant expression of the incapacitating emotions sex education controversies can produce.

Conservative Pat Buchanan had said in 1992 that the culture wars were a battle for the soul of America. They were also a battle for America's feelings. Local debates over sex education are often impassioned occasions. As we saw in Chapter 3, the Moral Majority's Jerry Falwell had urged conservative Christians to get mad and to speak harsh language in furthering their moral beliefs. In sex education debates, language and emotions could indeed be ugly. Community meetings have erupted in shouting matches and even physical violence. Neighbors scream at each other during meetings, overwrought residents faint, people shove and hit each other. School board members and prominent activists have received death threats, donned bulletproof vests, and after volatile meetings received police escorts to their cars. Residents often describe the degree of sudden acrimony and resentment in their communities as civic brawls or civil war. School board meetings go from sleepy affairs to late-night shouting matches. (One national network documentary on local sex education conflicts shows a grumpy school board member peering at her watch and announcing to the meeting that it was quarter to one in the morning.) After a particularly bitter public forum in one town, a sex education supporter said, "I now know what it felt like to be in Nazi Germany. I now know how it felt to be a black in Alabama."[3] Both sides of the sex education debate have decried the so-called McCarthyist tactics on the parts of their opponents.[4] Not simply hyperbole, these responses signaled the extent to which people came to feel under siege. Much is at stake and, for some, the heated emotions were welcome. One sex education opponent said about her allies, "I was glad they were strident. We really feel our children are under threat."[5] Sex education conflicts involve not merely which curriculum a public school adopts; rather, they are highly emotional public arguments about sexuality and young people.

The discursive politics of sex education are contests over the meanings and emotional culture of sexuality. Such explosive local battles are not spontaneous outbursts of support or resistance. Rooted in history and politics, they are occasions in which activists evoke in audiences intense feelings and encourage their public expression. Discursive politics frame issues and construct a collective mood which shapes the nature and outcome of national and local debates. Intense emotions can attract supporters to a social movement and galvanize them to action. In local sex education conflicts, emotional outbursts can influence whether a curriculum is adopted or voted down. Nationally, politicized emotions have helped stall the progress of comprehensive sex education. In this regard, then, feelings serve as a potential resource for social movements. However, political appeals to emotion are unpredictable and, like Brian Camenker, can collapse unexpectedly.

Part of the cultural power of sex education conflicts is that they are viewed as unmediated collective expressions of the attitudes and feelings of individual Americans in response to controversial issues such as sexuality. This is because, in the popular imagination, emotions seem perhaps the deepest, most natural expression of our core selves. But neither emotions nor culture wars are simply spontaneous reactions. Emotions are not just automatic, gut responses, although this is not to say that bodily sensations are trivial. Rather, sociologists argue that emotions are complex expressions of interpretations we make in response to cultural definitions and demands. They are socially constructed—yet another dimension in which we are deeply social beings.[6] Social constructionist research on emotion allows for understandings of emotion as contextual, interactive, and performative. These aspects of emotions suggest their importance in the political culture.

Emotions play a prominent role in political protest and social change. They have, however, received uneven attention from sociologists over the past several decades.[7] In the sixties, researchers of collective behavior saw emotions as key in phenomena such as "the panic," "the craze," and "the hostile outburst."[8] Often in such studies feelings were undertheorized as being simply, for example, (over)reactions to rumor or to "hysterical beliefs."[9] By the seventies, emotions dropped completely from the paradigms of resource mobilization theorists, who instead stressed the rationality of social movement activists.[10] At the same time, however, a radically different perspective on collective behavior emerged in British sociologist Stanley Cohen's concept of "moral panic,"[11] which some theorists extrapolated into the complementary notion of "sex panic."[12] Intense public hostility is an important characteristic of moral panic. The nature of emotions in moral panics has been the subject of some debate. While many theorists view the anger, paranoia, and intolerance expressed during moral panics as disproportionate—wherein "objective molehills have been made into subjective mountains"[13]—others object, saying that such an evaluation trivializes the concerns of protesters.

Meanwhile, since the mid-eighties, the study of emotions has moved to the foreground of social and cultural analysis.[14] Literary theorists have examined emotions in cultural politics—for example, Lauren Berlant's analysis of the rhetorics of affective persuasion in the transformation of the political public sphere to the intimate public sphere.[15] Linda Kintz shows how the Right creates "resonance" for its politics among a diverse public through the skillful use of intimate emotions.[16] Specific attention to the role of emotions in social protest emerged from several broad areas. New social movement theorists, particularly feminists, demonstrated how feelings such as love, fear, and anger can play a significant part in both the strategic actions and the internal dynamics of movements.[17] The political dimensions of shame emerged in the studies of both anthropologist Carole S. Vance and sociologist Arlene Stein.[18] Finally, in his call for a more comprehensive examination of feelings in protest movements, sociologist James Jasper argued that important analytic concepts such as identity and injustice frames have substantial emotional dimensions.[19] Jasper, however, noted the reluctance of many social movement theorists to include affective components in their models of protest. Oddly, this reluctance shows up in sociological debates over the culture wars. Emotions occupy a shadow existence in these debates, while instead sociologists focus on whether individual Americans are polarized in their attitudes about controversial issues.[20] In the next section I argue that the affective dimension is a significant arena of culture wars.

Emotions are central to the discursive politics of sex education. The term "discursive politics" typically refers to contests over meanings, because discourse, as critic Samuel R. Delany notes, "tells us what to pay attention to and what to ignore. It tells us what sort of attention to pay."[21] Discourse, I suggest, also tells us how to feel; it produces and shapes emotion. The social guidelines that define the emotional tone and expectations of a situation—what sociologist Arlie Hochschild calls "feeling rules"[22]—are embedded in discourse. Discourse authorizes and legitimates particular ways of thinking and talking as well as ways of feeling. Poststructuralist analysis further suggests how feeling rules and emotion management constitute important aspects of the governance of the self.[23] Social movements strive to use language, images, and symbols to establish particular cognitive meanings as well as emotional conventions. The affective power of discursive politics is possible because feelings are so responsive to social conventions and, by extension, to social control. Therefore, their production becomes an important, albeit unstable, resource for social movements. In her study of emotion management in service industries, Hochschild found that human feelings can be commercialized by the marketplace.[24] So too when emotions are triggered and managed as resources by social movements they become politicized.

Emotions become politicized in several ways during local sex education culture wars. On the simplest level, they heat up the climate and draw attention to the issue. Media coverage often intensifies when typically somnolent school board meetings explode. In turn, headlines and articles that emphasize explosions of feeling in the language of warfare not only sell newspapers, but they also coach citizens in the emotional expectations of town meetings. Moreover, emotions can amplify the symbolic power of language, thereby enhancing its potential to persuade and mobilize followers. For example, communities can be electrified by allegations that a school is teaching "pornography." Sex education opponents can, at least momentarily, galvanize a range of residents, including many who have never before been activists, by an evocative claim. Power inheres in emotions in that they can naturalize sexual hierarchies, establishing some sexualities as normal and others as disgusting or unspeakable. When conservative activists called a curriculum that mentions gay families "the sodomy curriculum," they recuperated historical meanings about the perversion of homosexuality while also tapping emotional expectations for fear or anger on the part of concerned parents. Activists seek the production of these emotions while relying on and reinscribing a popular notion that feelings are a core reflection of an inner truth or knowledge. They tap a taken-for-grantedness about what can be said and felt about sexuality. Finally, when a social movement strategically evokes strong feelings and encourages their expression in public debates, emotion is politicized. Therefore, in community culture wars, as we shall see, an important element of emotion work involves their public performance.

## EMOTIONS IN PRACTICE

Sex education debates are not inherently incendiary; they are flare-ups which have been ignited. This happens through a mix of factors. No one comes to sex education debates devoid of prior experiences which might shape an emotional response. Nor, conversely, is the particular reaction of anyone involved in a community dialogue fixed or determined.

Individual predispositions interact with contextual dynamics in a person's response to the emotional triggers which abound in local sex education debates. Predispositions might include factors such as strong political inclinations, personal experiences with sexual diversity, and the level of openness toward sexual pluralism. As this book suggests, religious commitments can mediate emotional responses in important ways. National evangelical and fundamentalist leaders such as Jerry Falwell have encouraged public demonstrations of anger and outrage among their followers. Values, then, can predispose an individual toward specific feelings, while the display of intense emotions can also be a means by which one demonstrates religious or political affiliation. Still, many people come to community debates without extreme predispositions. How is it, then, that these discussions become hostile, even violent events? I suggest that the polarization of debates stems from practices purposely intended to evoke passionate feelings.

When social movements "evoke" feelings, they do not tap into essences which are outside of discourse. Rather, they engage in strategic practices that will motivate individuals toward what Hochschild calls "emotion work"—the effort to produce "a desired feeling which is initially absent."[25] Emotion as political practice involves history, culture, and power. Social movements rely on two dimensions of emotional culture—background conventions and immediate dynamics—to foster emotion work and volatile community outbursts. Background conventions are Hochschild's "feeling rules"—the historically specific guidelines and expectations for how individuals will produce and manage affect.[26] In sex education debates, background conventions involve both ideologies about childhood sexuality and standards for public emotional styles. Immediate dynamics include contextual factors such as heated rhetoric. Background conventions and immediate dynamics interact. Provocative language provokes, for example, through what philosopher Judith Butler calls "the citational character of speech."[27] Language invokes and reinforces prior cognitive and affective conventions. Both background and immediate factors operate as cues to individuals and groups for the production of emotionally normative reactions. The taken-for-grantedness of feelings is crucial to the politicization of emotion.

Traditional affective conventions of sexuality are essential background features of impassioned community debates. Conservative opponents depend on a normative emotional climate of sexual shame. Strategic rhetoric draws on prior affective conventions in which sex is taboo and dangerous. Sexuality education, therefore, can be rendered suspicious with little difficulty, and educators themselves can be easily stigmatized by their association with sex. The emotions of sex education debates are intensified by long-standing conventions about children and sexuality. Sex education opponents hope to produce anger, fear, and disgust among parents by tapping those affective expectations inherent in our broad cultural narrative about the violation of childhood innocence. They may also tap, intentionally or not, what cultural theorist James Kincaid calls our "hard-core righteous prurience" about sexuality and children.[28] It is a powerful mix. This diffuse matrix of affective conventions regarding both sexuality and childhood—anger, titillation, fear, shame, disgust— constitutes an enormous strategic advantage for conservatives. The language and images, public arguments and allegations which sex education opponents employ are all designed to invoke this negative affective culture. When the opponents succeed, not only do they potentially win local battles, but they also reinscribe sexual stigma in the broader emotional climate.

Background conventions also entail historically shifting expectations for how emotions will be produced and expressed in public debates. Local sex education conflicts are not unique in their volatility. Small-town democracy can be messy. Moreover, as a particularly antagonistic style of civic engagement, local culture wars do seem to be consistent with other recently publicized types of emotional volatility, such as air rage, road rage, sports rage (when the parents of young athletes attack or, in extreme cases, murder their children's coaches or other parents), rock rage, and even concert rage (described as "classical-music fanatics who can no longer abide the coughing, muttering, shuffling, and fidgeting of their neighbors," wherein, for example, New York's "Lincoln Center [theater] has become a war zone of withering glances and hissed asides").[29] Historian Peter Stearns in *American Cool: Constructing a Twentieth-Century Emotional Style* argues that emotional conventions have evolved from a late nineteenth-century valorization of emotional intensity into a contemporary ethos of emotional restraint.[30] However, it may be useful to explore whether we are undergoing a broader historical shift in U.S. emotional culture toward what one journalist called "a culture of rage."[31] A wider emotional culture of rage would not simply give residents permission for hostile expressions during local events; rather, it would constitute a diffuse set of conventions under which rage was anticipated and therefore produced. Such expectations for conspicuous display of feelings, including shouting and shoving matches and attempts to dominate meetings, are built in to local sex education debates.

Shaped by background conventions of affect, the quality and expression of emotions in culture wars are also influenced by local cues. The fluidity of emotions and their responsiveness to social expectation render them keenly sensitive to context. In this sense, feelings can be seemingly "contagious" in mass settings. However, the individual and collective emotions of local culture wars are best viewed as contingent rather than as authentic. Next I examine several factors that shape the emotions of sex education debates: provocative speech and speakers, the physical setting, material deterrents such as police presence, the repetition of sexual speech, and media coverage. Background and immediate dynamics work interactively in local debates.

We have already examined many instances in which the evocative vocabularies of Christian Right sex education discourses foster particular emotional expectations. Speech about sexuality is used in a way to scare parents with threats to their children and to mobilize these parents, through overt emotional displays, to oppose comprehensive sex education. Language and images are strategically intended to frighten, outrage, and disgust. It should not be surprising that scary rhetoric often does scare and hateful images do evoke hatred. For example, one community activist told me,

What the Religious Right did was, they started to call up all the churches and they distributed a document that included pornographic information, graphic information that they said was in the curriculum. Of course we knew it wasn't in there. But people were going to this meeting with misinformation, and very angry. I mean, I would have been very angry seeing graphic pornographic literature in what was supposed to be a curriculum. And so then that discussion started from that point. It's very hard to discuss something when people are hysterical and angry about something that they didn't have any information about from the beginning and then here is something they got. That was a fierce fight.[32]

In another case, a father was polled after casting his vote on the 1992 Christian Right–sponsored Ballot Measure 9, which would have amended the Oregon state constitution to forbid state agencies and schools to allow any program that would "promote, encourage, or facilitate" homosexuality.[33] It had been a particularly ugly campaign in which conservative activists had routinely described gay people as sexually depraved. He said, "I voted yes on 9, and why? Well, maybe because I look at my kids growing up in the schools, and about the time that somebody tells my kid, my boy that is, that it's okay to suck cock, I'm gonna kill the son of a bitch."[34] When residents are introduced to the issue of sex education through highly charged sexual language, they may go looking for a fight. It can be difficult for them to absorb competing information. And because this has an impact on the progress of sex education, collective emotions can be mechanisms for the exercise of power.

The physical setting shapes the nature and expression of emotions in sex education debates. In particular, public meetings can be occasions for unrestrained emotional displays. This is not mindless, irrational collectivity. Emotions, rather, are interactive and the conventions of different settings produce different affective responses. Large numbers of people can exacerbate a collective mentality in which what seems called for are demonstrations of fury rather than an exchange of viewpoints. One school board president in Brooklyn said, "In the early meetings people were yelling 'Faggots out!' and stuff like that. We stopped that and tried to create a tone that didn't let any of that happen. But every once in a while people just went off the rails, and publicly—a thousand people in the audience."[35] He continued, "The thing I did understand is that you needed a mass to do that. The same people who were passionately and wildly furious in large group settings were different in smaller group settings. So it needed contagion and it needed support and it needed emotional resonance from large groups, and that was the way in which maybe it was a mistake to do the big hearings because they didn't succeed in moving the debate to another level. Where it succeeded, I think, was in polarizing large factions across the district."[36] A school board member in another town concurred that people could react very differently in mass settings than in individual conversations. She said, "People that I trusted and had good relationships with would at least engage me in dialogue and they never came out and verbally abused me except at public meetings where everybody was yelling and you couldn't figure out what they were calling you."[37] Media and word-of-mouth reports prompt some towns that have not even had such conflicts to take preventive measures such as assembling a police presence. At one town meeting, written warnings circled the auditorium like Burma Shave signs: "ALLOW SPEAKERS TO FINISH THEIR PRESENTATIONS; THIS MEETING IS NOT A DEBATE!; RAISE YOUR HAND AND STAY IN YOUR SEAT." Yet the very presence of these material deterrents sets an emotional tone. Telling people what is prohibited instructs them in what is possible.

As part of the politicization of emotions, speakers at public meetings can use fiery rhetoric to inspire gestures of allegiance. Such rhetoric may appeal to feelings of anger, fear, love, or all of these. For example, after recounting numerous depravity narratives criticizing sex educators, national right-wing activist Judith Riesman yelled to a crowd at a Newton public meeting that all those in the audience who would be willing to die for their children should leap to their feet. Nearly the entire audience immediately arose. Most were clapping, some were hissing and grumbling. Riesman was working to establish a set of collective meanings about how loving parents act concerning sex education. She urged the audience to put these feelings of love and concern on tangible display to others, making it difficult for any parents to remain seated. Riesman did make an impact, as the spectacle of a crowd in action, leaping to its collective feet, acted as a further emotional accelerant.

Politicized emotional appeals such as this one are part of how local culture wars can both mobilize and polarize those who might previously have been uninformed or ambivalent. In Newton, for example, one Jewish, pro-choice mother seemed an unlikely recruit to the sex education opposition. But she had basic concerns about the new curriculum. She was afraid the teachers would be untrained or biased. Although she described herself as tolerant of homosexuality, she did not want it taught in the schools. She thought children should learn that the nuclear heterosexual family was the foundation of society. Abortion posed a more difficult problem for her, since, unlike many anti–sex education activists, she was pro-choice. Perhaps the issue could be taught as a debate, she mused. In short, she described herself as having a complicated range of opinions not driven by unyielding ideological or religious convictions. She went to the community forum after seeing a flyer at the local school; she recalled, "I went by myself. I didn't know any of the people. I just sort of showed up. I had no agenda with me whatsoever."[38] A concerned and somewhat confused parent, this woman was galvanized by Riesman: "She looked like my mother, just like my mother. And I see this woman up there, and let's face it, that woman was not ignorant. And she gets up and in the middle of this just flips out. I mean, the woman, I don't think she went crazy but she was slamming her fists down and—do you remember how she was? She was 'Stand up if you would die for your children!' Wow, this is heavy. You know, I just thought, do we want to teach this or don't we?"[39] This mother joined the opposition right after the forum. Demonstrating how quickly locals can assume leadership positions, she soon emerged as the group's spokesperson. Although it is not foolproof, the evocation of strong emotions such as sexual anxieties and protectiveness among parents can be a trigger for Christian Right mobilization.

The media also play an important role in establishing meanings and expectations for local sex education debates. In general, drama and emotions drive the social production of news.[40] "Joy, sorrow, shock, fear, these are the stuff of news," said a former network president.[41] The passions of culture wars, particularly because they are negative and sensational, enhance news value. Headlines and articles emphasize explosions of feelings, particularly rage and hatred, often framed in the language of battle ("A Fight Rages . . . ," "Battlelines Drawn . . . ," "Amid the Uproar . . ."). Not only do they sell newspapers, but they also coach citizens in the emotional possibilities of town meetings ("Parents: Emotion Is Running High," "Parents Clash . . . ," "Outcry Grows . . ."). They can even instruct when emotional expectations fail, as in one headline that noted, "Quiet Sex Ed Hearings Disappoint Those Looking for Fiery Condemnation."[42]

Activists on both sides of the sex education debates view the media as a powerful forum for capturing public support. They are also alert to media bias and suspicious of their opponents for allegedly manipulating media coverage. During the course of my interviewing, both sides complained that their opponents had staged explosive events to win public sympathy. After a conservative school board chair had abruptly adjourned a volatile meeting, for example, one of his critics charged, "He's very good at spinning the press. And so in the news media that night and in the papers the following day, it looked as if the meeting had been so out of control, with protesters, sixties style, in-your-face protesters of aging flower children, as he put it, that he and the two women needed a police escort to guarantee their safety out of the meeting. Their safety had never been in question."[43] Media coverage of politics, as sociologist Gamson notes, can prompt people to feel angry at someone, even if such anger is displaced.[44] Neither side of the sex education debates wants to be the target.

Activists, therefore, are exquisitely attuned to distortions. In one case, the *New York Times* spotlighted the antagonisms of two antipathetic members of the city's AIDS advisory council in an article headlined "AIDS Curriculum: Fighting Words" and subtitled "Shapers of Teachers' Guidelines Are Hostile and Exhausted."[45] Militaristic metaphors dominated the article, which described the meetings as "trench warfare" and "a theater of anger in a culture war over sex and the public schools," while it described the council members as "opposing field commanders" who are "emotionally exhausted, but nursing hostilities. And both are girding for new battles." It went on to describe how a debate over one section of the curriculum had become so polarized that it "devolved into a shouting match over where to place the asterisk." The two advisory council members were pictured with captions in which one woman said of the other, "Louise is a killer. She's a very vicious person." This woman claims to have really said that her colleague was a killer in terms of how hard she worked, but that the journalist decontextualized the quotation to enhance the bitterness of the disagreements.[46] Even without purposeful distortions, however, these types of articles spread the message that community meetings are polarized by irreconcilable hostilities.

Public repetition of evocative speech can also heighten the emotional pitch of sex education debates. The reproduction of sexual material by critics who wish to censor or regulate sexuality—the type of dynamic Michel Foucault likely had in mind when he referred to "the pleasure of the surveillance of pleasure"[47]—is common not only in sex education battles but also in other sex-related political contests.[48] For example, Citizens for Decent Literature purveyed a sexually explicit filmstrip in the fifties called *Target Smut*, and since the seventies, feminist groups such as Women Against Pornography have exhibited slide shows of what they consider the most offensive pornographic images. In the late eighties, witnesses at the hearings of the U.S. Attorney General's Commission on Pornography (the Meese commission) frequently projected unconventional images such as bestiality and sadomasochism.

Likewise, sex education critics pursued tactics of repeating the unmentionable. National leaders, as we saw in Chapter 3, often excerpted (or invented) passages from curricular materials they found offensive, reproduced them in flyers or mass mailings, and distributed them throughout the country. Sex education opponents read explicit sexual materials aloud at public venues. We saw in Chapter 2 how late sixties critics organized reading relays so as to circumvent time limits at school board meetings. In the nineties, one community school board chair told me she had to warn a sex education opponent four times that he could not read explicit sections of a book at school board meetings, so he called various media and read them over the phone. Finally, at a public meeting he read a section on sexual foreplay and oral sex.[49] The repetition of sexually charged language and screenings of taboo images in such an anomalous public setting—for example, a school board meeting—might no doubt produce shock. It might also, as Carole Vance suggested about the Meese commission hearings, create an atmosphere of "excited repression," further complicating the collective mood.[50] In any case, this strategy was one by which conservative sex education opponents, while ostensibly trying to silence talk about sex, also contributed to the diffusion of detailed sexual speech.

The emotional texture of any particular local sex education conflict emerges from a complex mix of long-term dynamics and immediate triggers. One example of this involves structural inequalities in communities. In such cases, evocative rhetoric exacerbates already existing local fragmentation and breakdowns in civic debate. Sociologist Robert Putnam notes that "neighborliness," the proportion of Americans who socialize with their neighbors more than once a year, has shown a steady decline over the past twenty years, while the proportion of citizens reporting that most people can be trusted (37 percent in 1993 compared with 58 percent in 1960) has fallen by more than a third.[51] Moreover, inequalities in income and education lead to disparities in civic participation, fueling frustration among those who have less of a voice in American politics.[52] Together, the fraying of community engagement and trust, persistent social and economic inequalities, and inflammatory rhetoric in local sex education conflicts may allow for the expression of grievances not simply about sexuality but about other factors as well. Conflicts involving race and sexuality can manifest this tendency.

Racial dynamics in sex education debates have shifted since the sixties.

Then, for an emerging Christian Right infused with the racial politics of the Old Right, sex education provided an opportunity to exploit whites' sexual fears of blacks. Even by the late sixties, however, the widespread acceptability of such explicit appeals was waning. Sociologist Amy Ansell argues that the "new racism" of the Right,[53] now waged in four arenas of the culture wars—immigration, affirmative action, welfare, and traditional values—allows the movement to fight seemingly race-neutral battles while at the same time attempting to dismantle programs in the name of racial justice. By appropriating a language of equal opportunity and individual rights, these battles embody a less explicit racism than that of the Old Right. Sex education offers a unique platform for the staging of contemporary Christian Right racial politics. Because the movement is predominantly white and middle class, it typically targets schools in its own communities for sex education battles, while ignoring communities of color in curricula and outreach.[54] The movement's involvement in a New York City battle in the early nineties, however, marked its first major incursion into an important multiracial, multiethnic urban center.[55] The conflicts over the teacher's guide *Children of the Rainbow* dominated city politics and captured international attention. They serve as an important example of how the Christian Right uses sexuality and race to politicize emotions for its own purposes in local debates.

The *Rainbow* guide was a multicultural project intended to promote tolerance and facilitate appreciation for the diversity of families. It contained lessons for first-graders on the artifacts, folk songs, and holidays of many different cultures. The conflict centered on brief sections that discussed lesbian and gay families. One particularly controversial entry noted that "teachers should be aware of varied family structures, including two-parent or single-parent households, gay or lesbian parents, divorced parents, adoptive parents, and guardians or foster parents. Children must be taught to acknowledge the positive aspects of each type of household and the importance of love and care in family living."[56] The teacher's guide emphasized the recognition of lesbian and gay families within the context of cultural diversity. Nowhere was there any mention of sex.

Emotional responses to a particular political issue can be exacerbated by individuals' feelings about long-standing injustices in their lives. There is, as Gamson notes, a "coupling of the cognition of unfairness in the larger society with the emotion of indignation."[57] The volatile conflicts over

*Children of the Rainbow* exposed deep anger and resentment among city residents over long-standing inequalities in the public schools. Two groups in particular—communities of color and the gay community—responded on the basis of systematic structural exclusion. Lack of resources and poor school systems fueled resentment among communities of color about racial inequities in public education. Blacks and Latinos in the New York City school system are consistently slotted into lower tracks, have higher drop-out rates, and receive fewer services. Funding disparities are stunning. In the early nineties, for example, during the time period of the *Rainbow* controversies, the city's poorest districts received $.90 per pupil from legislative allocations, compared with $14 per pupil in wealthy districts.[58] One critic indicted public education as a "dual society,"[59] while another grimly warned that even keeping in mind "these doleful statistics," New York schools are "really worse than they seem."[60] Anti-gay discrimination in the public schools took the form of either forced invisibility or scapegoating. Gay educators saw *Children of the Rainbow* as an opportunity to be recognized in a multicultural program designed to teach tolerance and respect. As Andy Humm of the Hetrick-Martin Institute later said about the conflicts, "If [the guide] is going to be written, it's got to be inclusive. What are we supposed to say, 'No, go ahead, write it without us, we'll catch up later.'"[61] As the debates unfolded, the rhetoric of organized opponents polarized these two groups by mobilizing sexual and racial fears and resentments. Ways of talking about the *Rainbow* guide pitted (allegedly white) lesbians and gay men against (allegedly heterosexual) communities of color, separating the intersectional social categories of race and sexuality for political purposes.

On one level, the political opposition to the *Rainbow* guide assumed the dynamics common in other sex education battles. Both national and local conservative religious groups were deeply involved. Attorneys coordinating the legal opposition to the teacher's guide had long-standing associations with the archdiocese of New York. Observers reported the influence of the national Christian Coalition. Given the nature of stealth politics, it is unclear to what extent national activists were actually present. As in other community debates, however, the rhetoric of national Christian Right organizations inflected local politics, in this case through New York City's own groups such as the Family Defense Council and the newly developed Concerned Parents for Educational Accountability (CPEA).

On another level, the anti-*Rainbow* organizing demonstrated how, by the nineties, the Christian Right used opposition to homosexuality as a strategy for multiracial coalition building. Opponents of the *Rainbow* tapped a receptive cohort of what political historian Angela Dillard calls "multicultural conservatives"—African Americans and Latinos whose conservative religious traditions align closely with the Christian Right on issues such as homosexuality and abortion.[62] As one African American opponent of the *Rainbow* curriculum told me, "A lot of us from the Christian community don't want to see the ethics and the morals and the values that have sustained us as a people in the face of the worst kind of adversity abandoned in favor of some lifestyle that's guaranteed to take our kids right down the drain, destroy them. So we were militantly opposed to any kind of curriculum guide that was going to give our children a mind-set that was death-oriented."[63] As Dillard notes, national organizations such as the Christian Coalition use a language of seemingly shared values of moral and religious opposition to homosexuality as a way to mobilize within African American and Latino churches. This language, as we shall see in the next chapter, was one of aversion toward gay people.

As has been the case since the sex education battles of the sixties, local groups appropriated familiar rhetorical strategies of national Christian Right organizations. For example, CPEA produced a video called *Why Parents Should Object to the Children of the Rainbow* that reproduced, often word for word, the distortions and evocative language popularized by national groups. The video stressed that condoms have five-micron holes. It repeated verbatim familiar anti-gay accusations, such as that gay people are recruiting children, and associated homosexuality with pedophilia. The narrator read an out-of-context passage from a parody that was once printed in Boston's *Gay Community News*, with such lines as "we shall sodomize your sons" and "our only gods are handsome young men." She claimed that this sentiment represents the national agenda of "militant homosexuals."[64] CPEA claimed to have more than forty-eight thousand members, and although this figure more likely represents the length of its mailing list, the video was widely distributed and shown at meetings throughout the city. As the controversy escalated, the teacher's guide was called "homosexual/lesbian propaganda" that was "teaching sodomy to first graders." One assemblyman called gay people "a sin against mankind," while a state senator described them as "pure evil and wickedness."[65]

Oppositional rhetoric in the *Rainbow* controversy was designed to exploit historical tensions among groups and fan feelings of injustice and competition for resources. It stoked the fear among blacks that the recognition of gay people would somehow diminish blacks' social position or erode whatever legitimacy they have managed to garner from years of civil rights efforts. Playing to this fear, the white school board president Mary Cummins said, "I will not demean our legitimate minorities, such as Blacks, Hispanics and Asians, by lumping them together with homosexuals in that curriculum."[66] Her lawyer ridiculed the notion that gay people might rightfully be represented in a multicultural curriculum by claiming, "There are all sorts of groups and lifestyles in the world, but it's highly misleading and I think unhealthy to treat them as cultures in the same sense as Hispanic culture or Afro American culture or Italian American culture. . . . If diversity is to be worshipped without limit, then presumably we should have Ku Klux Klan clubs in high schools, or we should have cocaine clubs in high schools."[67] Such tactics, not surprisingly, touched many nerves. At one community school board meeting, an African American teacher said, "Where was the gay community when many of us were beaten at a lunch counter? Is this the only way we can be included in the curriculum—to allow the gay community to piggyback off our achievement?"[68] One African American mother claimed that gay people had been included in the multicultural curriculum so that black children "won't have enough time to learn to read, write, and count."[69]

Anger and distortion are often the currency of sex education debates. Eventually, open conflict erupted at meetings over the *Rainbow* guide, as when black parents yelled "white faggots" at ACT UP members and ACT UP men yelled back, "Black racists."[70] One school board member described having to be escorted out of the auditorium by police in the aftermath of voting on the curriculum: "I could see all this hate, all this unbridled, naked hate. That's all I could see. I was so scared."[71] Some groups, especially among lesbians and gay men of color and progressive whites, worked hard to bridge the divide and address the complex matrix of inequalities underlying the anger.[72] But fear, hatred, and intolerance are not unexpected community responses to rhetoric specifically designed to elicit it. Tensions were so heightened over the *Children of the Rainbow* controversy that scared parents saw homosexuality everywhere. Almost no accusation was too bizarre. One administrator said, "I was at a public meeting when someone objected because they indicated we were somehow or other subconsciously influencing kids to homosexuality by the fact that we had an example [in the curriculum] about gerbils. Some persons have gotten up and said that by saying that we are subconsciously advocating and promoting homosexuality."[73] Others claimed that the purple cover of the curriculum proved it was a gay plot, and they insisted that secret gay images were encoded throughout the text.[74] This conspiracist reading of supposedly hidden gay symbols flourishes in a context in which rhetorical strategies encouraged high anxiety among parents.

By the end of the conflicts in New York, although a Louis Harris poll showed that more than 70 percent of parents had supported the *Rainbow* guide,[75] the multicultural text was shelved in nearly all the city's thirty-two school districts. New York City public schools chancellor Joseph Fernandez had received two death threats and was eventually fired. As the *New York Times* concluded, "Invective has drowned out reasonable debate. Once opponents had transformed Mr. Fernandez into a Hitler and the curriculum's lessons about families into the ABC's of sodomy, it no longer really mattered what the curriculum actually said."[76] In this case, the resultant "firestorm of hostility"[77] was a production of collective emotion that worked to further the interests of conservative and right-wing religious groups through the elimination of the curriculum. Still, there is rarely a tidy, singular outcome to these local conflicts, and one openly gay teacher I interviewed suggested that the impact was more complicated:

> If they had just let that book go through without the big uproar that they created—I'm talking about the Right, okay?—there would have been a minuscule amount of [school] training around lesbian and gay issues compared to the explosive exposure of lesbian and gay issues in the press. . . . So the uproar was invented . . . and in fact, they did more for educating children about lesbian and gay issues than any curriculum that they could have let slide through. They had this giant uproar and it was on the news for months, and kids talked about it all the time. Even in elementary school they talked about it.[78]

As we shall see in the next section, the intense emotions of local sex education battles frequently prompt unanticipated outcomes.

The political mobilization of collective emotions is a crucial dynamic in local sex education debates. In this section, I have suggested that feelings are produced and shaped in response to both particular background conventions and to immediate contextual dynamics which serve as triggers or cues for emotional expectations. As several school board members noted, for example, individuals often reacted quite differently in large groups than when they were alone or in smaller, more intimate settings. Such shifts underscore the interactive and performative dimensions of emotions. Rather than being instinctual reactions, the expressions of anger and intolerance are often nurtured in sex education debates. As the teacher quoted earlier put it, the uproar was invented. Still, the instability that allows for the politicization of emotions also renders them fickle elements in local contests. As I have previously suggested, when sex education opponents succeed in recreating expressions of negative sexual affect in public debates, they reinforce these conventions. They take a risk, however, in seeking to evoke such emotions and their display.

## UNRULY FEELINGS

Social movements cannot count on inflammatory rhetoric and the production of collective emotions as stable resources. Discourse is unpredictable and may trigger unexpected counterreactions, taking "a wolfish turn on the activists who rely upon it," as sociologist Marc Steinberg points out.[79] Ultimately, emotions are no more under the control of activists than is speech. The "adrenaline of emotion" is unruly, [80] especially in a moment of social transformation. When the emotional demands of short-term events like local culture wars call for audiences to produce strong negative emotions, people may comply. But the target of those emotions is outside of a movement's control. Sociologist Joshua Gamson found such instability of emotion in his analysis of sexual nonconformity and tabloid talk shows. When episodes featured virulently anti-gay, right-wing experts, the audiences turned their wrath on them and not the lesbian, gay, or bisexual guests. Such experts served as "hateful embodiments of intolerance."[81] However, in the experts' absence, the audiences directed hatred and anger toward sexual minorities themselves in explosive attacks. This dynamic is not unlike that in community sex education debates. It shows how an audience's, and by extension a community's, response is not a fixed expression of the aggregate of individual beliefs but rather is a more fluid, collectively managed construction. Furthermore, this dynamic suggests that hatred and intolerance are not stable, immutable mental states residing within individual bodies. Instead, hatred and fear might well be viewed as interactional processes and community events which can be either mobilized or assuaged under specific strategic conditions.

Still, the outcome of attempts to politicize emotions is beyond the control of activists. Organizers who endeavor to evoke and harness collective feelings for political ends risk that audiences will exceed the organizers' expectations. Conservative activists want a moderate display of anger that will seem to ratify their oppostion to sex education. Instead they may incite a hostile insurrection. Conversely, harsh rhetoric and punitive policies can prompt a collective refusal altogether of emotional demands. In both cases, conservatives become vulnerable to charges of extremism and bigotry, which can cost them public support.

The combination of evocative sexual rhetoric, expectations for explosive feelings, and prior sensational media coverage can help foster events that spiral out of the organizers' control. For example, one local activist reflected on an especially volatile meeting her group had organized to fight the *Children of the Rainbow* guide. A lawyer and mother, she told me that most of those who worked the hardest against the guide were religiously motivated, noting, "What drives me fundamentally is my Christianity. It's the fact that I have certain values that I'm not willing to sacrifice and are worth fighting for."[82] This activist emphasized that her group deliberately adopted a more rational approach to opposing the teacher's guide: "We listed a whole bunch of point by point reasons why this was an intolerable form of education and tried to present it in a way that wasn't inflammatory, which did not make it an emotional appeal to anybody's baser instincts." She did, however, note the powerful emotional reactions among parents with whom the group spoke, reflecting that "they were really frothing at the mouth." In response, the organizers tried "to guide the force" by telling parents to attend meetings and write letters. Still, on the night when the school board was to vote on the guide, a "mob mentality" took over, the activist recalled.

It was an ugly scene. The gay people who had shown up to speak in favor of the curriculum were routinely shouted down by an unruly group of angry conservative parents as well as other groups ("the tattoo crowd showed up"). The activist complained, "These people just came in to yell and scream and carry on and could care less about the issue, but they know that there are gays in the room and they're just going to yell bad stuff. And so it makes it look like, hey, these are our supporters, when they weren't. They just came for a good fight." Meanwhile, church groups kept breaking into song in expressions of dominance over their opponents: "It was like kicking them when they were down. We were winning; the tide of public opinion was with us and this was like grinding them into the ground and there was no need to do that. And so in a way it was painful because it was like we had created something but it had gone beyond our control and we couldn't rein it back in. And there was a lot of residual resentment as a result of it."[83] The local conservative group felt unfairly blamed in subsequent media coverage. This activist recounted how she told a reporter, "I am not responsible for the people that showed up at that meeting. That is not who I recruited, so to lay this at our doorstep and say that we fanned the flames of hatred and riot and bigotry is irresponsible." She was particularly distressed since she believed her group had taken care to present their positions in a noninflammatory way. Community sex education debates are local affairs but they are also inflected by the emotional rhetoric of national culture wars. The anger, hatred, and bullying that have come to be associated with national sex education debates may well surface at local events, despite the stated intentions of the local organizers. Like this activist, the organizers may come to feel that their efforts backfired.

The Merrimack, New Hampshire, case shows how miscalculations by conservative activists counting on collective outrage ultimately cost them the battle. Communities nationwide felt the aftershocks of the intense animosities of New York's *Children of the Rainbow* conflicts. As a metaphor for the menace of sexual deviance, the issue of school discussion of homosexuality seemed to carry enormous cultural power for conservative Christian activists. In Merrimack, however, there had been little discussion about homosexuality in the schools. As one liberal teacher noted, it would be "a cold day in hell" before Merrimack implemented any of the progressive school programs on lesbian and gay issues that were proliferating to the south in Massachusetts.[84] A school board member said, "I had been attending board meetings for five years straight and I attended every meeting except one where I was on vacation. So I could say with some certainty that I know everything that came before that board in the past five years. Not one parent had ever brought out a complaint to the school board about anything to do with homosexuality. It never became an issue to the town. Homosexuality isn't even mentioned in the health curriculum."[85] But the conservative school board chair attempted to capitalize on the hostile climate triggered by the *Children of the Rainbow* conflicts in New York. As one school board member said, he "wanted to make it sound as if [the *Rainbow* curriculum] was on our doorstep unless he took some preventive action."[86] And so Merrimack passed Policy 6540—"Prohibition of Alternate Lifestyle Instruction"—the most restrictive public school anti-gay speech initiative in the nation.

Policy 6540 was sweeping in scope. It banned any instructional or counseling activity that had "the effect of encouraging or supporting homosexuality as a positive lifestyle alternative."[87] The policy exercised a chilling effect in the classroom, causing teachers to fear any mention of homosexuality at all. As one teacher put it, "If you walked out of my classroom and said, 'Well, [that teacher] thinks homosexuality is cool; I guess it's okay,' regardless of what the intent of my lecture was . . . if my words had that effect, I was in violation of the policy. So the policy really became a gag order."[88] Teachers claimed that they eliminated books and videos, such as one on Walt Whitman, from the classroom, dropped certain canonical works, such as Shakespeare's *Twelfth Night*, and deleted AIDS prevention material from the curriculum. A local paper reported that a math teacher "said he has even stopped the practice of asking kids to bring in newspaper or magazine clippings for data analysis, for fear the articles would be about homosexuality."[89] Counselors complained that they would be unable to talk to a student with concerns about homosexuality. According to the lawyer for Merrimack residents who filed suit against Policy 6540, it had "triggered a tidal wave of self-censorship."[90] The school board chair, however, described the policy as an initiative "to keep our Merrimack schools free from promoting homosexuality."[91]

The silences imposed by Policy 6540 were so loud they reverberated internationally. *CBS News*, the *London Times*, and *Time* magazine, among others, reported the news, as did many newspapers across the United States. Teachers discussed how they could not talk about what they were prohibited from speaking about. One said, "So of course the kids come to school the first day and what are we supposed to say? All they want to do is talk about it and we have to say, 'No, I'm sorry. We can't do that. We can't talk about any of that here.' And so that's what happened."[92] On the first day of classes, one teacher told the students in her advanced English class that "they would not be able to explore some of the literature as fully as they otherwise would have, because of the district's new policy banning discussion of homosexuality in a positive light."[93] Suddenly the town was riveted by a discussion of homosexuality. One newspaper proclaimed, "Homosexuality remained foremost on the minds of residents on Tuesday's raucous School Board meeting, the first since the board approved a landmark policy last month banning any mention of homosexuality in a positive light."[94] A group of students vowed to wear black armbands and pink buttons until the policy was repealed.[95] Silence itself became a spectacle.

By the ways in which emotions can simultaneously paralyze debate and trigger more talk about sex, they figure prominently in the paradox wherein conservatives prompt more talk about sex while attempting to curtail it. In Merrimack, visibility and support for gay issues further increased on the night of the school board vote. Protesters held the first gay rights rally in Merrimack's history in the school's parking lot. About 150 participants stood in peaceful protest outside the school, where speakers addressed them from the back of a pickup truck adorned with American flags.[96] A local newspaper covering the rally concluded that "the angry debate over a policy that seeks to limit discussion of homosexuality will have the opposite effect, making students more interested than ever before in talking about it in school."[97] And so Policy 6540 changed Merrimack. But not in the direction desired by the policy's supporters. Their bid for silence about homosexuality turned Merrimack into a town where, for some time, little else was discussed. It prompted pockets of resistance to the implicit expectation for intolerance. One teacher said the school board's conservative Christian majority "took out the smoking gun, which is homosexuality, and it backfired on them because it enraged the town."[98] One school board member reflected, "There was a larger body in the community that would ultimately reject all this, and they did. But the pain and the damage that was caused in the meantime was something no community should ever have to experience."[99] In the end, the anger that conservatives mobilized was directed back toward themselves. In Merrimack, conservative Christians lost their majority on the school board at the election held after they implemented Policy 6540, and the new school board eliminated the policy.

Emotions are unstable, and strategies which appeal to them can backfire on a social movement. Still, emotions were a powerful element in sex education debates throughout the nineties and into the new century. Intense feelings seemed like viruses, as ugly battles spread from community to community. Exhausted residents told me of how property values in their communities dropped as a result of highly publicized conflicts, and how they wanted more than anything else to be out of the news. Controversy itself became a factor in decisions about sex education programs, often exerting a conservatizing effect. One obvious way to avoid conflict was to scale back programs and limit what could be said in the classroom. This in fact happened, as a nationwide chilling effect resulted in the erosion of comprehensive sexuality education. Meanwhile, towns which were fighting about school discussion of sexuality often fought about programs that mentioned gay issues. In the next chapter we shall see how these contests demonstrated the conservative strategy of appealing to aversive feelings.

## Chapter 8 | THE POLITICS OF AVERSION

On April 30, 1997, before a record audience of forty-two million, Ellen came out. The character Ellen Morgan, played by Ellen Degeneres on her eponymous television show, publicly disclosed her lesbianism. Thus *Ellen* became the first show in television history with an openly gay lead character. The show pushed the envelope in many ways, including its depiction of a more expansive definition of "family." For example, after coming out, Ellen visits her disapproving father who is tinkering in the basement with an elaborate model train village he calls "Morganville." Gesturing toward the model family he is building of plastic homes and toy figures, he says, "I guess we don't need them anymore." Ellen retorts that just because she is gay, it does not mean she cannot have a family. Then, without missing a beat, she picks up the male toy and agrees, "I mean, I don't need *him*. We can put him with Edna over here." In one radical moment, Ellen and the medium of television recuperated the importance of family even while destabilizing its traditional heteronormativity. This move by the major network ABC, owned by Disney, was not without controversy. The Southern Baptist Convention passed a resolution to boycott Disney for what they termed its "anti-Christian and anti-family direction."[1] Christian Coalition founder Pat Robertson persistently called *Ellen* star Degeneres "Ellen Degenerate." From talk shows to tabloids, media coverage of Ellen's coming out made visible broad national debates about sexual identities and contemporary meanings of family.

If the visibility of the Sex Information and Education Council of the United States (SIECUS) in the sixties galvanized right-wing opposition to sex education, the prominence of the contemporary lesbian and gay rights movement catalyzed the pro-family movement to fight any mention of homosexuality in the classroom. Through the last half of the twentieth century, the gay movement had become an important presence in American cultural and political life. By the late eighties, prompted by concern that the educational system was, as one teacher described New York's public schools, "a breeding ground for intolerance,"[2] public education had taken its place alongside AIDS activism and various military and domestic partnership initiatives as a key site for lesbian and gay social reform. Many education reformers, gay and straight, urged the integration of lesbian and gay content into anti-violence education, diversity programs, or curricula on the family. Founded in 1995, the Gay, Lesbian, and Straight Teachers Network (now known as the Gay, Lesbian, and Straight Education Network, or GLSEN) symbolized the increasing importance of youth and public education to the gay movement. SIECUS and Planned Parenthood supported discussion of gay issues in comprehensive sexuality education. Public schools developed support groups, such as the increasingly common gay-straight alliances. All of these initiatives met with controversy. Discussion about homosexuality in the public schools was fiercely debated and resisted. SIECUS noted that during the 1996–97 school year, almost 20 percent of community sex education conflicts concerned policies over sexual orientation.[3] As a result, although thousands of young people could watch Ellen come out on national television, many of them could not talk about it with their teachers the next day in the classroom.

Cultural theorist Lauren Berlant has described the national climate of the nineties as "a state of sexual emergency."[4] Emotions ran high in debates such as those over abortion, contraceptive accessibility, sexuality in the media, AIDS policies and pedagogies, and the visibility of lesbians and gay men to young people in public schools. The tensions about Ellen's coming out on a major television network signaled national ambivalence toward myriad challenges in the dominant sexual culture. Capturing public sentiment and politicizing emotion was crucial in such a moment of instability. As anthropologist Mary Douglas has noted, fears of the "harmful consequences of a pollution" can fortify unstable moral codes by galvanizing public opinion "on the side of the right."[5] Toward this end, conservatives highlighted homosexuality and, by extension, talk about homosexuality in the classroom as symbols of dangerous contagion. In moral contests over gay school reform, they developed national rhetorics intended to mobilize support for their movement through evoking fear, anger, and disgust toward gay people. Through the process of trying to persuade the public that there should be silence in the schools about gay issues, conservatives themselves became the most vocal discussants of gay sexuality.

## NATIONAL EMOTIONS AND GAY RIGHTS

Like the controversy around Ellen's coming-out show, battles over lesbian and gay school reform are the crises of a unique historical moment. Public school programs that include discussion about a range of sexual practices and identities are of a piece with broader trends such as the increasingly open popular culture, the growing public acceptance of alternative sexualities, and the erosion of the idealized nuclear family. Sex education has a long history as, in part, a project to prepare young people for citizenship in a democratic society. This was perhaps most noticeable in fifties versions of the Family Life Education program, which sought to ready students for marriage and parenting.[6] Talk about homosexuality alongside discussions of traditional marriage and parenting is destabilizing precisely to the degree that it suggests to children that legitimate sexual citizenship is possible outside of the heterosexual norm. Programs that discuss lesbian and gay identities are pedagogies of sexual alternatives, and the conflicts over them are far more than local school wars; rather, they constitute a version of citizenship politics.[7] They are battles not simply about homosexuality, but over which sexualities and which citizens are valued as legitimate. The Christian Right, which opposes the discussion of lesbian and gay issues in public schools as the quintessential manifestation of a secular humanist educational system, was consistently on the frontlines of the efforts to dismantle such programs.

Opposition to gay rights is a cornerstone of the Christian Right's political strategy. In one study from the early nineties, conservative evangelical activists ranked gay rights first on their list of opponents, placing it even above Planned Parenthood.[8] Opposition to gay rights is a priority for more than thirty-five major groups. It is a highly condensed symbol at a time of transition in the sexual culture. Preservation of sexual morality, traditional gender relations, and the nuclear family are at the center of contemporary Christian Right religious beliefs and cultural politics. Furthermore, the matrix of concerns over sexuality, gender, and the family occupy not just the Christian Right but many mainstream Americans. Thus, anti-gay initiatives, like opposition to comprehensive sex education, are a vehicle by which the Christian Right attempts to draw in new supporters. It can best do so in a broader climate of moral disapproval.

Yet ambivalence and change best describe trends through the nineties in how individual Americans described to researchers their attitudes and feelings about homosexuality. Public opinion research showed that although Americans increasingly favored equal rights for gay people, widespread moral antipathy against homosexuals persisted.[9] For example, in his highly publicized study on middle-class Americans, sociologist Alan Wolfe declared homosexuality to be the ultimate test of tolerance in a country divided into "two genuinely different moral camps" over the issue.[10] Political scientists Clyde Wilcox and Robin Wolpert reported that although Americans' emotional reactions toward lesbians and gays were changing, they still voiced significantly negative affect. Thirty-six percent of respondents to the 1993 National Election Study Pilot Survey reported feeling "strong disgust" toward lesbians and gays.[11] Still, social surveys showed that from the late eighties until 1996, the number of Americans reporting moral censure of homosexuality dropped from a high of 75 percent to 56 percent.[12] In addition to this rapid decline in disapproval, support rose for equal treatment under the law. For example, public support for lesbian and gay teachers, one of the most contested employment areas, rose significantly by the nineties.[13] Even many religious Americans did not hold absolutist values about gay issues. The National Health and Social Life Survey found significant differences among cohorts in their willingness to describe "same-gender sex" as "always wrong": 96.4 percent of a cohort of "traditional/conservatives," compared with only 6.4 percent of "contemporary religious" who belonged to more liberal denominations.[14] This meant that while a substantial number of religious Americans would always oppose gay sexuality, another large cohort was more tolerant. Communities involved in debates over public education were at the center of this unstable climate.

Emotions would play a significant role in the moral politics of lesbian and gay education reform in the public schools. Because contemporary Western societies consider feelings as core to the self, emotions are seemingly a site of truth and ethics. Hence feelings, as Michel Foucault has argued, are "the main field of morality."[15] They were therefore key to the political conflict over gay school reform. Wilcox and Wolpert claim that affect about lesbians and gays is the likely source of a person's position on a range of anti-discrimination policies.[16] Whether such a linear causal relationship exists, ideology and emotional conventions are bound up in powerful ways concerning homosexuality. As well as being a battle for justice and equality, the struggle for gay rights is also a political contest over the national emotional culture. Conservative organizations sought to keep alive conventions of intolerance so that their language and images would trigger strong feelings of fear, anger, and disgust in local battles. Even episodic outbreaks of such passionate feelings in local debates could stall gay education reform.

## CONVERSION ANXIETY

The gay movement had come late to youth issues. This could have been predicted, since sexual stigmatization has historically shaped the direction of gay politics. As one education activist acknowledged, "Youth has traditionally been seen as the third rail of gay and lesbian politics because it brings up the whole pedophilia issue."[17] Stereotypes about homosexuals as child molesters would make school reform seem unthinkably dangerous. Public schools not uncommonly fired teachers who were even suspected of being gay. A gay teacher who later became an activist told me that he would meet informally with other gay teachers in his high school

to commiserate about the difficulties we had as gay educators and how crippled we were in being able to advocate for gay youth, and yet none of us felt empowered at that point to do that. There were two teachers who in the late seventies were out about their homosexuality and were embroiled in a lot of controversies and really hit the brunt of the worst kind of homophobia possible. I watched the difficulties that they went through and it really frightened me. If anything, I held on to my being closeted even more. They were falsely accused of just really terrible things.[18]

Anxieties about children and sexuality flourished in public schools. The first educators who came out and advocated for gay reform not only broke a silence; they also violated a taboo. In turn, they were exceedingly careful.

Gay education reform programs so assiduously excluded sex that, aside from advocating respect for a stigmatized constituency, they might easily have been written by the most chaste Adolescent Family Life Act (AFLA) grantee. Reform initiatives generally fell into two categories, which I have elsewhere described as the public health model and the culture-based model.[19] The public health model was structured around health promotion and risk prevention. For example, Project 10, the first major school-based program to address gay concerns, was prompted by the harassment of an openly gay male student who eventually dropped out of school. Project 10, along with many of its progeny, emphasizes protecting gay youth from school victimization as well as from the ancillary effects of self-hatred such as substance abuse. The image of the suicidal gay youth haunted the public health model, inspiring prevention initiatives such as teacher trainings, student support groups, and policy reforms. The *Children of the Rainbow* teacher's guide was an example of the culture-based model, wherein gay issues were braided into multicultural programs. The culture-based model considers lesbians and gay men to be a minority, like racial and ethnic groups. It teaches tolerance and respect for diversity. Although they have different emphases, both models stressed ending bias, challenging hatred and hate crimes, promoting safety, and enhancing the health of young people. They talked about human rights, suicide prevention, anti-violence, and multiculturalism. Neither model talked about sex.[20] Even basic discussion of sexual orientation was, as SIECUS reported in the late nineties, "rare."[21]

It is, of course, not so easy to desexualize the topic of homosexuality. And while some of these programs avoided outright warfare, none sidestepped opposition. Gay reformers disavowed any mention of sexuality so their programs would not be reduced to sex in the public's eyes. But conservative opponents consistently reinserted sex. They characterized gay reform initiatives as "sex clubs" or "sodomy curricula." They described any mention of homosexuality—for example, in the context of anti-suicide programs—as "deviant sex practices," "sodomy," "anal sex," "sodomythology," and "homosexology." One conservative activist responded as though discussion of gay families was discussion about deviant sex: "Kids shouldn't be subjected to sexual subject matter before they're mature enough to handle it."[22] An education reform activist described to me how opponents would say to him, "You're talking about homosexuality. You're talking about what you do in bed."[23] In their insistence on reframing homosexuality as exclusively about sex, conservatives were more active than sex educators themselves in keeping explicit discussions of sex prominent in the culture.

One way in which opponents of gay school reform mobilized to keep the sex in homosexuality, at least in their own rhetoric, was to play to the public's uncertainty about sexuality itself. Gay education initiatives implicitly raise questions about sexual desires and identities, about how people come to be straight or gay. Those who opposed classroom discussion of homosexuality contended that childhood sexuality is infinitely malleable, homosexuality is contagious, and the innocent child—who could and should be heterosexual—was imperiled by lesbians and gay men preying in the public schools. One school board president described how anti-gay rhetoric fostered community anxiety that there was "something sexual and deviant penetrating the school."[24] Pollution anxieties can best be mobilized, however, when the potential offender is actually thought to be contagious. From this point of view, contact with gay people or talking about homosexuality in the classroom could make kids gay. For example, Christian Right leaders Beverly and Tim LaHaye warned that "every homosexual is potentially an evangelist of homosexuality, capable of perverting many young people to his sinful way of life."[25] Language, however, "tastes of the context in which it has lived its socially charged life."[26] The LaHayes's use of the term "evangelist" is one with deep resonance within their own evangelistic cosmology. It is a biblical mandate that Christians should go forth and seek the conversion of nonbelievers, winning them for Christ. One evangelist estimates that 75–90 percent of Christian converts are the direct result of witnessing by friends, relatives, or close associates.[27] The conversion experience—a sudden, intensely emotional transformation in beliefs and personality known to Christians as being "born again" and to psychologists as "snapping"[28]—is a familiar one to evangelicals. For them, therefore, it is a powerfully evocative model for childhood sexual development. Conversion anxiety was their fear that if exposed to education about a range of sexual possibilities, their children would snap on a sexual level.

In a broader sense, conversion anxiety is powerful because it taps one pole of contradictory popular understandings of sexuality. Recent years have witnessed the resurgence of a strong biological determinism in the form of genetic or neurological theories of sexuality,[29] and yet this view coexists with both a "folk constructionism"[30] in which sexuality is a willful choice, and a "universalizing"[31] perspective in which sexual identities are viewed as highly mutable. Rhetoric at the far end of this continuum of malleability and choice plays on terrors of the vulnerability of innocent children to the contagion of perversion. One school board president in New York said, "We hit over and over again the sense that children were that old cliché, blank vessels or blank tablets onto which you could imprint anything, and therefore what we were advocating was an imprinting of something that would direct them inevitably into deviance. . . . There was this notion that sexuality is responsive to secrets and that if somehow you let this out then, whoops, there go your kids. And I would think, What is your notion of sexual development?"[32] It is not that these parents lacked "correct" knowledge of sexuality, however; it is that there are multiple perspectives about sexuality. National conservative organizations circulated those which were conducive to the production of fear.

Fears about sexual instabilities were also bound up with anxieties about gender in school reform. Opponents voiced fears that programs which challenge gender stereotypes also potentially disrupt normative heterosexuality. For example, New York's *Children of the Rainbow* teacher's guide said, "Men and women need not hold restricted work or family roles."[33] This prompted criticism by conservative Christians. As one anti–sex education activist said, "There are people in our society who refuse to acknowledge that there are differences between the sexes . . . and the average parent who takes a more biblical view, perhaps a more faith-inspired view, knows that there are differences and the reasons for those differences."[34] One evangelical minister complained: "One of the teachings was to take the girls in the classroom and give them trucks and take the boys and give them dolls. They switch the patterns so that boys will learn how to tolerate girls and girls will learn how to tolerate boys. That's nonsense. That was educating girls to being lesbians and boys at being homosexual."[35] In this view, homosexuality is both the cause and the effect of gender differences, and programs that encourage children in a wider range of gender-acceptable behaviors are a dangerous experiment in social engineering. One anti-*Rainbow* curriculum activist said

> Part of the whole agenda of sexual liberation is to get kids out from under this bondage of thinking that there isn't this interchangeability between the sexes. I believe it's part of the whole movement behind the gay and lesbian and bisexual agenda, that they do not want people to think of their sexuality as being inherently male or inherently female. On one level it seems harmless, but if you know what it leads to, what it's a stepping-stone to, you sound the alarm early on and you say, No, we're not going to let you break down this notion because this will lead you to this, this, and this.[36]

In this activist's way of thinking, challenges to traditional gender relations are a vehicle by which to convert children to homosexuality.

Mobilizations of conversion anxiety had been common in earlier anti-gay campaigns. Jerry Falwell, in his early Moral Majority fund-raising efforts, wrote, "Many practicing homosexuals are militant recruiters and allowing them to teach might be an open invitation for them to subvert our young and impressionable children into their lifestyle."[37] Anti-gay campaigns in the seventies, such as Anita Bryant's Save Our Children Crusade and California's Proposition 6 (the Briggs Initiative), were dominated by recruitment rhetoric. Bryant rehabilitated long-standing myths about the homosexual recruitment of children, saying that since gay people cannot have children, they can only recruit children. One of her advertising men, Mike Thompson of the Florida Conservative Union, got to the heart of the issue: the fear that children could be converted to homosexuality not just through "molestation" but through positive role modeling. Thompson noted:

> It's the homosexual who is blatant in his profession of his preferences and who gives the impression to young people that this lifestyle is not odd or to be avoided, but just an alternative. All the evidence indicates that homosexuals aren't born; they're made. They choose. We believe that homosexuals can become heterosexual and that heterosexuals could become homosexuals. But even if they can't change what they are, at least they can keep it hidden, or suppress their drive to express their proclivities.[38]

Similarly, the language of California's Proposition 6 suggested the need to shelter children even from any discussion about homosexuality for fear of the consequences. Following closely in Bryant's wake, Proposition 6, which was defeated, would have required the dismissal of any school employee (gay or straight) who engaged in "advocating, soliciting, imposing, encouraging, or promoting of private or public homosexual activity directed at, or likely to come to the attention of, school children and/or other employees."[39] The intense conflicts over Bryant's campaign and Proposition 6 reveal the power of symbolism suggesting the seduction of innocent children to fuel anti-gay initiatives.

Decades later, despite a radically changed cultural climate regarding lesbian and gay issues, the same arguments recirculated. Recruitment rhetoric—playing to fears that children will be converted to homosexuality—dominated conservative discourse, with explicit suggestions that a growing acceptance of homosexuality would lead children to become gay. For example, Beverly LaHaye, whose influential evangelical group Concerned Women for America has been at the forefront of fighting gay rights and sexuality education, wrote: "The homosexual movement poses the most serious threat to families and to our children. They want their depraved 'values' to become our children's values. . . . Worse yet, they are looking for new recruits!"[40] She describes how such "recruiting" occurs by gay Boy Scout troop leaders, homosexual superhero characters in comics, and gay-related programs in the schools. On the local level, activists used recruitment rhetoric to depict gay education reformers as sexual deviants who prey on youth. One New York African American activist said about the multicultural guide on families, "It was the first time that someone was probably trying to woo our children into a lifestyle that we didn't even deal with because we didn't think anybody in our community—I mean, we use the word 'queer'—they were a group apart so you didn't have to worry about anybody trying to get your kids to become a homosexual. The curriculum for the first time was systematically going to recruit them and going to make them accepting of that lifestyle."[41] A Massachusetts activist complained, "They are teaching about a felony lifestyle and promoting it."[42] Conversion anxiety depends on gay people occupying a reviled social category; otherwise there would be no threat. As we shall see, sexual stigma was one way for the Christian Right to maintain this threat.

Meanwhile, contentions that homosexuality could be contracted inevitably led to assertions that it could be cured. Christian Right activists embarked on such a strategy. Since homosexuality could be cured, the opposition claimed, ex-gay groups were the more effective alternative to gay-supportive school reform programs. The ex-gay movement is both a grass-roots ministry and a significant network in the Christian Right's infrastructure. Launched in the early seventies, it has gained momentum over the decades.[43] Ministries such as Love in Action, HOPE Ministries, P-Fox, and Exodus International were typically started by gay men (or the parents of gay people, in the case of P-Fox) who became fundamentalists and resolved to convert to heterosexuality. Although the American Psychiatric Association condemned interventions such as "reparative therapy" which claims to "cure" gay people, the ex-gay movement in practice combines quasi-therapeutic premises with religious convictions that God can "heal" homosexuality. The conversion entails elaborate lifestyle changes to help "the overcomer manage the most annoying and discouraging aspects of homosexuality."[44] These include changes such as adopting "gender-appropriate clothes, appearance, talk and behavior."[45] Those who work with gay people adopt an evangelistic mode of prayer and counseling to help the overcomer eschew all gay friendships, colleagues, or casual contacts. Since overcomers are often already evangelicals, they need only be recruited back to heterosexuality.

The ex-gay movement is significant for several reasons. First, like the AFLA-sponsored abstinence-only sex education curricula, it allows the Christian Right to offer an alternative to lesbian and gay educational programs. As Donald Wildmon, president of the American Family Association, said, "A national 'Coming Out of Homosexuality Day' provides us a means whereby to dispel the lies of the homosexual rights crowd who say they are born that way and cannot change."[46] Instead of a program like Project 10, they argue, schools should sponsor ex-gay initiatives that can help convert young people back to heterosexuality. In addition, the ex-gay movement is crucial because it has spawned a network of ministries with direct ties to national Christian Right organizations.[47] By the late nineties, Exodus International had more than one hundred individual chapters in the United States and abroad.[48] The national organizations provide resources and organizational support to the local ministries. National ex-gay organizations are directly linked to major Christian Right groups like Focus on the Family, Concerned Women for America, and the Family

Research Council. Combined, the extensive abstinence-only sex education network and the web of ex-gay ministries constitute a service-oriented infrastructure by which the Christian Right can recruit new members and mobilize supporters on behalf of their causes. As with AFLA and sex education, the development of the ex-gay movement has enabled the Christian Right to further broaden its infrastructure through a network of service organizations that are by and large linked to national organizations.

Finally, the ex-gay movement helps the Christian Right try to manage the incongruity between Christ's command to love all people and the movement's condemnation of lesbians and gay men. As Alan Wolfe notes in *One Nation, After All*, his interviewees reconciled their rejection of gay people with their strong support for moral individualism in other contexts by claiming that they reject homosexual *acts*, not people.[49] However, even Jerry Falwell admitted that "many of us pastors like to talk about loving the sinner but hating the sin," but "unfortunately that statement has often become a meaningless cliché" because "we too often fall short of the mark of . . . truly loving the sinner."[50] Nevertheless, the ex-gay movement allowed activists to claim love (for the sinner) instead of hate (for the sin) while still playing to the confusions and anxieties parents might have about their children's sexuality. However, after launching a national ex-gay ad campaign in 1998, Robert Knight of the Family Research Council said, "This is the Normandy landing in the larger cultural wars."[51] His language of war suggested that, in practice, the ex-gay initiative did not fully interrupt the antagonistic position of national movement leaders.

## THE RHETORICS OF AVERSION

The national debate over lesbian and gay school reform highlights the role of aversive feelings in moral politics. What sociologist James Jasper calls the "moral shock" can be a powerful impetus for involvement in social movements.[52] The galvanizing outrage of a moral shock occurs either from a sudden incident or when a citizen receives some type of threatening news. Since fear and anger are highly mobilizing emotions, the construction of moral shock works to the advantage of social movements. Yet in order for protest to arise from moral shocks, there must be a target of blame. Demonization of an enemy is common in moral protest movements, in part because this strategy triggers strong feelings of hatred and anger that bind together activists in opposition to the threatening Other, who is cast as a legitimate and deserving target. Through the nineties, the national Christian Right constructed gay school reform as a moral shock for communities. Perhaps even more so than in its characterizations of SIECUS sex educators, opponents used sexual language and repellent images to stigmatize gay education reformers. These national rhetorics sought to evoke negative feelings, in particular, disgust.

Moral judgment, as legal scholar William Miller notes, demands "the idiom of disgust."[53] And that is what conservatives sought to evoke, by depicting gay lives in the most aversive light. They made claims that gay people are diseased and die early, comparing homosexuals to ax murderers, drug addicts, and Nazi skinheads. One common strategy was to link gay sexuality to historically stigmatized sexual activities. Anti-gay videos, which began to proliferate throughout the nineties, were crucial to the diffusion of this sexually stigmatizing rhetoric. These videos usually featured an authoritative-looking, older white male (sometimes a physician), such as Dr. Stanley Monteith in the video *The Gay Agenda*. Monteith, who once headed his local John Birch Society chapter,[54] recites a list of statistics about the percentages of "homosexuals" who supposedly engage in stigmatized behaviors. His serious demeanor holds throughout the discussions of "rolling around in feces" and "rimming," giving way to a higher-pitched tone of incredulity with, "And what are golden showers? Why, a man lies on the ground naked and other men stand around and urinate on him!"[55] Anti-gay materials from national organizations routinely associated gay sexuality with eating and smearing feces, drinking and bathing in urine, and other fetishes such as boot-licking and sadomasochism. Sometimes these materials implied, such as in a second video, *The Gay Agenda in Public Education*, that educators proposed to teach about these activities in the classroom.

These videotapes were an important vehicle by which national Christian Right rhetorics went local. In March 1993, the producers of the video *The Gay Agenda* claimed that sales had exceeded sixty thousand.[56] Many of those videos were supplied to states and towns embroiled in disputes over sexuality or AIDS education, and provocative claims were easily woven into depravity narratives in those local conflicts. For example, during Oregon's 1992 bitter fight over a ballot initiative that, among other things, would have prohibited any mention of homosexuality in the classroom, an anti-gay activist regaled a crowd with tales of how gay men smear feces on each other and throw it on the walls: The way you can tell they are in there engaged in such activities, he claimed, is when you see feces flying out the windows.[57] One critique of *The Gay Agenda* notes that it is so filled with graphic footage that its distribution would be illegal in some jurisdictions. Nevertheless, excerpts were aired on Christian television, such as Pat Robertson's *700 Club*, perhaps supporting Miller's contention that disgust can attract as well as repel.[58]

Two related developments enhanced the Christian Right's production of this rhetoric: the growth of a research infrastructure and the capacity to secularize moral arguments. Paul Cameron's Family Research Institute exemplifies these developments. Established in 1982, the Institute is a small, specialized anti-gay organization that makes a powerful impact by generating quasi-scientific research for the opponents of lesbian and gay educational reform. Cameron noted that one of his goals in founding the Institute was opposing homosexuality, and he describes it as "the wellspring of right-wing data in that area."[59] Other right-wing groups like the Family Research Council "use [his] data all the time" in their anti-gay and anti–sex education projects.[60] To reach a much broader nonreligious base, research institutes like Cameron's fostered the secularization of moral discourse into a medicalized idiom. One way they did so was to use medical language and scientific studies that present gay people as dangerously unhealthy. Unsubstantiated or methodologically weak statistical data were braided together to purportedly prove the depravity of homosexuals. The AIDS epidemic fueled the secularization of moral rhetoric, since activists could leave out any mention of God and simply equate homosexuality with a deadly disease. For example, one opponent of gay education reform charged, "Homosexuality is just as dangerous as drug abuse . . . it's a very unhealthy, self-destructive lifestyle. It should really be called a deathstyle."[61] Secularized rhetoric backed by often questionable statistical data spread to the local level.

The Family Research Institute demonstrates the capacity of even a small Christian Right national organization to widely disseminate resources. It funnels statistical information to grassroots activists who deploy these data, often without knowing their source, typically extracting a kernel of information or an out-of-context statistic to formulate an argument.

Cameron and his work have been the subject of controversy for years, however. He was dropped from the American Psychological Association in 1983 for ethical violations related to his distortions of gay-related research and denounced by the American Sociological Association for having "consistently misinterpreted and misrepresented sociological research."[62] Scholars have time and again criticized his methodology, such as one research psychologist who wrote, "Six serious errors are identified in the Cameron group's sampling techniques, survey methodology, and interpretation of results. The presence of even one of these errors would be sufficient to cast serious doubts on the legitimacy of any study's results. In combination, they make the data virtually meaningless."[63] Claims made in the highly publicized video *The Gay Agenda* were the subject of an exposé by the *Los Angeles Times,* which reported that the highly inflammatory statistics were derived from Cameron's study of only forty-one men.[64] Even the profoundly anti-gay California Congressman William Dannemeyer distanced himself from Cameron, claiming discomfort with Cameron's "obsessive preoccupation with homosexuality."[65] Nonetheless, sex education opponents nationwide use Cameron's statistics.

Even when inaccurate, after enough repetition, statistical data often diffuse into communities to become the accepted wisdom of education debates. This was true with Cameron's research. One popular claim—that lesbians and gay men generally die in their forties—comes from his "lifespan study." Cameron's article, "The Longevity of Homosexuals: Before and After the AIDS Epidemic," which compares obituaries from gay newspapers to those of mainstream newspapers, concludes that lesbians and gay men have an abbreviated lifespan.[66] Despite serious methodological shortcomings in this study, the allegation now turns up everywhere.[67] For example, Moral Majority cofounder Tim LaHaye criticized the coming-out episode on the television show *Ellen,* saying, "It is the most unhappy lifestyle in the world, and the average age [of death] is about forty-one. And yet the intellectuals of our day and in the media and the Hollywood types, they want to present it as a wonderful lifestyle. Well, sure, Ellen is maybe at her prime right now. I'd like to take a look at Ellen about twenty years from now."[68] In local communities, many use that age without knowledge of its source, as when I asked a New Hampshire sex education opponent about her assertion that homosexuals have a life expectancy of forty-two years. She replied, "That is just a national statistic. It's well known. The Centers for Disease Control will back that statistic."[69] Routinely used by both national and local activists, the fallacious statistic simply became common knowledge circulated in the argument that any classroom discussion about homosexuality is too dangerous.

Disgust can be a powerful tool in moral politics. It evokes deeply unpleasant sensory images so that, as Miller says, "no other emotion, not even hatred, paints its object so unflatteringly."[70] Disgust reinforces social boundaries about which citizens are worthy and acceptable and which are not. When used to portray gay people as polluted and polluting, disgust reinscribes a hierarchy of good and bad sexualities. In debates involving children, such as those over educational reform, sexual disgust can be particularly powerful in mobilizing parents. However, conservatives' widespread use of these rhetorics of aversion made visible a dark side of moral protest. While negative emotions can mobilize activists' strong feelings, they can also be hard to control and may lead to entrenched political hatred and antagonism.[71] A movement always risks that it cannot finely calibrate the emotions that might be produced among followers in response to its discourse. In the late nineties climate of anti-gay violence, murders of abortion providers, and bombings of abortion clinics, the Christian Right faced scrutiny and criticism even by its own activists.[72] For example, evangelical leaders such as Ed Dobson, a founding board member of the Moral Majority, condemned the harsh rhetoric of his movement because it "gives permission to an already unstable person to take the next deadly step."[73] After her gay son, Bobby, committed suicide, fundamentalist Christian Mary Griffith became an outspoken critic of what she called the "dishonest and deceitful" rhetoric of anti-gay fundamentalists engaged in a school reform battle.[74] Although few in number, these dissenting voices broke the silence which sexual demonization requires to succeed. Like sexuality educators, however, gay education reformers found it difficult to fight sexual scapegoating.

THE POLITICS OF RESPECTABILITY (REVISITED)

As had happened since the sixties with sex educators, advocates of gay school reform were sexually stigmatized by their opponents, regardless of the actual content of the programs they developed. Unlike sex educators, however, gay reformers had a progressive movement behind them. Long before reform initiatives in public education, lesbians and gay men suffered the rhetorics of disgust and pollution. In response to a social universe which forced them to either silently hide or face discrimination, they had built a movement. And yet the broader lesbian and gay rights movement had itself been vexed since its earliest days about how, or even whether, to develop a politics of sex.[75] In the face of stigmatization, some gay activists disavowed any mention of sex. They pursued identity politics which assert the normalcy of homosexuality, rather than challenge the actual political hierarchies that regulate sex as either normal or deviant, healthy or disgusting. Their vision was that assimilation would bring equality, and their strategies involved talk about gay families, gay marriage, and gay culture—not talk about sex. As cultural theorist Michael Warner notes, "The movement in too many ways has chosen to become a politics of sexual identity, not sex."[76] This distinction was important. It is a question of which strategies were most effective in challenging discrimination. Which would undermine rather than reinforce hierarchies of sexual respectability and shame?

Although this debate emerged in many movement initiatives, it was virtually absent throughout the actual development and implementation of school reform programs. The unspoken consensus to avoid sexuality and stress safety, health promotion, and tolerance emerged for several reasons. For one thing, program planners were careful to observe the taboo regarding sexuality and children. The bitter conflicts involving sex educators had already made visible how much trouble teachers could face as a result of any discussions about sexuality in the classroom. Talk about homosexuality—which opponents had dubbed "emotional molestation"— would prove even more troublesome. As a gay teacher insisted during the *Children of the Rainbow* controversies, "Nobody is talking about sex. Believe me, I don't want to talk about sex to kids."[77] And trouble did result whenever there was a mention of gay sexuality. For example, after a state-sponsored workshop for gay youth in Massachusetts (held at a local university, not in a high school), conservatives complained that the educators spoke too explicitly about sexuality. In response, the Department of Education fired the educators, and in the 2000 budget the state legislature dictated that no money could be used in gay youth programming for sex education. In this climate, simply introducing the notion of gay identity seemed a radical enough step.

Moreover, discussions of sexuality were not always appropriate or relevant in school programs. Program planners, in avoiding any mention of sex, hoped to undermine the conflation of sexual orientation and actual sex. They wanted to achieve the normalization of homosexuality that would come with its routine inclusion in the curriculum. Kevin Jennings, the founder of GLSEN, told me,

> We need to incorporate gay and lesbian people into the curriculum by formal English exercises. There should be, "Robert wants to date Pierre," where being gay is not the issue. The issue is what's the correct conjugation of the verb "to date." We're simply a part of the society and we should be treated like we're part of the society. Now secondly, we do need to specifically address gay and lesbian concerns, but I think I want to see the first one happen first, almost because I think then, when the kids are used to just conjugating "to love" with Robert and Pierre, they learn to accept gay people in a way that is very different as part of the landscape of our society.[78]

None of the many different approaches to gay educational reform are mutually exclusive; they can coexist. And yet except for extremely circumscribed inclusion in HIV education programs, discussion of gay sexualities remained relatively rare in public school programs. Gay education reformers were in the awkward position of balancing an active pursuit of anti-discrimination with a passive strategy to hide sexuality.

This balance did not hold. When communities erupted into controversy over gay education reform, the familiar movement tensions over sexuality emerged. In fact, such disagreements surfaced over education policy even before the advent of school programs. California's 1978 ballot initiative Proposition 6 had directly targeted public schools. Had it passed, any gay or straight public school employee could have been fired for any activity—either at work or at home—that was construed as "advocating" homosexuality.[79] The initiative was winning in the polls prior to the election. Gay activists fought bitterly over how to oppose Prop 6. Some activists wanted to so circumscribe any discussion of homosexuality they insisted that only professional heterosexual consultants should run the campaign. David Goodstein, the publisher of the national gay magazine *The Advocate*, was adamant on this point. Sounding like conservatives in his depiction of gay lives, he (wrongly) forecast that addressing gay issues would exacerbate public disapproval of homosexuality and lead to passage of the ballot initiative: "This problem is seriously compounded by some of our gay activists who believe we should use elections to put our most unacceptable stereotypical faces forward: intergenerational sex, drag, leather, public sexuality, Marxism, lesbian separatism, and the rest of the familiar liturgy of our extremists. . . . The election gives us an opportunity to manifest an image. If we continue to put forward the most bizarre, it will take that much longer to gain acceptance for the rest of us."[80] But there were some activists who disagreed that direct discussion of gay issues would evoke universal revulsion.

Gay school reform, and controversies about it, unfold within a broader matrix of ignorance, uncertainty, and terror about sex, desire, and pleasure. To ignore this and to maintain silence about sexuality and homosexuality, some activists argued, was to risk leaving intact the hierarchies of disgust and shame that allow anti-gay initiatives to succeed. Organizers like Amber Hollibaugh traveled to small towns in rural areas throughout California speaking about sexuality and against Proposition 6. In later reflections she said

> People are really terrified of having sexuality, especially children's sexuality, discussed as a primary issue. . . . If you can refocus it like that, it also avoids making us, homosexuals, the enemy, but points to the whole question of sexuality. People are not just terrified of gay people, but of sexuality and sexual forces that they cannot easily understand. . . . If you don't address it as a complex issue, you can't even begin to have a good discussion. That's what some of us discovered through the campaign, though we never came up with a complete answer."[81]

The desexualization of homosexuality, from this point of view, is a mistake despite the intense emotional pitch of controversies over school programs.

Still, regardless of whatever shifts parents might undergo in relation to their own sexual understanding, their position on their children's sexuality is often considerably less flexible. The power of the rhetorics of recruitment and disgust derives less from their appeal to parents closely aligned with conservative and right-wing cultural politics and more from how such rhetorics tap commonplace fears among a much broader cohort. Many parents fear what they perceive as the sinfulness, deviance, danger, or merely the social anomaly of being lesbian or gay. For many parents, it is simply that, as journalist Anne Roiphe put it during the *Rainbow* controversies, "when it comes to their own little Heather's fate they would rather keep gender choice on the straight path."[82] Education reformers found it difficult to confront conservative rhetoric and the fear of contagion it might tap, and many of them chose to argue that sexual orientation is fixed, so therefore young people would not become gay by hearing about gay issues.[83] It was simple and direct, whereas an argument that addressed sexual development and desires lent itself to distortion. This is precisely what happened in one of only a few instances I found wherein an activist confronted recruitment rhetoric head-on by publicly arguing that gay education programs might indeed make an impact on young people's sexuality.

It was perhaps not the most auspicious moment—at the height of the New York City conflicts about *Children of the Rainbow* in the early nineties—for a nuanced political argument. Nonetheless, journalist Donna Minkowitz, who had been bothered by how gay activists had responded to recruitment rhetoric, instead formulated different arguments. In a series of articles and media appearances, she made it clear that she completely rejected the accusation that gay people seduce and abuse children to make converts. She nonetheless affirmed the sexual rights of young people, insisted that sexual identity is fluid not fixed, and dared to imagine that gay activism might indeed make homosexuality look more socially attractive. Why, after all, would education reformers otherwise be working so hard to teach about gay concerns if such discussion had no impact? Minkowitz refused the basic premise of recruitment rhetoric—that it would be disastrous if young people became gay. Instead, she affirmed "the morality of teaching kids that gay is OK even if it means that some will join our ranks," and she suggested that it could be positive for children to "try on different forms of sexuality as they now try on musical styles, career choices, and haircuts."[84]

Minkowitz was blasted from all sides. Conservatives quoted her as proof of the gay agenda. One local conservative activist said, "Donna Minkowitz—what she says in this particular article is, 'why not say it's recruitment?'"[85] In her widely distributed anti-gay videotape *Why Parents Should*

*Object to the Children of the Rainbow, HIV K–6 Curricula*, activist Dolores Ayling said Minkowitz admitted on television that gay people recruit.[86] Conservative gay activist Bruce Bawer, well known for his complaint that "countercultural" gay people disrupt the mainstreaming efforts of those who are more assimilationist, condemned Minkowitz as simply on a "reckless quest for celebrity."[87] At an appearance on the Montel Williams show, the host announced Minkowitz by saying, "Next we'll hear from a gay woman who says it's all about recruiting."[88] It simply was not possible for Minkowitz, who later told me she felt "a little sensitive" about the issue, to be understood as both disavowing recruiting and acknowledging the cultural power of the gay movement.

This speaks to how both the dominant conservative and the gay discourses narrowed the fields of engagement over education reform. Not only was it politically difficult to argue against the grain. Any argument was simply incoherent outside of the structuring terms in which conservatives claimed gay people recruit children, while many gay reformers insisted that sexuality is fixed and that they were not talking about sex anyway. Minkowitz's claim, in which was embedded questions about the complex nature of sexuality and the potential impact of cultural representation, was worthy of broader public debate. Its mischaracterization and condemnation reflected the entrenched dynamics of the culture wars over sex. There was virtually no room for arguments which could not be expressed in sound bites. In addition, there was no latitude in the oversensitized public conversation about sexuality and children. Minkowitz had touched the third rail.

As the new century began, those who were speaking most about gay issues were the gay rights movement, specific community health and AIDS service organizations, television programs, and anti-gay conservatives. Those who were speaking the most openly in the public arena specifically about gay sexuality were largely the anti-gay conservatives. The national gay movement, afraid of attack, had chosen to focus on issues such as military service and marriage. Many community-based AIDS service organizations fought to stave off controversy and hold on to their funding in order to bring safer-sex information to adults. Television, with its bevy of gay characters, had no gay sex. Although *Ellen* was off the air by then, the 2000–2001 season featured seventeen recurring or leading gay characters. But as one critic observed, gay TV characters were isolated and stereotyped, "never finding community and never getting laid."[89] Albeit trendy, gay characters lacked sex lives. So although conservatives vehemently denounced the alleged gay agenda, it was they who were most vocal about gay sex. In communities nationwide, they narrated their own version of gay sexuality, speaking of disease, death, and activities such as anal sex, oral sex, urine drinking, rolling in feces, sadomasochism, and boot-licking. They did so to frighten and disgust residents deciding on ballot questions or public education programs. It was another example in which conservatives themselves were most responsible for making visible the sexualities they claimed to despise.

One sex educator, responding to the embattled climate she faced in the late nineties, predicted, "My guess is that if [SIECUS founder] Mary Calderone were sitting here, she'd say, 'It's déjà vu all over again.'"[90] It was true; the divisive battles over teaching about sexuality in the public schools seemed like clones of the sixties conflicts. There were palpable differences, since earlier battles had diminished after a year. They had, however, served as a bridge in the establishment of a right-wing Christian political movement that would eventually target a range of sexual issues. Years later, scores of national organizations were committed to furthering conservative sexual politics. By then, debates about whether to talk in the classroom about sexuality and homosexuality unfolded in the context of myriad bitter conflicts over sexuality, such as abortion and gay rights. Conservatives sought to change minds and hearts, mobilizing collective emotions in service of opposing specific initiatives such as school reform and abortion access. Their rhetoric about these issues, and others such as President Clinton's impeachment, proliferated public talk about sexuality. Their success was uneven. While on some fronts conservatives felt beleaguered, even beaten, they had nonetheless scored significant victories in limiting what could be discussed in the classroom. Not only were gay-related school programs desexualized, but so was much of sexuality education itself.

## Chapter 9 | IF ASKED, DON'T TELL

*A Final Comment*

The culture war is over, some conservative Christians lamented in 1998, and they had lost. Instead of being removed from office, instead of resigning in disgrace, President Bill Clinton received approval ratings that soared despite his extramarital affair and impeachment. This apparent death of collective outrage provoked disgust among several Christian Right leaders such as Paul Weyrich, one of the founders of the Moral Majority, who claimed that a moral majority no longer existed and suggested that Christian fundamentalists retreat from the political arena back into separatism.[1] James Dobson of Focus on the Family complained that the greatest problem was not with Clinton but with "the people of this land."[2] Told to feel outraged, the people had largely declined.

Yet on another front of the culture war—sexuality education in the public schools—the Christian Right had fared far better. At the turn of the twenty-first century, most public schools offered sex education. But at a time in which their access to sexual imagery in popular culture was unprecedented, very few students received the type of comprehensive sexuality education advocated by the Sexuality Information and Education Council of the United States (SIECUS). Some students might have a semester-long course, while some heard only one or two sessions from an outside group like Planned Parenthood. Most students underwent a few class periods of instruction sometime between the seventh and twelfth grades.[3] However, since abstinence-only education had grown in prominence from the late eighties, many students only heard about abstinence. While in 1988 only 2 percent of teachers taught abstinence as the *sole* means of pregnancy and disease prevention, 23 percent did so in 1999. A study of public schools revealed that among all districts in the United States, 10 percent had a comprehensive sexuality education policy, 34 percent promoted abstinence as the preferred option for teenagers but allowed for discussion of contraception, and 23 percent required the sole promotion of abstinence.[4] Thirty-three percent of districts had no policy on sexuality education. The abstinence-only-until-marriage districts either completely prohibited any instruction in contraception or required that teachers only emphasize its failures. The researchers concluded that of all U.S. students who attended a public school including grades six and higher, only 9 percent were in districts with a comprehensive sexuality education policy. The chilly climate in sex education classrooms was a success for conservatives, who since the sixties had been criticizing comprehensive sexuality education as pornographic, dangerous, and immoral. It had proven to be one of their most powerful issues.

A decided conservative victory was that "comprehensive" sex education atrophied, coming to increasingly resemble abstinence-only programs. The term no longer implied the integrated, K–12 course of instruction SIECUS had recommended. "Comprehensive" had become a code for programs that stress abstinence but also teach about contraception. Even so, 37 percent of students in so-called comprehensive courses reported getting no information on how to use birth control and where to get it.[5] Virtually all public school sex education, including comprehensive programs, stressed abstinence as the wisest and most effective course for young people. There was a move, as Martha Kempner at SIECUS put it, toward "abstinence as anti-controversy."[6] It seemed to work. During the 1999–2000 school year, SIECUS documented one hundred and twenty-two conflicts in thirty-one states. There were seventy-five in 2000–2001.[7] Widespread restrictions in what could be taught in sexuality education produced course content which was less controversial, resulting in fewer conflicts compared with previous years. Although the controversies had been painful, the silence was ominous for comprehensive advocates. Abstinence-only programs were increasingly being accepted and implemented in communities without public debate.[8]

Teacher training is meager as well. Most public school sexuality education takes place in health education courses, but a prospective health education teacher can finish a program without ever taking a single course on human sexuality. One study of 169 teacher-education programs in the United States found that few of them required their students to take sex education.[9] In fact, there was so little structured opportunity for teachers to undertake sexuality education training that an interested educator would have found it extremely difficult to arrange a course of study. Such determination would be unlikely when there was so little incentive and so much risk for teaching sex education.

The turn of the new century marked a widespread erosion of what could be said about sexuality to young people in many classrooms. In 1999, only 59 percent of teachers explained that condoms can be effective in preventing HIV and other diseases, compared with 87 percent who did so ten years earlier. Reports from across the country described how pages were ripped from books and teachers forbidden to utter certain words or answer particular questions. Six percent of teachers operated under a policy in which they were forbidden to teach or even answer students' questions about birth control. Twenty-two percent of teachers said that school policy restricted them from answering questions on topics outside of the regular curriculum.[10] In some communities, teachers were silenced in dramatic ways. For example, after passage of a state law requiring that school districts in North Carolina teach abstinence-only-until-marriage, three chapters covering HIV, contraception, and sexual behavior were sliced out of the ninth-grade health textbook in one district. After teachers balked, one mother volunteered to cut out the offending chapters.[11] In Van Buren, North Carolina, public schools, several pages of an advanced biology text were torn out because they discussed abortion as part of family planning.[12] Schools in Burbank, California, removed the videos *Girl to Woman* and *Boy to Man* after a handful of parents complained about references to masturbation.[13] The videos had been shown without complaint for the previous twenty years. Even nocturnal emission was the subject of debate. In Fairfax, Virginia, puberty videos were edited so that information on tampon insertion was removed from the copy shown to boys and the section on nocturnal emission was removed from the girls' version.[14] Some schools simply gave up, such as one Los Angeles school that abandoned sex education completely rather than teach about contraception.[15]

Sexual language was a predictable magnet for controversy. For example, parents in Oregon fought over which vocabulary words could be used in sex education classes. One mother complained when anatomical terms such as "penis," "vagina," "testicles," and "fallopian tube" were used in a third-grade class, saying, "You don't have to learn the name of everything under the hood just to learn to drive."[16] The school moved all reproductive terms from third to fourth grade and all "sensitive" language such as masturbation, clitoris, and ejaculation from fifth grade to sixth and seventh grade. Still, this Oregon school ranks as liberal compared with the many across the United States which remained silent about topics deemed controversial, in particular masturbation, homosexuality, abortion, and contraception.[17] In the wake of Surgeon General Joycelyn Elders's firing in 1994, many schools were terrified to discuss masturbation. A typical example was the director of curriculum at the Utah Office of Public Instruction, who said masturbation is excluded from their programs because "it's not worth it. It becomes too big of an issue."[18] In Charlotte, North Carolina, teachers received a list of words which they were forbidden to use in human development classes. Dubbed by one teacher "the dirty dozen," this list included abortion, bisexual, gay, homosexual, lesbian, masturbation, orgasm, transsexual, and transvestite.[19] Meanwhile, in one Florida middle school, school board members voted five to two to allow teachers to say "condom" in health classes, but only to students whose parents had signed permission forms.[20]

Conservatives had been enormously successful at establishing structural support for their programs. By the late nineties, there were three major sources of federal funding for abstinence-only education programs. In addition to the Adolescent Family Life Act (AFLA), Section 510(b) of Title V of the Social Security Act in 1996 (Public Law 104-193) provided states with $50 million per year for five years, starting in 1998. States that accepted this funding were required to match every four federal dollars with three state dollars. Combined with this rich source, at the end of 1999, conservatives secured an additional $50 million in funding for abstinence-only education programs over a two-year period. This money, available through a competitive grant process from Maternal and Child Health Bureau, could only be used for programs which met the narrow definitions of abstinence education as set out by Section 510(b).[21] For example, in addition to prohibiting discussion of any topics outside of abstinence until marriage, these programs mandate instruction that sexual activity outside of marriage is physically and psychologically harmful. Such hefty federal funding for one particular type of sexuality education—abstinence programs—constituted state legitimation of restricted programs as the normative pedagogical standard. Made possible because of the budding Christian Right sex education infrastructure generated by AFLA through the eighties, the funding provided by Section 510(b) promoted an even more vibrant conservative sexuality industry of curricula, speakers and trainers, and abstinence products. As the founder of the Abstinence Clearinghouse acknowledged in the fall of 2000, "All of a sudden, abstinence has become a business," which she estimated had grown by nine hundred new programs in recent years, coincident with federal funding.[22]

Having achieved such success in the nineties under a Democratic president, the swing to the right effected by George W. Bush's administration brought conservatives the prospect of an even friendlier climate. At the beginning of his presidency, they signaled their ambitions to expand their own programs and curtail those with which they disagreed. Both Bush and conservative activists pressed for even more federal support for abstinence-only programs. Bush administration officials declared their intent to increase federal spending on abstinence-only education to $135 million annually.[23] (In March 2001, Bush's brother, Jeb, sought to shift $1 million in Florida funding for family planning services into abstinence-only programs.) Meanwhile, the evangelical organization Focus on the Family began urging Health and Human Services Secretary Tommy Thompson to restrict Title X–funded family planning programs, and the administration proposed no increase for such programs in its 2001 budget.[24] In addition to promoting abstinence-only education and restricting family planning services as domestic policy, the Bush administration moved to export that position through U.S. foreign policy.[25] One of Bush's first acts as president was to reinstitute a ban on abortion counseling at overseas health clinics. And in preparations for the September 2001 United Nations General Assembly on Children, the administration insisted on abstinence-only education and rejected language such as "reproductive health services," which might imply abortion or contraception education. Leslie Unruth of the National Abstinence Clearinghouse confirmed that they were getting "nothing but support from the Bush administration."[26]

Meanwhile, nine days into his term, Bush created an Office of Faith-Based and Community Initiatives. The president proposed the broad implementation of "charitable choice"—provisions by which the government contracts with religious organizations for services. Although the initiative had stalled by the end of 2001, these faith-based proposals signaled the administration's willingness to formally relax the boundaries between church and state. In fact, evangelical Christian and Catholic groups already receive much of the federal money for sex education.[27] Among the recipients of federal sex education funding are Mid-South Christian Ministries in West Memphis, Arkansas, Roseland Christian Healthy Ministries in Chicago, and the Catholic Archdiocese of New York. Federal money from AFLA in the eighties had already spawned the Christian sex education industry, and under AFLA, Catholics and evangelicals had demonstrated a strong tendency to integrate Christian messages into public school programs. Religious groups, post–*Kendrick v. Heckler*, are supposed to be restricted in how they implement programs, although there is little, if any, enforcement of this policy. The current national climate is a congenial one for conservative Catholic, evangelical, and fundamentalist sex education organizations to use taxpayers' money for program development and implementation.

The battle is not over, however. Comprehensive sex education advocates did have some successes during this time. SIECUS had many esteemed allies who joined them in support of comprehensive school programs, including the American Medical Association, the American Public Health Association, and the American Academy of Pediatrics. In addition, a new wing of advocacy emerged in the late nineties. Prompted by the funding of abstinence-only programs embedded in the 1996 welfare law, the National Coalition Against Censorship (NCAC) along with other free speech activists took up sex education as a First Amendment issue. In broad public education campaigns, the NCAC argued that federal funding of abstinence-only education represented censorship in that it is state restriction on what teachers can or cannot teach about sex. In June 2001, the NCAC launched opposition to the planned 2002 reauthorization of funding under Section 510(b), saying that abstinence-only programs are government control over what students were allowed to "read, see, hear, think, and say."[28] Since 54 percent of sex education teachers use standard curricula,[29] many of which are abstinence-only programs developed by conservative Christian groups, classrooms were thus censored through a narrowing of what could be said about sexuality. This argument can be extended. Censorship is not only explicit, as when laws and policies prohibit teachers from certain kinds of speech. It also operates when acceptable and unacceptable boundaries of speech are implicitly determined.[30] It is unclear what will be the eventual impact of advocates such as the NCAC on the dynamics of the sex education debates. However, their entrance into the public conversation helps break the isolation from progressive groups which sex educators have historically suffered. It introduces a constitutional rather than a reproductive health argument and, by expanding the debate, will almost certainly shape its terms.

On other fronts, comprehensive programs showed strength. By 2000, Planned Parenthood affiliates employed over seven hundred staff educators and trainers, who reached one and a half million people annually.[31] Polls consistently showed that a large majority of the public believed sex education should be expanded beyond abstinence-only messages.[32] Parents filed and sometimes won lawsuits challenging abstinence-only programs on the basis of medical inaccuracy. And although politicians who promoted abstinence-only legislation were more successful than comprehensive supporters, in 1999 sixteen legislative measures were enacted to promote or mandate comprehensive sexuality and/or HIV education, compared with only four such measures in 1998.[33] (This contrasts, however, with the twenty abstinence-only measures enacted in 1999.) Some individual states fought off conservative challenges. For example, despite allegations that teachers were teaching "promiscuity," New Jersey—which since 1980 has had a state mandate for family life education—overcame legislative challenges in both 1993 and 2001 attempting to restrict instruction in contraception and safer sex.[34] In 2001, another surgeon general, David Satcher, spoke out in favor of comprehensive sex education, this time by issuing a report advocating that schools teach about contraception in addition to abstinence. (However, the immediate demand for his resignation by Focus on the Family suggested that it was, indeed, déjà vu all over again.[35]) Finally, in the fall of 2001, a coalition of advocates introduced federal legislation to appropriate $100 million of funding for comprehensive sex education for each fiscal year over a five-year period. Although estimating its chances of passage under the new administration as "slim to none,"[36] these proponents hoped to open a national conversation about the merits of comprehensive versus abstinence-only programs.

Should it occur, such a conversation might certainly include the issue of effectiveness. Despite federal support, difficult questions remained unanswered concerning whether abstinence-only programs actually work. In 1996, when Section 510(b) was enacted, an independent review of the evaluations conducted by the various AFLA programs had found that the evaluations were all inadequate and concluded that there were no solid data to demonstrate the effectiveness of abstinence-only curricula.[37] In May 2001, an independent meta-review of sexuality education program evaluations reaffirmed this conclusion, adding that "early results are not encouraging."[38] Evaluations of three prominent curricula—Sex Respect, Teen-Aid, and Values and Choices—did not support advocates' claims that the programs delayed sexual initiation among young people. Despite the paucity of supporting research, Section 510(b) initially included no evaluation component, although when pressured, Congress appropriated $6 million to conduct such research. Currently an independent researcher holds the contract to conduct thorough evaluations of the programs funded through Section 510(b), with a preliminary report due to Congress by late 2002. However, participation in the broad evaluation is voluntary, which will affect the overall quality of program review data. One prominent program had already withdrawn from the evaluation process by the fall of 2000.[39] If congressional hearings should transpire, it is ultimately unclear whether legislative backing of abstinence-only curricula will be directly affected by effectiveness data or will remain politically motivated.

Sexuality education deserves a broad national conversation. It involves sexual knowledge and citizenship and therefore is a civic matter of wide significance. This book has shown that conservatives have dominated the public conversation about sexuality education. Both AFLA and Section 510(b) were enacted without legislative debate. Community discussions, as we have seen, often become explosive affairs. I have suggested that several factors account for this. Sexuality issues, in particular sex education, facilitated the Christian Right's rise to political power. The movement's broad infrastructural expansion since the seventies, in particular the development of its own alternative sexuality industry, plus its strategic emphasis on social issues afforded it significant cultural power in community sex education debates. National conservative organizations have been instrumental in impeding the progress of comprehensive sexuality education through rhetoric that escalates conflict. Local activists adopted national ways of thinking and talking about sex education for a variety of reasons, including resonance and expediency. All of these factors worked to constrain dialogue.

Perhaps most important, the negative affect culture of sex holds in place the volatile sex education conflicts. Conservatives stigmatized and silenced their critics. As journalist Judith Levine points out about sex education, "The Right won, but the mainstream let it. Comprehensive sex educators had the upper hand in the 1970s, and starting in the 1980s, they allowed their enemies to seize more and more territory, until the Right controlled the law, the language, and the cultural consensus."[40] This book has recounted the many obstacles since the sixties facing those who advocated for sex education. Much of the symbolic power of aversive rhetorics derives from the stigma historically attached to sex. Conservatives have drawn on the tenacious power of sexual shame and fear to galvanize residents to oppose comprehensive programs. Their success depends on maintaining the risk in speaking out for sex education. They are frequently successful. Fear of stigma silences potential supporters of sex education and, in turn, their silence suggests a consensus for the opposition. Parents or school board members who have stood up to conservative sex education opposition report that they have been made to feel "dirty." Teachers and other sex education advocates (even a former surgeon general) have lost their jobs or reputations. These strategies can only succeed in the type of sexual culture which conservatives have worked to hold in place, wherein sex is largely shameful and stigmatizing rhetoric is acceptable. Yet an important theme of this book is that culture and discourse operate in unpredictable ways. So what is the potential for reworking the historical associations of evocative speech and thereby undermining the power of conservatives in battles over sex education?

Only a successful challenge to this culture of stigma could meaningfully shift the dynamics of the sex education debates. The conditions for such disruption would require the voices of not only sex educators themselves, but also those of a wider range of advocates. More sexual speech does not inevitably bring more sexual freedom, as its proliferation by the Christian Right proves.[41] However, broad discussion about sexuality allows for opportunities to interrupt provocative speech strategies. In different contexts comes the potential for disruption of entrenched local culture war dynamics. As philosopher Judith Butler suggests, with the repetition of provocative speech may come an erosion of prior associations, allowing for the possibility of reworking and resistance.[42]

The dynamics surrounding President Clinton's impeachment offer some insight into how public reaction might undermine the intentions of conservative speakers. Rather than singularly reinforcing sexual shame and reticence, Clinton's affair prompted such widespread sexual dialogue that one headline proclaimed, "In a matter of days, a change in culture" in which "Americans have actually debated the definition of adultery, made 'oral sex' part of the public conversation, and speculated about the most private elements of the President's life in ways that would have been inconceivable as recently as New Year's Day, to say nothing of Harry Truman's day or even Ronald Reagan's."[43] One psychotherapist predicted, "This is a defining moment in terms of how we talk about sexuality."[44] Pundits mused that "such public talking about private sexual acts" might enhance a general comfort with sex and in particular could loosen up parents in dealing with their children's sexuality.[45] Joking at work became commonplace, along with satiric depictions of the impeachment proceedings. Independent counsel Kenneth Starr's politics of shame invited parody. *Screw* magazine ran an "illustrated" version of the "Starr Report" with doctored photos of Clinton and intern Monica Lewinsky, while *Hustler* publisher Larry Flynt threatened to publish the names of prominent Republicans who had had affairs. When the repetition of terms like "oral sex" and "semen" failed to provoke the citizenry, it may have been from the empathic realization that, as one sex educator mused, "even the blandest sexual acts can, if described in progressive detail, be made to sound mildly pornographic."[46] Conversely, the repetition of "pornographic" speech, such as that in the "Starr Report," could come to sound bland.

It is important not to overstate the cultural resistance to provocative sexual rhetoric during the impeachment process. Yet even a measure of public equanimity was a challenge to the assumption that explicit sexual speech would inevitably outrage. The response to the impeachment may have signaled a collective resistance to perceived political manipulation, a refusal to obey the emotional demands that conservatives attempted to impose on the situation. When people are not provoked by incendiary rhetorics, conservatives risk encountering ambivalence and indifference or even fostering the circumstances for public resistance wherein provocative speech casts suspicion upon the speakers rather than the targets. A cultural climate in which sexual stigmatization—like stigmatizing rhetoric toward other social groups—is discredited might prompt conservatives to rethink its use. The Old Right had to reinvent itself, in part to gain distance from its use of racial appeals after such tactics had lost public acceptance. Public repudiation of sexual stigmatization would necessitate another strategic shift.

Still, sex education battles are resistant to resistance. Joycelyn Elders's firing showed how little latitude there is in our public dialogue about sexuality and children. Appeals to protect innocent children, especially their sexual innocence, wield enormous emotional power. Parents in particular are vulnerable to the Christian Right's allegations that their children are being taught deviant sex or that sex education is mental molestation. Even if parents do not believe these charges, it can be enormously difficult to publicly resist or challenge them. Since the sex education culture wars are not simply polarized disagreements among firmly committed cohorts, conservatives depend on mobilizing ambivalent or uncommitted citizens in order to prevail. Much of the cultural power of sexual speech—its capacity to spark battles over what to say in the classroom—derives from the ideal of Romantic childhood.

Riddled with contradictions and inflected by adult anxieties, the lingering image of the Romantic child is nonetheless a politicized and highly exploitable icon. It demands that we ignore the complexities of real children while policing their exposure to sexual knowledge in ways that are impossible, even undesirable, in contemporary culture. The image of the Romantic child keeps us vulnerable to political rhetoric by groups that count on provoking strong feelings by placing terms such as "children" and "masturbation" in the same sentence. Under such circumstances, sex education can only be, at best, an uncomfortable prospect, and sex educators themselves remain susceptible to suspicions that because they talk with children about sexuality, they are unsavory if not outright dangerous.

In 1967, well before Reverend Billy James Hargis discovered the potential to expand his movement through battling sex education, *Newsweek* magazine rightly situated classroom courses as simply one more expression of a broadly sexualized society. Sex education then was an opportunity for children "to bring to the teacher the 'dirty words' heard on the playground for a discreet explanation."[47] Open sexual discussion, the article made clear, was an irrevocable feature of modern culture. It rightly assumed that whether or not sex education exists, young people would talk about sex. Decades later, an unremarked upon aspect of Clinton's impeachment process was how it momentarily pierced a collective denial about how young people, simply by way of popular culture, are already participants in a textured national conversation on sex. "Phone sex. Oral sex. Masturbation. The stain on the dress. How do you explain these things to your children?" worried two reporters at the height of the sex scandal.[48] The earnest tone of the commentary about children's exposure to the details of Clinton's affair prompted a lacerating series in cartoonist Garry Trudeau's "Doonesbury" strip in which a "scandal facilitator" comes to school to help students talk. In one episode, the balding bespectacled facilitator tells the children, "There may even be certain words or phrases that puzzle you, words like . . . um. . . ." Into the silent discomfort, a youngster asks if he means the semen-streaked dress. And the hapless facilitator says, "Uh . . . right. Good example. We'll come back to it. If there's time.[49] Trudeau lampooned the cultural fiction that children are ignorant of the adult sexual world. The butt of the joke is the unhelpful adult helper. His irrelevance in the classroom destabilizes complacency about what kinds of discussions might be useful to students.

This is a long transitional moment in our cultural understanding of childhood. SIECUS founder Mary Calderone was criticized back in the sixties for suggesting that young peoples' bodies, pleasures, and sexual awareness can coexist with their innocence. We still face the challenge of redefining childhood in order to more fully meet the needs of contemporary young people. Can we fashion an image of childhood in which innocence and a need for protection do not depend on a complete repudiation of some level of sexual understanding? These may seem like irreconcilable notions from the point of view of the Romantic child, but an ideal of children that depends on their complete asexuality and ignorance will inevitably shape, even distort, the meanings of sexual protection. And the culture wars over sex education cannot readily abate until this construct of childhood has been reinvented.

Sex education and the conflicts about it signal broader shifts in the cultural visibility of sex and our historical definition of childhood. Meanwhile, two things are certain: both culture and childhood are in motion. And the changes in each are likely to be as multiple, complicated, and discomfiting as those changes that have unfolded over the past forty years since SIECUS's birth. This book describes a series of countervailing tendencies: that a majority of parents support comprehensive sex education amid widespread community conflict over it; the narrowing of classroom sexual speech in an era of expanding cultural accessibility to sexual discussion; the Christian Right's speech that is both stigmatizing and therapeutic; and provocative speech that both incites and flattens in community debates which are blandly scripted and strikingly unpredictable. Nowhere is this seeming incompatibility of tendencies more evident than in the Christian Right's sexual speech itself. The movement that has vowed to circumscribe public talk about sex is itself a loud voice in the sexualized society. But these all bespeak the discontinuities of the sexual culture in which seeming contradictions coexist, however uneasily. And the uneasy coexistence of the expansion of a visible sexual culture and the increasing momentum to shut down classroom discussion about sexual topics will undoubtedly fuel debates well into the future. The ways we talk in these debates will shape the sexual culture and childhood itself.

# ON METHODS AND TERMINOLOGY

This book began with a deceptively simple question. How can we explain the bitter battles over sex education given that, since the sixties, most people have reported to pollsters that they support it? Answering this question required a range of interpretive approaches, in particular historical, cultural, and discourse analyses. The first half of the book examines the role of sex education in the rise of the right wing since the sixties. Chapters 1 through 4 chronologically trace the founding of the Sexuality Information and Education Council of the United States (SIECUS), the subsequent backlash against sex education which bridged the Old Right and the New Right, the visible emergence of the pro-family movement in the mid-seventies, and the development of a Christian evangelical sexuality industry in the eighties and nineties. The second half of the book is a cultural analysis of how national sex education discourses operate in local community conflicts. In particular, it emphasizes the roles of language and emotions in local battles. These two emphases on historical and cultural analysis are interconnected throughout, although the balance shifts in particular chapters.

The book is based on interviews, oral histories, participant observation, court records, and other primary documents. I interviewed over seventy-five people who have been actively engaged in sexuality education battles, either in the sixties or more currently. These were national leaders or local activists.[1] In addition, I directly observed sex education battles in several communities of Massachusetts, New Hampshire, and New York. I closely followed conflicts in other cities across the country through telephone conversations, media coverage, discussions with activists on both sides, and analysis of primary documents. I garnered essential primary documents, such as personal correspondence, minutes from meetings, organizational statements, and political tracts of key groups such as the Christian Crusade and the John Birch Society, from the archives of the Schlesinger Library at Radcliffe College, SIECUS, the American Civil Liberties Union, the Center for Reproductive Law and Policy, and Political Research Associates. In addition, a number of generous organizations and individuals sent me their own files. Chapter 4 makes extensive use of legal documents. In particular, I use these documents to discuss the implementation of the Adolescent Family Life Act (AFLA) and the content of abstinence-only programs as they were developed after passage of AFLA. Interviews and oral histories were crucial to my narrative. I interviewed early SIECUS associates, anti–sex education activists, prominent Old and New Right leaders, and legal counsel from both sides, supplementing my own interviews with those conducted by others. Researcher Deb Tolman gave me access to her extensive oral history with SIECUS founder Mary Calderone, which she conducted in the late eighties. Lumiere Productions allowed me to use several transcripts of interviews they conducted with activists for their series on the rise of the Christian Right, *With God on Our Side: The Rise of the Religious Right in America.* This documentary also featured important media clips, such as news coverage of the Anaheim battles in 1968. These excerpts, along with other journalistic accounts, offered me a glimpse into both the cultural dialogue about sex education and the media construction of the controversies.

The second half of the book closely examines local battles over sex education. Chapters 5 through 8 look at the discursive strategies of both sex education advocates and opponents and explore the powerful impact that rhetorics of national organizations can have in local communities. These chapters emphasize contemporary ways of thinking, talking, and feeling about sex education. I weave together my interviews, field notes, and primary documents (such as educational texts as well as political tracts and videotapes) as the bases for this part of the book. I analyze journalistic coverage as a primary source of data for my discussion of how media shape the emotions of local culture wars. I use interviews not as a representation of the unmediated truth of a person or event discussed, especially in light of my central arguments about how opinions and attitudes are fluid and contextual. Rather, in a book about sexual speech, interviews represent ways in which local and national activists talk about sexuality during a particular controversy. With local activists in particular, interviews offer a glimpse of how national Christian Right sexual discourses produce certain ways of talking and feeling, and constrain other possibilities. My interpretations of these interviews and the many documents of the battles over sex education can be described as a form of discourse analysis, but not in the sense the term is used by linguists. I am less concerned with a formal reading of texts and their structural organization and more interested in the historical and social production of national sex education discourses, their diffusion into local communities, and the ways in which they operate in community debates.

The focus of this study is specifically on the debates over sexuality education in the public schools. Sex education programs have been developed in a range of other settings, such as private schools and community organizations. As a public institution, however, the public schools represent a unique historical site for disputes over values and ideologies. Sex education is one facet of a broader debate about the role of public education in a democratic society. In addition, my analysis is limited to what has come to be called comprehensive sexuality education. Comprehensive programs began to include discussion of HIV/AIDS some years after the AIDS epidemic began. But, although there is some overlap, this book does not tell the unique story of HIV/AIDS education programs. The history of such programs, with their associations to a stigmatized epidemic and community, deserves special attention.[2] The gay educational reform programs I discuss in Chapter 8 are limited to those aimed at safety, tolerance, and anti-bias.

.    .    .

This book examines conflicts throughout the course of four decades over sex education in the public schools. The story begins in the early sixties with the founding of SIECUS and, while controversies will likely continue well into the future, my narration of them ends in 2001. These forty years mark major transitions in U.S. national politics, as well as transformations in the social organization and cultural history of sexuality. Since terminology has also evolved and changed, I want to clarify the terms I use in relation to the individuals and social groups involved in the story I tell here.

In the eighties, sex educators initiated a shift from the term "sex education" to "sexuality education." SIECUS, in response to this transition, changed its name in the early nineties to the Sexuality (rather than Sex) Information and Education Council of the United States. Since my book begins in the early sixties, I use the term "sex education" and the name Sex Information and Education Council of the United States, both of which are historically accurate for that period. The date of the shift is imprecise, and for this reason, and also for consistency and brevity, I generally use "sex education" throughout. However, I want to acknowledge the importance of this shift in terminology, since it is a statement about sexuality educators' recognition of the broader nature of their field.

The subset of programs and curricula that have emerged as a result of AFLA are variously known as "abstinence-only," "abstinence-until-marriage," and "abstinence-only-until-marriage" programs. Both supporters and detractors occasionally call these programs "chastity curricula." For consistency and brevity, I usually refer to them throughout as "abstinence-only."

The Christian Right is an umbrella term that refers to conservative Catholics, conservative evangelicals, and Christian fundamentalists. When I refer to specific cohorts, I employ definitions that are consistent with sociologist Nancy Ammerman's usage in "North American Protestant Fundamentalism."[3] In brief, conservative Christians share a supernatural interpretation of events such as the virgin birth and the resurrection of Jesus. Evangelicalism consists of a broad group of people who have undergone a born-again experience of salvation through Jesus Christ, and who share the mandate to win souls to Christ. Although there is a long and important tradition of liberal evangelicalism, I use the term in this book to refer to conservative evangelicals. Fundamentalists are a subgroup of evangelicals. While they share with evangelicals the conversion experience and mandate to witness, fundamentalists also believe in an inerrant Bible. Consistent with sociologist Christian Smith's research, I also found that few of those I interviewed who fit this definition of fundamentalism either understood the term or identified with it.[4] Therefore, I generally use the term "evangelical" since it encompasses both groups, unless I am referring to a particular belief system or to a group or a person who has embraced a fundamentalist identity. Often throughout the text I refer to the combined cohorts of sex education opponents as "conservatives." This is mainly for brevity. However, the term underscores that social conservatism is generally what links comprehensive sex education opponents, who might otherwise come from diverse religious and political locations.

Finally, I approach the culture wars over sex education as a form of discursive politics. Although I discuss sexual speech throughout the book, I use the term discourse not in the tradition of linguistic analysis wherein discourse refers to spoken or written language. Rather, I use the term to mean broad, socially produced ways of structuring and circulating meaning and knowledge. In this way, discourse is not interchangeable with rhetoric and speech, on the one hand, or culture, on the other hand. In my use of the various terms, rhetoric (the persuasive use of language), language, speech, and talk are all expressive elements of discourse as social action. I argue, as well, that emotional conventions are part of discourse. I consider discourses to be linked to particular social institutions or organizations, for example, the Christian Right's sex education discourses.

# OPPONENTS OF
# COMPREHENSIVE SEX EDUCATION

Below is a sampling of the most prominent organizations which oppose comprehensive sexuality education.

American Center for Law and Justice
Virginia Beach, Va.

American Family Association
Tupelo, Miss.

Campus Crusade for Christ
   International
Orlando, Fla.

Christian Coalition
Chesapeake, Va.

Christian Womanity Educational
   Fund
Pleasant Hill, Calif.

Committee on the Status of Women
Golf, Ill.

Concerned Women for America
Washington, D.C.

Eagle Forum
Alton, Ill.

Educational Guidance Institute
Arlington, Va.

Educational Research Analysts
Longview, Tex.

Family Research Council
Washington, D.C.

Focus on the Family
Colorado Springs, Colo.

Free Teens USA
Westwood, N.J.

Heritage Foundation
Washington, D.C.

Human Life International
Front Royal, Va.

Institute for the Scientific Investigation of Sexuality/Family Research Institute
Madison, Wis.

John Birch Society
Appleton, Wis.

Josh McDowell Ministry
Dallas, Tex.

Medical Institute for Sexual Health
Austin, Tex.

National Abstinence Clearinghouse
Sioux Falls, S.Dak.

National Association for Abstinence Education
Falls Church, Va.

National Association of Christian Educators/Citizens for Excellence in Education
Costa Mesa, Calif.

National Coalition for Abstinence Education
Colorado Springs, Colo.

Research Council on Ethnopsychology
Santa Monica, Calif.

Rutherford Institute
Charlottesville, Va.

STOP Planned Parenthood International
Stafford, Va.

Traditional Values Coalition
Anaheim, Calif.

Unification Movement
New York, N.Y.

# NOTES

## INTRODUCTION

1.  Paul Richter and Marlene Cimons, "Clinton Fires Surgeon General over New Flap," *Los Angeles Times*, 10 December 1994, A36.

2.  The Communications Decency Act (CDA) of 1996 criminalized sending minors "indecent" Internet communications, such as those that describe sexual activities. For an analysis of the CDA, see Marjorie Heins, *Not in Front of the Children* (New York: Hill and Wang, 2001). For a letter of Christian Right leaders in support of the CDA, see Ed Meese, Donald Wildmon (American Family Association), Phyllis Schlafly (Eagle Forum), Louis Sheldon (Traditional Values Coalition), Paul Weyrich (Free Congress Foundation), Len Munsil (National Family Legal Foundation), Kenneth Sukhia (former U.S. Attorney), Ralph Reed (Christian Coalition), Alan Sears (former executive director of the Attorney General's Commission on Pornography), Beverly LaHaye (Concerned Women for America), Jay Sekulow (American Center for Law and Justice), Paul McGeady (Morality in Media), and Robert Peters (Morality in Media), letter to the Honorable Thomas J. Bleley Jr., Chairman of the Committee on Commerce, 16 October 1995; also "Christian Right Asks Stronger Cyberporn Controls," *Communications Daily* 15, no. 214 (6 November 1995). See also Chip Berlet, "Clinton, Conspiracism, and the Continuing Culture War," *The Public Eye* 13, no. 1 (spring 1999); Jean Hardisty, *Mobilizing Resentment* (Boston: Beacon Press, 1999); Family Research Council, "FRC Applauds Efforts to

Protect Our Families from Porn on the Internet" (Washington, D.C.: Family Research Council, July 26, 1995, press release).

3. I refer to sex education conflicts as "culture wars" and consider them a form of discursive politics. This approach to the culture wars differs from that of many sociologists, some of whom emphasize polarized attitudes of Americans while others dismiss the existence of culture wars altogether. In Chapter 7 I advance a model for thinking about discursive politics of the culture wars which acknowledges the central role of emotions, on both the individual and collective levels. Intense and episodic controversies involving sexuality have also been called "moral panics" or "sex panics." Although these terms are useful, I have decided not to use them. By the inclusion of the word "panic," these concepts do flag the significance of emotions. However, there are aspects of these terms that are inconsistent with my model of local culture wars. For one, "panic" suggests a collectively overpowering emotion, and I argue that culture wars are occasions for the production of a more complicated range of feelings, such as anger, disgust, and shock. Moreover, the term "moral panic" generally implies a disproportionate, misguided, even irrational response, which is an assumption I challenge in my discussion of conspicuous displays of emotion. See James Davison Hunter, *Culture Wars: The Struggle to Define America* (New York: Basic Books, 1991); Rhys Williams, ed., *Cultural Wars in American Politics* (New York: Aldine De Gruyter, 1997); and for a review of these debates, see Amy Binder, "Culture Wars in American Politics," *Contemporary Sociology* 27, no. 4 (1998): 386. On discursive politics, see Mary Katzenstein, *Faithful and Fearless* (Princeton, N.J.: Princeton University Press, 1998); and Ernesto Laclau and Chantal Mouffe, *Hegemony and Socialist Strategy* (London: Verso, 1985), although these authors use the term to refer to contests over cognitive meanings.

4. Samuel R. Delany, "The Rhetoric of Sex, the Discourse of Desire," in *Heterotopia: Postmodern Utopia and the Body Politic*, ed. Tobin Siebers (Ann Arbor: University of Michigan Press, 1994), 242.

5. "Sex O'Clock in America," *Current Opinion* 55 (1913): 113–14.

6. S. Robert Lichter et al., *The Rude and the Crude: Profanity in Popular Entertainment* (Washington, D.C.: Center for Media and Public Affairs, 1999).

7. Dale Kunkel et al., "Sex on TV" (University of California, Santa Barbara, Henry J. Kaiser Foundation, February 2001). Available on the Internet at www.kff.org/content/archive/1457/sex_rp .html.

8.  Michael Carrera et al., "Knowledge about Reproduction, Contraception, and Sexually Transmitted Infections among Young Adolescents in American Cities," *Social Policy* (spring 2000): 41–50.

9.  Esther D. Schulz and Sally R. Williams, *Family Life and Sex Education: Curriculum and Instruction* (New York: Harcourt, Brace and World, 1968), see chap. 4, "Questions Children Ask," pp. 25–46.

10. Ibid., chap. 4.

11. This question was asked by a high school student at a Massachusetts Department of Education workshop held on 25 March 2000 at Tufts University.

12. Susan Wilson, "Learning from Teens' Questions," *Family Life Matters* no. 41 (fall 2000): 2, a publication of Network for Family Life Education.

13. Alan Hunt, *Governing Morals: A Social History of Moral Regulation* (Cambridge: Cambridge University Press, 1999); Nicola Beisel, *Imperiled Innocents* (Princeton, N.J.: Princeton University Press, 1997); Allan Brandt, *No Magic Bullet: A Social History of Venereal Disease in the United States since 1880* (New York: Oxford University Press, 1985); David Pivar, *Purity Crusade* (Westport, Conn.: Greenwood Press, 1973).

14. John D'Emilio and Estelle Freedman, *Intimate Matters: A History of Sexuality in America* (New York: Harper and Row, 1988), 155.

15. Ibid.

16. Lester Kirdendall, "The Journey Toward SIECUS: 1964," *SIECUS Report* 12, no. 4 (March 1984): 1.

17. SIECUS describes comprehensive sexuality education as comprised of four basic objectives: information; attitudes, values, and insights; relationships and interpersonal skills; and responsibility. See Debra Haffner and Diane de Mauro, "Winning the Battle: Developing Support for Sexuality and HIV/AIDS Education" (New York: SIECUS, 1991).

18. Hunter, *Culture Wars*, 43.

19. There is a difference in how researchers view this phenomenon, which is aptly described by William Gamson as "whether the glass is half-empty to half-full." In response to data which consistently show low levels of political knowledge and social scientists who emphasize how Americans are uninformed, Gamson argues that "people are not so passive, people are not so dumb." See William Gamson, *Talking Politics* (New York: Cambridge University Press, 1992); John R. Zaller, *The Nature and Origins of Mass Opinion* (New York: Cambridge University Press, 1992); Benjamin Page and Robert Shapiro, *The Rational Public* (Chicago: University of Chicago Press, 1992).

20.    Among some critics, a fixed, essentialist model of attitudes has given
       way to one in which attitudes are not internal "ghostly entities," but
       rather are fluid and culturally mediated. Popular opinion surveys of
       the type generally used during culture wars measure attitudes as seem-
       ingly stable mental constructs that determine the individual's "true"
       responses to a range of often controversial topics such as abortion and
       gay rights. Many survey researchers consider individual attitudes to be
       stable structures. Even from this point of view—that attitudes are rel-
       atively fixed mental states—measurements of these attitudes are com-
       plicated and often flawed. For example, polls often show Americans
       holding inconsistent, contradictory views. And citizens demonstrate a
       willingness to proffer opinions to pollsters on topics about which they
       admit to knowing little or nothing. These methodological dilemmas
       raise the conceptual question of what exactly is being measured and
       what specifically, if anything, survey data on controversial issues tell us
       about Americans. Political scientist John Zaller argues that individuals
       hold not one but multiple opinions on an issue, depending on which
       interpretive schema they mobilize in the moment. He further suggests
       that "attitudes" as such do not exist; rather, people make "attitude
       reports" or "survey responses." Survey research captures a particular
       response at a particular moment, as evidenced by the pronounced
       inconsistency of Americans' reported attitudes.
           Attitudes have an important affective component. They are situa-
       tional expressions in which the respondent is in both an internal and
       external dialogue shaped by multiple factors such as the particularities
       of the researcher, the order of questions, the amount and type of prior
       information on the topic, the predispositions of the respondent
       (which might be religious beliefs), and even the current mood. Frames
       and emotional expectations operating in local culture wars exacerbate
       this matrix of contingencies. These perspectives, which allow us to see
       the discursive existence of attitudes and therefore their cultural con-
       tingency, help us understand how communities can erupt into some-
       times violent conflict even though most residents tell pollsters that
       they support sex education programs. See, for example, Zaller, *Nature
       and Origins of Mass Opinion;* George Bishop et al., "Pseudo-Opinions
       on Public Affairs," *Public Opinion Quarterly* 44, no. 2 (summer 1980):
       198–209; John Shotter and Michael Billig, "A Bakhtinian Psychology,"
       in *Bakhtin and the Human Sciences,* ed. Michael Bell and Michael Gar-
       diner (Thousand Oaks, Calif.: Sage Publications, 1998), 13–29; Carroll
       Glynn et al., *Public Opinion* (Boulder, Colo.: Westview Press, 1999);

and Anna Greenberg, "Public Opinion Makes Better Sense without the Opinion Makers," *Chronicle of Higher Education*, 14 May 1999, B8–B9. See also Edward Laumann et al., *The Social Organization of Sexuality* (Chicago: University of Chicago Press, 1994).

21. In very different studies, James Davison Hunter and Arlene Stein describe this polarizing process. See Hunter, *Culture Wars;* and Arlene Stein, *The Stranger Next Door* (Boston: Beacon Press, 2001).

22. Tina Hoff et al., *Sex Education in America* (Menlo Park, Calif.: Henry J. Kaiser Foundation, September 2000); Hickman-Brown Public Opinion Research Survey, March 1999. Commissioned by SIECUS and Advocates for Youth, available from SIECUS (130 W. 42nd Street, Suite 350, New York, N.Y. 10036) and Advocates for Youth (1025 Vermont Avenue N.W., Suite 200, Washington, D.C. 20005). Hickman-Brown surveyed 1,050 adults nationwide in February through March 1999. See also "The Thirtieth Annual Phi Delta Kappa/Gallup Poll of the Public's Attitudes toward the Public Schools," *Phi Delta Kappan*, September 1998, 54; and Kaiser Family Foundation, *National Survey of Public Secondary School Principals: The Politics of Sex Education* (Menlo Park, Calif.: Henry J. Kaiser Family Foundation, December 1999); Planned Parenthood Federation of America, "Public Attitudes toward Teenage Pregnancy, Sex Education, and Birth Control" (Louis Harris and Associates, 1988); A. M. Gallup and D. L. Clark, "The Nineteenth Annual Gallup Poll of the Public's Attitudes toward the Public Schools," *Gallup Polls* 69, no. 1 (September 1987); Stanley Elam, ed., *Gallup Polls of Attitudes toward Education, 1969–1984: A Topical Summary* (Bloomington, Ind.: Phi Delta Kappa, 1984).

23. Kaiser, *Sex Education*, 4.

24. Hickman-Brown Public Opinion Research Survey, "Thirtieth Annual Phi Delta Kappa/Gallup Poll," 54.

25. See Chip Berlet and Matthew Lyons, *Right-Wing Populism in America: Too Close for Comfort* (New York: Guilford, 2000); Hardisty, *Mobilizing Resentment*; and Rick Perlstein, *Before the Storm: Barry Goldwater and the Unmaking of the American Consensus* (New York: Hill and Wang, 2001).

26. See Berlet and Lyons, *Right-Wing Populism;* Ellen Messer-Davidow, "Manufacturing the Attack on Liberalized Higher Education," *Social Text* 36 (1993): 40–80; and Barbara Cruikshank, "Cultural Politics: Political Theory and the Foundations of Democratic Order," in *Cultural Studies and Political Theory*, ed. Jodi Dean (Ithaca, N.Y.: Cornell University Press, 2000), 63–79.

27. Pat Buchanan, 17 August 1992, Republican National Convention Speech, "Buchanan Urges His Brigade to Stand Beside the President," *Congressional Quarterly*, 22 August 1992, 2,543.

28. Institute for Cultural Conservatism/Free Congress Research and Education Foundation, *Cultural Conservatism: Toward a New Agenda* (Washington, D.C.: Institute for Cultural Conservatism/Free Congress Research and Education Foundation, 1987).

29. Robert Bork, *Slouching towards Gomorrah* (New York: Regan Books, 1996).

30. Stein, *Stranger Next Door*.

31. On the importance of discourse and language for social movements, see, for example, Norman Fairclough, *Discourse and Social Change* (Malden, Mass.: Polity Press, 1992); Michel Foucault, *The History of Sexuality, Vol. 1: An Introduction* (New York: Random House, 1978); Dominique Masson, "Language, Power, and Politics: Revisiting the Symbolic Challenge of Movements," *Alternate Routes* 13 (1996): 67–99; Marc Steinberg, "Tilting the Frame: Considerations on Collective Action Framing from a Discursive Turn," *Theory and Society* 27, no. 6 (December 1998): 845–72; Pierre Bourdieu, *Language and Symbolic Power* (Cambridge: Harvard University Press, 1982); and Jacob Torfing, *New Theories of Discourse* (Malden, Mass.: Blackwell, 1999).

32. William Gamson, *Talking Politics* (New York: Cambridge University Press, 1992).

33. Ann Swidler, "Cultural Power and Social Movements," in *Social Movements and Culture*, ed. Hank Johnston and Bert Klandermans (Minneapolis: University of Minnesota Press, 1995).

34. See the classic essay on this topic by Gayle Rubin, "Thinking Sex: Notes for a Radical Theory of the Politics of Sexuality," in *Pleasure and Danger*, ed. Carole S. Vance (Boston: Routledge and Kegan Paul, 1984), 267–319.

35. Michael Warner, *The Trouble with Normal* (New York: Free Press, 1999), 21.

36. Anne Higonnet, *Pictures of Innocence: The History and Crisis of Ideal Childhood* (New York: Thames and Hudson, 1998). See also Phillipe Aries, *Centuries of Childhood: A Social History of Family Life*, trans. Robert Baldick (New York: Knopf, 1962); and James Kincaid, *Child-Loving: The Erotic Child and Victorian Culture* (New York: Routledge, 1992).

37. Higonnet, *Pictures of Innocence*.

38. Richter and Cimons, "Clinton Fires Surgeon."

1.  Mary Breasted, *Oh! Sex Education!* (New York: Praeger, 1970), 241.

2.  Unlike Planned Parenthood Federation of America (PPFA), which is a provider of a broad range of reproductive health services, SIECUS focuses strictly on sexuality education. However, sex education in the public schools was never SIECUS's primary mission, despite the many attacks directed at the organization for this. In contrast, PPFA founded an education department in 1979, and its educators went directly into school classrooms to provide sexuality education.

3.  Jeffrey Moran, *Teaching Sex* (Cambridge: Harvard University Press, 2000), 160.

4.  Michel Foucault, *The History of Sexuality, Vol. 1: An Introduction* (New York: Random House, 1978).

5.  Moran, *Teaching Sex*, 160.

6.  Oregon and Michigan had had mandatory programs since the late 1940s. Evanston's (Illinois) Family Life Education program was an interdisciplinary course integrated into the overall curriculum starting in kindergarten. In Anaheim, California, school nurse Sally Williams was embarking on a broad Family Life and Sex Education program that proposed to teach high school students not only about anatomy and physiology, but also about pregnancy, parenting, and controversial topics including masturbation, homosexuality, and abortion. See Moran, *Teaching Sex*; Walter Goodman, "The New Sex Education," *Redbook*, September 1967, 63–142; Joseph N. Bell, "Why the Revolt against Sex Education?" *Good Housekeeping*, November 1969, 93–193; Leonard Gross, "Sex Education Comes of Age," *Look*, 8 March 1966, 21–24; and James Whitely, "Sex Education," *Report*, October 1966, 16–21.

7.  Whitely, "Sex Education," 19.

8.  Sally Williams, telephone interview with author, 11 June 1996.

9.  Ira Reiss, telephone interview with author, 9 May 1995.

10. Rose Somerville, "Family Life and Sex Education in the Turbulent Sixties," *Journal of Marriage and the Family* 33, no. 1 (February 1971): 11–35.

11. See Somerville, "Family Life"; Harold Lief, "What Your Doctor Probably Doesn't Know about Sex," *Harper's Magazine*, December 1964, 92–96.

12. Esther Schulz, telephone interview with author, 20 January 1997.

13. Goodman, "New Sex Education," 63.

14. Bernhardt Gottlieb, *What a Girl Should Know about Sex* (1961), cited in Patricia J. Campbell, *Sex Education Books for Young Adults, 1892–1979* (New York: R. R. Bowker Company, 1979), 110.

15. Campbell, *Sex Education Books,* 110.

16. John D'Emilio and Estelle Freedman, *Intimate Matters: A History of Sexuality in America* (New York: Harper and Row, 1988), 256.

17. Rickie Solinger, *Wake up Little Susie: Single Pregnancy and Race before Roe v. Wade* (New York: Routledge, 1992), 211.

18. See Rickie Solinger, *The Abortionist* (New York: Free Press, 1994); Rosalind Petchesky, *Abortion and Woman's Choice* (New York: Longman, 1984).

19. Solinger, *Wake Up Little Susie,* 206.

20. Lilli Vincenz, quoted in Rodger Streitmatter, *Unspeakable: The Rise of the Gay and Lesbian Press in America* (Boston: Faber and Faber, 1995), 62.

21. "The Second Sexual Revolution," *Time,* 24 January 1964, 54.

22. See, for example, Susan J. Douglas, *Where the Girls Are: Growing up Female with the Mass Media* (New York: Times Books, 1994); D'Emilio and Freedman, *Intimate Matters;* and Todd Gitlin, *The Sixties: Years of Hope, Days of Rage* (New York: Bantam Books, 1987).

23. "The Morals Revolution on the U.S. Campus," *Newsweek,* 6 April 1964, 54.

24. Lillian Faderman, *Odd Girls and Twilight Lovers* (New York: Penguin, 1992).

25. Streitmatter, *Unspeakable,* 55.

26. D'Emilio and Freedman, *Intimate Matters.*

27. Anthony Lewis, "Sex . . . and the Supreme Court," *Esquire Magazine,* June 1963, 82.

28. James Skinner, *The Cross and the Cinema: The Legion of Decency and the National Catholic Office for Motion Pictures, 1933–1970* (Westport, Conn.: Praeger, 1993). See also Charles Lyons, "The Paradox of Protest," in *Movie Censorship and American Culture,* ed. Francis G. Couvares (Washington, D.C.: Smithsonian Institution Press, 1996), 277–318.

29. Gitlin, *Sixties.*

30. Barbara Ehrenreich, Elizabeth Hess, and Gloria Joseph, *Remaking Love: The Feminization of Sex* (New York: Anchor Press, 1986), 6.

31. Douglas, *Where the Girls Are,* 81.

32. A survey from Purdue University cited in Campbell, *Sex Education Books,* 113. In *Sexual Behavior in the 1970s* (Chicago: Playboy Press,

1974), Morton Hunt describes his own survey in which school programs account for 3 percent of sexual information for males and 5 percent for females. Friends are the most frequently cited source of information for young people.

33. Mary Calderone, oral history conducted by Deborah Tolman, 2 July 1987.

34. Calderone, oral history conducted by Tolman, 6 July 1987.

35. Nat Lehrman, "Playboy Interview: Dr. Mary Calderone," *Playboy*, April 1970, 63–78, 154, 236–40.

36. Esther Schulz, telephone interview with author, 20 January 1997.

37. Letter to Mary Calderone, 11 March 1971. #179, Box 14, Folder 230. Mary Steichen Calderone Papers. Schlesinger Library, Radcliffe Institute, Harvard University.

38. David Allyn, *Make Love, Not War: The Sexual Revolution, an Unfettered History* (New York: Little, Brown, 2000), 108–18.

39. Ibid.

40. John Gagnon, interview with author, New York City, 2 April 1995.

41. Mary Calderone, oral history conducted by James Reed. Family Planning Oral History Project, 7 August 1974. Schlesinger Library, Radcliffe Institute, Harvard University.

42. Allyn, *Make Love, Not War*.

43. Elliot Bernstein, producer, "Dirty Old Woman," *60 Minutes* 14, no. 4 (CBS Television Network, transcript of episode that aired on Sunday, 25 October 1981).

44. Calderone, oral history conducted by Tolman, 1 July 1987.

45. "The SIECUS Purpose," *SIECUS Report* 1, no. 1 (February 1965): 2.

46. For example, in a telephone interview with the author on 23 May 1995, Peggy Brick discussed her early work that emphasized social sciences. Williams, interview.

47. Calderone, oral history conducted by Tolman, 22 July 1987.

48. Gagnon, interview.

49. Lehrman, "Playboy Interview."

50. Calderone, oral history conducted by Tolman, 6 July 1987.

51. Debra Haffner, interview with author, New York City, 3 March 1992.

52. Reiss, interview.

53. Calderone, oral history conducted by James Reed. Family Planning Oral History Project.

54. Janice M. Irvine, *Disorders of Desire* (Philadelphia: Temple University Press, 1990).

55. Douglas, *Where the Girls Are*, 66.

56.     James W. Ramey, "Dealing with the Last Taboo," *SIECUS Report* 7, no. 5 (May 1979): 4; "Attacking the Last Taboo," *Time*, 14 April 1980, 72; George Will, "A Researcher Puts in a Good Word for Incest," *Washington Post*, 22 May 1980, A17; Susan Sawyer, "Lifting the Veil on the Last Taboo," *Family Health* 12, no. 6 (June 1980); Benjamin DeMott, "The Pro-Incest Lobby," *Psychology Today* (March 1980): 11–18; John Leo, "Cradle-to-Grave Intimacy," *Time*, 7 September 1981, 69.

57.     Deborah Roffman, telephone interview with author, 18 July 1995. Schulz, interview.

58.     Lehrman, "Playboy Interview."

59.     Schulz, interview.

60.     Calderone, oral history conducted by Tolman, 22 July 1987.

61.     Bernstein, "Dirty Old Woman."

62.     Calderone, oral history conducted by James Reed. Family Planning Oral History Project.

63.     Calderone, oral history conducted by Tolman, 22 July 1987.

64.     Ibid.

65.     Bernstein, "Dirty Old Woman."

66.     Calderone, oral history conducted by Tolman, 23 July 1987.

67.     Mary Calderone, "SIECUS: Its Present and Its Future," *SIECUS Report* 1, no. 2 (summer 1965): 1.

68.     Mary Calderone, Letter to Sec. Califano, 27 July 1978. #179. Mary Steichen Calderone Papers.

69.     Letter to Mary Calderone, 19 March 1969. #179, Box 14, Folder 230. Mary Steichen Calderone Papers.

70.     Letter to Mary Calderone. 7 May 1970. #179, Box 14, Folder 230. Mary Steichen Calderone Papers.

71.     This and related quotes in this paragraph from Mary Calderone, "Sex and Social Responsibility," *Journal of Home Economics* 57, no. 7 (September 1965): 500.

72.     See, for example, Lehrman, "Playboy Interview."

73.     Mary Calderone, personal correspondence, 5 March 1979. From SIECUS archives.

74.     Laura Kipnis, *Bound and Gagged: Pornography and the Politics of Fantasy in America* (New York: Grove Press, 1996), 131.

75.     Calderone, oral history conducted by Tolman, 1 July 1987.

76.     Ibid.

77.     Calderone, oral history conducted by Tolman, 6 July 1987.

78.     Bernstein, "Dirty Old Woman."

79.     Calderone, oral history conducted by Tolman, 14 July 1987.

80. Calderone, oral history conducted by Tolman, 23 July 1988.

81. Lester Kirkendall, Letter to SIECUS Board, SIECUS archives, n.d.

82. Isadore Rubin, Letter to SIECUS Board, SIECUS archives, n.d.

83. Foucault, *History of Sexuality.*

84. Calderone, oral history conducted by Tolman, 23 July 1987.

85. See Rick Perlstein, *Before the Storm: Barry Goldwater and the Unmaking of the American Consensus* (New York: Hill and Wang, 2001); Mary C. Brennan, *Turning Right in the Sixties: The Conservative Capture of the GOP* (Chapel Hill: University of North Carolina Press, 1995). See also William Martin, *With God on Our Side: The Rise of the Religious Right in America* (New York: Broadway Books, 1996); and Allen Hunter, "Virtue with a Vengeance: The Pro-Family Politics of the New Right" (Ph.D. diss., Brandeis University, 1985).

86. Gary K. Clabaugh, *Thunder on the Right: The Protestant Fundamentalists* (Chicago: Nelson-Hall Company, 1974).

87. Gagnon, interview.

88. Mary Calderone, oral history conducted by James Reed. Family Planning Oral History Project.

## 2. DAYS OF RAGE

1. Leonard Gross, "Sex Education Comes of Age," *Look*, 8 March 1966, 21.

2. Joseph N. Bell, "Why the Revolt against Sex Education?" *Good Housekeeping*, November 1969, 93.

3. Mary Calderone, oral history conducted by James Reed. Family Planning Oral History Project, August 7, 1974. Schlesinger Library, Radcliffe Institute, Harvard University.

4. Todd Gitlin, *The Sixties: Years of Hope, Days of Rage* (New York: Bantam Books, 1987), 341.

5. Beth Bailey, *Sex in the Heartland* (Cambridge: Harvard University Press, 1999).

6. John D'Emilio and Estelle Freedman, *Intimate Matters: A History of Sexuality in America* (New York: Harper and Row, 1988).

7. Dick Kagan, "Movies Are Gayer Than Ever," *Women's Wear Daily*, 29 April 1969, 30.

8. Billy James Hargis, telephone interview with author, 13 March 1997.

9. Beatrice Gudridge, *Sex Education in Schools, Education U.S.A. Special Report* (Washington, D.C.: National School Public Relations Association, 1969).

10. Esther Schulz, telephone interview with author, 20 January 1997.

11. Mary Calderone, "Planning for Sex Education," *NEA Journal* (January 1967): 29.

12. "Public Opinion Study Concerning Sex Education in Junior and Senior High Schools" (conducted during November 1963 for the Citizens' Advisory Committee of Anaheim Union High School District, mimeographed document).

13. Tom Newsom, "Students: How They Are Reacting," *Times-Democrat* (Davenport, Iowa), 7 May 1969.

14. Sally Williams, telephone interview with author, 11 June 1996.

15. Mary Breasted, *Oh! Sex Education!* (New York: Praeger, 1970). Also, Eleanor Howe, interview conducted for *With God on Our Side: The Rise of the Religious Right in America*, prod. Calvin Skaggs, Lumiere Productions, 1996, videocassette.

16. See, for example, Gudridge, *Sex Education in Schools;* American School Health Association, Committee on Health Guidance in Sex Education, "Growth Patterns and Sex Education: A Suggested Program, Kindergarten through Grade Twelve," *Journal of School Health* 37 (1967): 1–136.

17. "Facing the 'Facts of Life,'" *Life*, 19 September 1969, 34.

18. From the Illinois guidelines passed in 1965, see pp. 6–12 in Gudridge, *Sex Education in Schools*.

19. Ibid., 8.

20. Breasted, *Oh! Sex Education!*, 111.

21. Ibid.

22. Ibid.

23. "Facing the 'Facts of Life,'" 34.

24. "A Fight Rages over Sex Education," *National Observer*, 9 June 1969, 1.

25. Williams, interview.

26. William Martin, *With God on Our Side: The Rise of the Religious Right in America* (New York: Broadway Books, 1996), 88.

27. Mary Brennan, *Turning Right in the Sixties: The Conservative Capture of the GOP* (Chapel Hill: University of North Carolina Press, 1995).

28. Allen Hunter, "Virtue with a Vengeance: The Pro-Family Politics of the New Right" (Ph.D. diss., Brandeis University, 1985), 83. See also Rick Perlstein, *Before the Storm: Barry Goldwater and the Unmaking of the American Consensus* (New York: Hill and Wang, 2001).

29. Martin, *With God on Our Side*, 76.

30. Ibid., 91.

31. Sara Diamond, *Roads to Dominion: Right-Wing Movements and Political Power in the United States* (New York: Guilford Press, 1995), 92.

32. Many scholars have noted the vital importance of an infrastructure to the political rise of the New Right and the Religious Right. See, for example, Diamond, *Roads to Dominion;* Martin, *With God on Our Side;* Nancy Ammerman, "North American Protestant Fundamentalism," in *Fundamentalisms Observed,* ed. Martin E. Marty and R. Scott Appleby (Chicago: University of Chicago Press, 1991), 1–65; and Jean Hardisty, "The Resurgent Right: Why Now?" *The Public Eye* 9, nos. 3–4 (fall–winter 1995): 1–13.

33. For a discussion of racism, see Diamond, *Roads to Dominion;* Martin, *With God on Our Side;* Gary Clabaugh, *Thunder on the Right: The Protestant Fundamentalists* (Chicago: Nelson-Hall Company, 1974); and Peter Schrag, "America's Other Radicals," *Harper's Magazine,* August 1970, 35–46.

34. See, for example, Emile Durkheim, *The Elementary Forms of the Religious Life* (New York: Free Press, 1965); Daniel Bell, *The Winding Passage* (Cambridge, Mass.: Abt Books, 1980); and Peter Berger, *The Sacred Canopy* (Garden City, N.Y.: Anchor Books/Doubleday, 1969). In particular, see Andrew Greeley, *Religious Change in America* (Cambridge: Harvard University Press, 1989), for a discussion of data related to secularization.

35. See Ammerman, "North American Protestant Fundamentalism," 39; and Harvey Cox, *Fire from Heaven: The Rise of Pentecostal Spirituality and the Reshaping of Religion in the Twenty-First Century* (Reading, Mass.: Addison-Wesley, 1995).

36. Martin, *With God on Our Side*, 91.

37. "Roof Leaks, Sex Courses Are Taken up by Board," *Niagara Falls Gazette,* 15 April 1969.

38. "Sex Classes Arouse Sudden Opposition," *Springfield Ohio News,* 14 May 1969.

39. Schulz, interview.

40. Mary Calderone, oral history conducted by Deborah Tolman, 1 July 1987.

41. Clabaugh, *Thunder on the Right*, 120–22.

42. Diamond, *Roads to Dominion*. See also p. 83 in Martin, *With God on Our Side*, where Mark Hatfield estimated that one-third of Republican delegates at the 1964 Goldwater convention were John Birch Society members.

43. Diamond, *Roads to Dominion*, 55.

44. Richard Hofstadler, *The Paranoid Style in American Politics* (New York: Random House, 1965), 131.

45. John George and Laird Wilcox, *Nazis, Communists, Klansmen, and Others on the Fringe* (Buffalo, N.Y.: Prometheus Books, 1992), 204.

46. Clabaugh, *Thunder on the Right,* 87.

47. On the question of racism on the Right at that time, see Diamond, *Roads to Dominion;* Martin, *With God on Our Side;* Schrag, "America's Other Radicals," 35–46; and John Redekop, *The American Far Right: A Case Study of Billy James Hargis and Christian Crusade* (Grand Rapids, Mich.: William Eerdmans, 1968).

48. Martin, *With God on Our Side,* 78.

49. James Morris, *The Preachers* (New York: St. Martin's Press, 1973), 274.

50. Vyacheslav Nikitin, *The Ultras in the USA* (Moscow: Progress Publishers, 1971), 55.

51. See Morris, *Preachers,* 267. John Kohler, "Sex Invades the Schoolhouse," *Saturday Evening Post,* 29 June 1968, 23.

52. See George and Wilcox, *Nazis, Communists, Klansmen,* 210; Morris, *Preachers,* 269.

53. Reference to *Hustler* (May 1976) in George and Wilcox, *Nazis, Communists, Klansmen,* 212.

54. Ibid., 204–5.

55. *Christian Crusade Weekly,* August–September 1969, 29.

56. Lisa McGirr, *Suburban Warriors: The Origins of the New American Right* (Princeton, N.J.: Princeton University Press, 2001).

57. Jerry Buck, "Attacks Developed Suddenly on Sex Education Courses," *Royal Oak* (Michigan) *Tribune,* 14 May 1969, 5.

58. "A Fight Rages," 1.

59. Ibid.

60. Benwah Sparkes, "Sex Study Declared Not in Christian Framework," *Nashville Banner,* 21 March 1969.

61. Tom Newsom, "Parents: Emotion Is Running High," *Times-Democrat* (Davenport, Iowa), 5 May 1969, 19.

62. Ibid.

63. Walter Goodman, "The Controversy over Sex Education," *Redbook,* September 1969, 79.

64. American Education Lobby, "Sex Education: Assault on American Youth" (Washington, D.C.: American Education Lobby, special publication, n.d.).

65. John Leo, "Objections to Sex Education Not Confined to Right Wingers," *Warrensburg, N.Y., News,* 29 May 1969, 5.

66. Goodman, "Controversy over Sex Education," 195.

67. Eleanor Howe, telephone interview with author, 10 March 1997.

68. Ibid.

69. See Nancy MacLean, *Behind the Mask of Chivalry* (New York: Oxford University Press, 1994); and Kathleen Blee, *Women of the Klan* (Berkeley: University of California Press, 1991).

70. Athan Theoharis, *J. Edgar Hoover, Sex, and Crime* (Chicago: Ivan R. Dee, 1995).

71. Barry Werth, *The Scarlet Professor* (New York: Doubleday, 2001).

72. John Gagnon, interview with author, New York City, 2 April 1995.

73. Michael Warner, *The Trouble with Normal* (New York: Free Press, 1999), 23.

74. Claire Chambers, *The SIECUS Circle: A Humanist Revolution* (Belmont, Mass.: Western Islands, 1977), 98.

75. *Pavlov's Children: (They May Be Yours)*, pamphlet and video (Los Angeles, Calif.: Impact Publishers, 1969).

76. Billy James Hargis, interview conducted for *With God on Our Side: The Rise of the Religious Right in America,* prod. Calvin Skaggs, Lumiere Productions, 1996, videocassette.

77. Gordon Drake, *Is the School House the Proper Place to Teach Raw Sex?* (Tulsa, Okla.: Christian Crusade Publications, 1968).

78. See Clabaugh, *Thunder on the Right,* for a discussion of this history.

79. Drake, *School House,* 20.

80. Richard Cohen, "Foes Fail to End Sex Education Spread," *Washington Post,* 3 June 1969, C1.

81. Article by Frank Cappel in the *Herald of Freedom* inserted into the *Congressional Record,* 22 October 1969, 31147–48.

82. Chambers, *SIECUS Circle,* 128.

83. William Welt, "Sex Courses Tied to Red Plot by Area Decency Group Chief," *Utica Daily Press,* 25 February 1969, 11.

84. Eric Cavaliero, "Birchers Suspicious of Sex Educators," *Honolulu Advertiser,* 15 March 1969, A5.

85. Howe, interview.

86. Ibid. See also Breasted, *Oh! Sex Education!*

87. McGirr, *Suburban Warrior,* 6.

88. Roland Barthes, "The Reality Effect," in *French Literary Theory Today: A Reader,* ed. T. Todorov (Cambridge: Cambridge University Press, 1982), 11–17.

89. James Townsend, telephone interview with author, 10 March 1997.

90.    Christian Defense League, *Special Report*, No. 6., P.O. Box 493, Baton Rouge, La.

91.    Goodman, "Controversy over Sex Education," 194.

92.    Gordon Drake, *SIECUS—Corrupter of Youth* (Tulsa, Okla.: Christian Crusade Publications, 1969), 47. Emphasis in original.

93.    Renee Romano, *Erosion of a Taboo: Black-White Marriage in the United States from World War II to the Present* (Cambridge: Harvard University Press, 2003).

94.    Ibid.

95.    Drake, *SIECUS*, 46.

96.    Frank Sutherland, "Smears, Ignorance Cloud Issue of Sex Education," *Nashville Tennessean,* 30 March 1969, 1B.

97.    Sally Williams, telephone interview with author, 11 June 1996.

98.    Nat Lehman, "Playboy Interview: Dr. Mary Calderone," *Playboy*, April 1970, 66.

99.    Harold Lief, telephone interview with author, 16 June 1995.

100.   Lloyd Shearer, ed., "Intelligence Report," *Parade Magazine*, 2 November 1969, 26.

101.   Thomas J. Foley, "Attack on Sex Education Has Shaky Foundation," *Omaha World-Herald*, 1 May 1969.

102.   Ibid.

103.   Ibid.

104.   Townsend, interview.

105.   Clabaugh, *Thunder on the Right*, 46.

106.   From Episode One of *With God on Our Side: The Rise of the Religious Right in America,* prod. Calvin Skaggs, Lumiere Productions, 1966, videocassette.

107.   Mary Calderone, oral history conducted by James Reed. Family Planning Oral History Project.

108.   Howe, interview. See also Martin, *With God on Our Side*.

109.   See Goodman, "Controversy over Sex Education."

110.   Mike Hammer, "Teachers Using Pornographic Sex Material, Woman Claims," *Oklahoma City Times*, 23 January 1969.

111.   John Steinbacher, "Parent Reads Textbooks, Causes Gasps and Giggles at Sex Education Hearing," *Anaheim Bulletin*, 15 November 1968, 1.

112.   Calderone, oral history conducted by Tolman, 14 July 1987.

113.   Drake, *School House*, 2.

114.   See Lehman, "Playboy Interview," 66. See Breasted, *Oh! Sex Education!*, for other examples of selective quoting and distortion.

115. Chip Berlet, "Following the Threads," in *Unraveling the Right,* ed. Amy Ansel (New York: Westview Press, 1998), 17–40.

116. Goodman, "Controversy over Sex Education," 193.

117. Konstance McKaffree, telephone interview with author, 28 August 1996.

118. Calderone, oral history conducted by Tolman, 14 July 1987.

119. Martin, *With God on Our Side,* 116.

120. Hargis, interview.

121. Schulz, interview.

122. Richard Cohen, "Despite Opposition, Sex Education Spreads in Schools," *Washington Post,* 3 June 1969, C3.

123. James Hottois and Neal Milner, *The Sex Education Controversy: A Study of Politics, Education, and Morality* (Lexington, Mass.: Lexington Books, 1975).

124. Mary Calderone, oral history conducted by James Reed. Family Planning Oral History Project.

125. Douglas Robinson, "Sex Education Battles Splitting Many Communities across U.S.," *New York Times,* 14 September 1969, 77.

## 3. BORN-AGAIN SEXUAL POLITICS

1. William Martin, *With God on Our Side: The Rise of the Religious Right in America* (New York: Broadway Books, 1996), 211.

2. Ibid.

3. In their study of American extremist groups, John George and Laird Wilcox note that although distorting or actually fabricating quotations is commonly employed by extremists, "American leftists have used spuriosities of that sort sparingly, [while] groups and individuals on the far right have raised such utilizations to a high art form." George and Wilcox appended a series of such notable lies and distortions to their study. Recently, some evangelical Christians have launched critiques of their own movement. Two prominent Christian Right leaders, Ed Dobson and Cal Thomas, charged that in the political arena the movement as a whole plays fast and loose with the facts. Dobson said, "It puzzles me that the leaders of the Religious Right, who are most careful and precise in their theology when they speak in the church, are most careless and loose in their theology when they deal with politics. Many of their favorite ideas and statements are, at best, partially true and at worst, completely untrue." And a member of the Christian Coalition wrote of his dismay not only at discovering that "the religious right has exhibited the lower standard of scholarship"

but also that several leaders continued to use fabricated quotations even after being corrected. See John George and Laird Wilcox, *Nazis, Communists, Klansmen, and Others on the Fringe* (Buffalo, N.Y.: Prometheus Books, 1992), 415; Cal Thomas and Ed Dobson, *Blinded by Might: Can the Religious Right Save America?* (Grand Rapids, Mich.: Zondervan Publishing, 1999), 185; and Everette Hatcher III, "Questionable Quotes," *Freedom Writer Magazine*, May–June 1997, 9. See David Brock for an account of his duplicity on behalf of the right. David Brock, *Blinded by the Right* (New York: Ground Publishers, 2002)

4.   Susan Harding, *The Book of Jerry Falwell* (Princeton, N.J.: Princeton University Press, 2000).

5.   See Robert Wuthnow and Matthew Lawson, "Sources of Christian Fundamentalism in the United States," in *Accounting for Fundamentalisms: The Dynamic Character of Movements*, ed. Martin E. Marty and Scott Appleby (Chicago: University of Chicago Press, 1994), 18–56; and Nancy Ammerman, "Accounting for Christian Fundamentalisms: Social Dynamics and Rhetorical Strategies," in ibid., 149–72.

6.   This discussion draws on Sara Diamond, *Roads to Dominion: Right-Wing Movements and Political Power in the United States* (New York: Guilford Press, 1995); and Chip Berlet and Matthew Lyons, *Right-Wing Populism in America: Too Close for Comfort* (New York: Guilford Press, 2000).

7.   Martin, *With God on Our Side*, esp. 197 for a discussion of cobelligerency.

8.   Robert Liebman and Robert Wuthnow, eds., *The New Christian Right* (New York: Aldine De Gruyter, 1983).

9.   Lyman Kellstedt, John Green, James Guth, and Corwin Smidt, "Religious Voting Blocs in the 1992 Election" (paper presented at the annual meeting of the American Political Science Association, Washington, D.C., 1–4 September 1993).

10.  Gertrude Himmelfarb, *One Nation, Two Cultures* (New York: Knopf, 1999), 45.

11.  See Nancy Ammerman, "North American Protestant Fundamentalism," in *Fundamentalisms Observed*, ed. Martin E. Marty and R. Scott Appleby (Chicago: University of Chicago Press, 1991); and also Nancy Ammerman, *Bible Believers: Fundamentalists in the Modern World* (New Brunswick, N.J.: Rutgers University Press, 1987).

12.  Rosemary Ruether, *Christianity and the Making of the Modern Family* (Boston: Beacon Press, 2000).

13.  Martin, *With God on Our Side*, 163.

14.  For the text of the full plan, see Appendix C in Alice Rossi, *Feminists in Politics: A Panel Analysis of the First National Women's Conference* (New York: Academic Press, 1982).

15.  Lucy Komisar, "Feminism as National Politics," *The Nation,* 10 December 1977, 624–27.

16.  Kaye Northcott, "At War with the Pink Ladies," *Mother Jones,* November 1977, 21–28.

17.  Rossi, *Feminists in Politics.*

18.  Jo Ann Gasper, telephone interview with author, 21 July 1997.

19.  Allen Hunter, "Virtue with a Vengeance: The Pro-Family Politics of the New Right" (Ph.D. diss., Brandeis University, 1985), 185. This IWY discussion draws on ibid.; Martin, *With God on Our Side;* and Rossi, *Feminists in Politics.*

20.  Quoted in Hunter, "Virtue with a Vengeance," 157.

21.  Northcott, "At War with the Pink Ladies," 23.

22.  Nadine Brozan, "White House Conference on the Family: A Schism Develops," *New York Times,* 7 January 1980, D8.

23.  Ibid.

24.  Quoted in Hunter, "Virtue with a Vengeance," 257.

25.  Martin, *With God on Our Side,* 178.

26.  For example, Concerned Women for America, at 565,000 members, claims to be the largest women's organization in the United States but counts as a member anyone who has *ever* paid the membership fee. A *New York Times* exposé charged the Christian Coalition with inflating its membership rolls by listing dead people or anyone who had ever signed a petition or sent in a contribution. Christian Right leaders Cal Thomas and Ed Dobson admitted that most of the Moral Majority state chapters were simply a separate telephone line in the pastor's office. See Corwin Smidt, Lyman Kellstedt, John Green, and James Guth, "The Characteristics of Christian Political Activists," in *Christian Political Activism at the Crossroads,* ed. William Stevenson Jr. (Lanham, Md.: University Press of America, 1994), 141; Laurie Goodstein, "Coalition's Woes May Hinder Goals of Christian Right," *New York Times,* 2 August 1999, 1; and Thomas and Dobson, *Blinded by Might.*

27.  Robert W. Klous, ed., *The Traditional Values in Action Resource Directory: Family/Homeschool Edition* (Concord, Va.: Christian Values in Action Coalition, 1997).

28.  Robert W. Klous, ed., *The Traditional Values in Action Resource Directory* (Concord, Va.: Christian Values in Action Coalition, 1997–98).

29.  Klous, *Family/Homeschool Edition,* 2.

30. Robert Putnam, "Bowling Alone: America's Declining Social Capital," *Journal of Democracy* 6, no. 1 (1995): 65–78; James Coleman, "Social Capital in the Creation of Human Capital," *American Journal of Sociology* 94 (suppl.) (1988): 95–120. Also Robert Putnam, *Making Democracies Work* (Princeton, N.J.: Princeton University Press, 1993); and Robert Putnam, *Bowling Alone: Civic Disengagement in America* (New York: Simon and Schuster, 2000).

31. Beth Bailey, *Sex in the Heartland* (Cambridge: Harvard University Press, 1999), 6.

32. Theda Skocpol and Morris Fiorina, "Making Sense of the Civic Engagement Debate," in *Civic Engagement in American Democracy*, ed. Theda Skocpol and Morris Fiorina (Washington, D.C.: Brookings Institution Press, 1999), 1.

33. Theda Skocpol, "Advocates without Members: The Recent Transformations of American Civic Life," in *Civic Engagement*, ed. Skocpol and Fiorina, 471. Skocpol's analysis informs this section. See also Putnam, "Bowling Alone: America's Declining Social Capital," 65–78; John Ehrenberg, *Civil Society: The Critical History of an Idea* (New York: New York University Press, 1999); Everett Ladd, *The Ladd Report* (New York: Free Press, 1999); Robert Wuthnow, *Loose Connections: Joining Together in America's Fragmented Communities* (Cambridge: Harvard University Press, 1998).

34. See Jean Hardisty, *Mobilizing Resentment* (Boston: Beacon Press, 1999).

35. Rebecca Klatch, *A Generation Divided* (Berkeley: University of California Press, 1999).

36. Janet Benshoof, "Countering the Religious Right on Reproductive Rights: Legislative and Legal Strategies" (paper presented at the Third Annual Blackmun Lecture, Washington, D.C., 5 March 1999).

37. Planned Parenthood Federation of America, the National Abortion Rights Action League, and People for the American Way have all monitored sex education controversies at different periods, although this has entailed only a small arena of their work.

38. Frederick Clarkson, "Takin' It to the States: The Rise of Conservative State-Level Think Tanks," *Public Eye* 13, nos. 2–3 (summer–fall 1999): 1–13.

39. Theda Skocpol, "The Tocqueville Problem: Civic Engagement in American Democracy," *Social Science History* 21, no. 4 (winter 1997): 455–79.

40. Smidt et al., "Characteristics of Christian Political Activists," 133–63.

41. Julia Lesage, "Christian Coalition Leadership Training," in *Media,*

*Culture, and the Religious Right,* ed. Linda Kintz and Julia Lesage (Minneapolis: University of Minnesota Press, 1998), 295–325. See also Robert Boston, *The Most Dangerous Man in America? Pat Robertson and the Rise of the Christian Coalition* (Amherst, N.Y.: Prometheus Books, 1996).

42. Clarkson, "Takin' It to the States."

43. Allan Mayer et al., "A Tide of Born-Again," *Newsweek,* 15 September 1980, 29.

44. Quoted in Greg Goldin, "The 15 Per Cent Solution," *Village Voice,* 6 April 1993, 19.

45. Robert L. Simonds, *How to Elect Christians to Public Office* (Costa Mesa, Calif.: Citizens for Excellence in Education, rev. 1996).

46. Ibid., unpaginated introduction.

47. Ibid.

48. See Sara Diamond, *Roads to Dominion: Right-Wing Movements and Political Power in the United States* (New York: Guilford Press, 1995), 92. Also see Francis A. Schaeffer, *A Christian Manifesto* (Westchester, Ill.: Crossway Books, 1981); and Gary North and Gary DeMar, *Christian Reconstructionism? What It Is, What It Isn't* (Tyler, Tex.: Institute for Christian Economics, 1991).

49. Diamond, *Roads to Dominion,* 248–49.

50. See Lesage, "Christian Coalition."

51. Donna Minkowitz, "Brooklyn Dodgers," *Village Voice,* 6 April 1993, 21.

52. Pat Hoffman, Coordinator, Christian Coalition of Worcester County, Massachusetts, Letter, 25 February 1993.

53. James Dobson and Gary Bauer, *Children at Risk* (Dallas, Tex.: Word Publishing, 1990), quoted in John Detweiler, "The Religious Right's Battle Plan in the 'Civil War of Values,'" *Public Relations Review* 18, no. 3 (fall 1992): 247–55.

54. David Bennett, *The Party of Fear* (New York: Vintage Books, 1990).

55. There is vast scholarship on this but see, for example, Richard Hofstadter, *The Paranoid Style in American Politics* (New York: Knopf, 1965); Seymour Lipset and Earl Raab, *Politics of Unreason* (New York: Harper and Row, 1970); and Berlet and Lyons, *Right-Wing Populism.*

56. Berlet and Lyons, *Right-Wing Populism,* 226.

57. Rosalind Petchesky, *Abortion and Woman's Choice: The State, Sexuality, and Reproductive Freedom* (New York: Longman, 1984).

58. Ammerman, "Accounting for Christian Fundamentalisms," 150.

59. Jerry Falwell, quoted in Harding, *Book of Jerry Falwell,* 16, 163.

60. William Marshner and Enrique Rueda, *The Morality of Political*

*Action: Biblical Foundations* (Washington, D.C.: Free Congress Research and Education Foundation, 1984), 35.

61.  Ibid., 38.
62.  James Dobson, "Why I Use 'Fighting Words,'" *Christianity Today*, 19 June 1995, 28.
63.  Jerry Falwell, quoted in Harding, *Book of Jerry Falwell*, 16, 163.
64.  Roger Craver, president of the direct mail firm Craver, Mathews, and Smith of Washington, D.C., quoted in James Davison Hunter, *Culture Wars* (New York: Basic Books, 1991), 166.
65.  "From the Desk of Jerry Falwell," fund-raising letter, Lynchburg, Va., 1 November 1980.
66.  Falwell reported that the textbook *Life and Health* made statements such as "Contrary to past belief, masturbation is completely harmless and in fact can be quite useful in training oneself to respond sexually and to learn which particular forms of stimulation are most enjoyable." To establish the context Falwell intended, in the event that readers might not actually be shocked by such an excerpt, the top of the page featured a warning in large, bold type: "THIS MATERIAL DID NOT COME FROM PLAYBOY OR PENTHOUSE—BUT FROM A HIGH SCHOOL TEXTBOOK."
67.  Moral Majority, "Is Our Grand Old Flag Going down the Drain?" fund-raising letter, Washington, D.C., n.d.
68.  Moral Majority, "How Do We Stack Up?" ad run in *Conservative Digest*, quoted in *Group Research Report* 28, no. 2 (summer 1989).
69.  Harding, *Book of Jerry Falwell*, 15.
70.  Randy Engel, *Sex Education: The Final Plague* (Gaithersburg, Md.: Human Life International), 204.
71.  Quoted in Robert Boston, *The Most Dangerous Man in America? Pat Robertson and the Rise of the Christian Coalition* (Amherst, N.Y.: Prometheus Books, 1996), 176–77.
72.  Debra Haffner, interview with author, New York City, 3 March 1992.
73.  Petchesky, *Abortion and Woman's Choice*, 267.
74.  For an excellent analysis of the racist rhetoric of white supremacists, see Abby Ferber, *White Man Falling* (Lanham, Md.: Rowman & Littlefield, 1998).
75.  See Christian Smith, *Christian America?* (Berkeley: University of California Press, 2000); Christian Smith, *American Evangelicalism* (Chicago: University of Chicago Press, 1998); Judith Stacey, *Brave New Families* (New York: Basic Books, 1991); and Christel Manning,

*God Gave Us the Right* (New Brunswick, N.J.: Rutgers University Press, 1999).

76. Reuben Diaz, interview with author, New York City, 15 November 1994.

77. Harding, *Book of Jerry Falwell*, 275.

78. See Stacey, *Brave New Families*; and Manning, *God Gave Us the Right.*

79. See Smith, *Christian America?* and *American Evangelicalism;* and Mark Shibley, *Resurgent Evangelicalism in the United States* (Columbia: University of South Carolina Press, 1996).

80. Smith, *Christian America?*

81. Ibid.

82. See Smith, *Christian America?* and *American Evangelicalism.*

83. Stacey, *Brave New Families*, 145.

## 4. THE NEW SEXUAL REVOLUTION

1. Tim LaHaye, *The Battle for the Mind* (Old Tappan, N.J.: F. H. Revell Co., 1982).

2. Tim and Beverly LaHaye, *The Act of Marriage: The Beauty of Sexual Love* (Grand Rapids, Mich.: Zondervan Publishing, 1976).

3. Ibid. Also Tim LaHaye, telephone interview with author, 19 June 1997.

4. William Martin, *With God on Our Side: The Rise of the Religious Right in America* (New York: Broadway Books, 1996), 156.

5. LaHaye and LaHaye, *Act of Marriage*, 98–99.

6. See Thomas C. Fox, *Sexuality and Catholicism* (New York: George Braziller, 1995); Geoffrey Parrinder, *Sex in the World's Religions* (New York: Oxford University Press, 1980); Peter Gardella, *Innocent Ecstasy: How Christianity Gave America an Ethic of Sexual Pleasure* (New York: Oxford University Press, 1985); and *The Book of Common Prayer*, quoted in Gardella, *Innocent Ecstasy*, 5.

7. See Jeffrey Weeks, *Sexuality and Its Discontents: Meanings, Myths, and Modern Sexualities* (London: Routledge and Kegan Paul, 1985).

8. Gardella, *Innocent Ecstasy.*

9. Marabel Morgan, *The Total Woman* (New York: Pocket Books, 1973).

10. Lewis Smedes, *Sex for Christians* (Grand Rapids, Mich.: Eerdmans, 1976); and M. O. Vincent, *God, Sex, and You* (Trumpet Books, 1976).

11. Barbara Ehrenreich, Elizabeth Hess, and Gloria Jacobs, *Re-Making Love: The Feminization of Sex* (New York: Anchor Press, 1986), 135. See also Michael Campion, "Christian Sex Books: Countering Some Sincere Simplicity," *Christianity Today*, 12 June 1991, 28–31; and Lionel

Lewis and Dennis Brissett, "Sex as God's Work," *Society* (March–April 1986): 67–75.

12. Focus on the Family, *Sex, Lies, and the Truth* (Wheaton, Ill.: Tyndale House, 1994), 72.

13. Howard Moody, "Pleasure, Too, Is a Gift from God," *Christianity and Crisis*, 10 June 1985, 228.

14. Darlene Hayes-Tharpe and Shari Singer, prods., and Ron Weiner, dir., *The Phil Donahue Show*, WGN Continental Broadcasting Company, 1979.

15. LaHaye and LaHaye, *Act of Marriage*, 288.

16. Ibid., 21.

17. There are some differences among groups; for example, the LaHayes assert that birth control is acceptable as long as it is only used temporarily and not in order for a couple never to have children.

18. LaHaye and LaHaye, *Act of Marriage*, unpaginated introduction.

19. Lewis and Brissett, "Sex as God's Work," 69.

20. LeHaye and LeHaye, *Act of Marriage*, 11.

21. Ibid., 85.

22. Ibid.

23. See Lewis and Brissett, "Sex as God's Work." Also, the LaHayes's did their own survey and compared the results to a survey in *Redbook* magazine. See also Focus on the Family, *Sex, Lies, and the Truth*.

24. Marabel Morgan, telephone interview with author, 12 June 1997.

25. Ibid.

26. Ibid.

27. Ibid.

28. Ibid.

29. Barbara Harrison, "The Books That Teach Wives to Be Submissive," *McCalls*, June 1975.

30. Ehrenreich, Hess, and Jacobs, *Re-Making Love*, 159.

31. Mary S. Calderone, "Total Woman—Menace or Manna?" *SIECUS Report* (January 1976): 11.

32. Ibid.

33. See Martin Marty, "Fundies and Their Fetishes," *Christian Century*, 8 December 1976, 11.

34. LaHaye, interview.

35. Ibid.

36. See Nancy Tatom Ammerman, *Bible Believers: Fundamentalists in the Modern World* (New Brunswick, N.J.: Rutgers University Press, 1987); Martin E. Marty and R. Scott Appleby, eds., *Fundamentalisms*

*Observed* (Chicago: University of Chicago Press, 1991); Martin E. Marty and R. Scott Appleby, eds., *Fundamentalisms and Society* (Chicago: University of Chicago Press, 1993); and Martin E. Marty and R. Scott Appleby, eds., *Accounting for Fundamentalisms: The Dynamic Character of Movements* (Chicago: University of Chicago Press, 1994).

37. Marilyn Morris, *Abstinence: The New Sexual Revolution* (book series) (Dallas, Tex.: Aim for Success, 1995).

38. See Martin, *With God on Our Side;* and Sara Diamond, *Roads to Dominion: Right-Wing Movements and Political Power in the United States* (New York: Guilford Press, 1995).

39. This discussion of abortion draws on Rosalind Petchesky, *Abortion and Woman's Choice* (New York: Longman, 1984).

40. Martin, *With God on Our Side.*

41. U.S. Department of Health and Human Services, *Surgeon General's Report on Acquired Immune Deficiency Syndrome* (Washington, D.C., 1986), 31.

42. John Leo, "Sex and Schools," *Time,* 24 November 1986, 54.

43. Nan Hunter, interview with author, New York City, 5 March 1992.

44. Janet Benshoof, "The Chastity Act: Government Manipulation of Abortion Information and the First Amendment," *Harvard Law Review* 101 (1988): 1,916–37. See also Petchesky, *Abortion and Woman's Choice;* and Kristen Luker, *Dubious Conceptions: The Politics of Teenage Pregnancy* (Cambridge: Harvard University Press, 1996).

45. Janet Benshoof, interview with author, New York City, 1 March 1995.

46. Charles Moritz, ed., "Denton, Jeremiah A., Jr.," in *Current Biography Yearbook* (New York: H. W. Wilson Company, 1982), 92–95.

47. Ibid.

48. Ibid.

49. Jerome Chandler, "A Funny Thing Happened on the Way to Washington," *Saturday Evening Post,* January–February 1982, 32.

50. Ibid.

51. Ibid. See also Reauthorization of the Adolescent Family Life Demonstration Projects Act of 1981. Hearings before the Subcommittee on Family and Human Services of the Committee on Labor and Human Resources, United States Senate. Ninety-Eighth Congress. 24 and 26 August 1984. U.S. Government Printing Office, Washington, D.C., 1985.

52. James Perry, "Alabama Admiral Sails into Capital and Isn't Impressed," *Wall Street Journal,* 4 December 1980, 1.

53. Ibid.

54. Martin, *With God on Our Side*, 220.

55. Reauthorization of the Adolescent Family Life Demonstration Projects Act of 1981, p. 185.

56. Jo Ann Gasper, telephone interview with author, 21 July 1997.

57. Benshoof, interview.

58. Ibid.

59. These include the Hyde Amendment of 1977, which curtailed Medicaid funding for abortion, and *Harris v. McRae,* which upheld these restrictions. Also included are a range of state and local prohibitions, such as those which require parental approval for teenage women.

60. Benshoof, "Chastity Act," 1,916.

61. Patricia Donovan, "The Adolescent Family Life Act and the Promotion of Religious Doctrine," *Family Planning Perspectives* 16, no. 5 (September–October 1984): 222–28.

62. Benshoof, interview.

63. Reauthorization of the Adolescent Family Life Demonstration Projects Act of 1981, p. 2.

64. Ibid., 36.

65. Ibid., 36–37.

66. See Donovan, "Adolescent Family Life Act."

67. Reauthorization of the Adolescent Family Life Demonstration Projects Act of 1981. Also see Donovan, "Adolescent Family Life Act."

68. Hunter, interview; Benshoof, interview; see also Civil Action No. 83–3175, United States District Court for the District of Columbia. *Chan Kendrick et al. v. Margaret Heckler, Secretary of Department of Health and Human Services.* Memorandum of Points and Authorities in Support of Plaintiffs' Motion for Summary Judgement, p. 3. This document also stipulates a six-volume appendix of documents and depositions. These facts were undisputed in the litigation. Also, the document Plaintiffs' Opposition describes that of these 1,215 facts, 97.8 percent are "admitted or deemed admitted." Facts in dispute are generally immaterial. Given the admission by defendants of these facts, several of the descriptions of AFLA programs are drawn from the ACLU facts and sometimes supported by secondary sources or interviews.

69. Civil Action No. 83–3175, *Kendrick v. Heckler.*

70. See Diamond, *Roads to Dominion;* and Martin, *With God on Our Side.*

71. Gasper, interview.

72. Hunter, interview. Also Susan Faludi, *Backlash: The Undeclared War against American Women* (New York: Anchor Books, 1991), 259.

73. Hunter, interview.

74. Stipulated in Facts, *Kendrick v. Heckler*, p. 36.

75. Ibid., 38.

76. Ibid., 42.

77. Ibid., 41.

78. Gasper, interview.

79. St. Margaret's Facts, unpublished document, p. 2. Available from the Reproductive Freedom Project of the ACLU, part of the ACLU's legal documents.

80. Ibid. One adolescent who was refused information and told to go elsewhere for it "chose" to have the child and place it up for adoption, a goal of AFLA, p. 12.

81. Stipulated in Facts, *Kendrick v. Heckler*, p. 23.

82. Ibid., 24.

83. Donovan, "Adolescent Family Life Act," 224.

84. Ibid.

85. Ibid., 225.

86. Stipulated in Facts, *Kendrick v. Heckler*, 31.

87. Donovan, "Adolescent Family Life Act," 225.

88. Ibid., 226.

89. Memorandum of Points, Civil Action No. 83–3175, *Kendrick v. Heckler*, p. 57–58.

90. Marjory Mecklenburg, Letter to Sister Kathleen Natwin, St. Margaret's Hospital, 16 April 1984.

91. National sex educator, telephone interview with author, 10 June 1997.

92. National sex educator, telephone interview with author, 25 June 1997.

93. Benshoof, interview.

94. Donovan, "Adolescent Family Life Act," 225.

95. Stipulated in Facts, *Kendrick v. Heckler*, p. 57.

96. Ibid., 15. "Continuing Violations," within *Kendrick v. Heckler*.

97. National sex educator, telephone interview with author, 25 June 1997.

98. Brian Wilcox and Jennifer Wyatt, "Adolescent Abstinence Education Programs: A Meta-Analysis" (paper presented at the Joint Meeting of the Society for the Scientific Study of Sexuality and the American Association of Sex Educators, Counselors, and Therapists, Arlington, Va., 16 November 1997); also Brian Wilcox, telephone interview with author, 25 March 1998. See also National Abstinence Clearinghouse, *Directory of Abstinence Resources* (Sioux Falls, S.Dak.), for a list of evaluators.

99.     LeAnna Benn, "A Successful Teen Sexuality Program for Your Com-
        munity," *Concerned Women*, February 1990, 7.
100.    Hunter, interview.
101.    Ron Haskins, staff for the U.S. House of Representatives Ways and
        Means Committee, telephone conversation with author, 28 June 1999.
102.    In Title V of the Social Security Act, Section 510(b) Abstinence Edu-
        cation Program.
103.    National Abstinence Clearinghouse, *Directory of Abstinence Resources*, 2.
104.    Leslie Kantor, "Scared Chaste? Fear-Based Educational Curricula,"
        *SIECUS Report* 21, no. 2 (December 1992–January 1993): 1.
105.    See Christian Smith, *American Evangelicalism: Embattled and Thriving*
        (Chicago: University of Chicago Press, 1998), for a discussion of atti-
        tudes toward fundamentalists.
106.    Molly Kelly, telephone interview with author, 25 June 1997.
107.    LaHaye and LaHaye, *Act of Marriage*, unpaginated introduction.
108.    *Onania; or, the Heinous Sin of Self-Pollution*, 8th ed. (London: Printed
        by E. Rumbal for T. Crouch, 1723).
109.    Morgan, interview.
110.    Human Life International, "A Catholic Critique of Molly Kelly's Let's
        Talk to Teens about Chastity and 'Teens and Chastity' Programs on
        Sex Ed" (Gaithersburg, Md.: Human Life International, 1992), 2.
111.    Ibid.
112.    Ibid.
113.    Melvin Anchell, quoted in Randy Engle, *Sex Education: The Final
        Plague* (Gaithersburg, Md.: Human Life International, 1989), 122.
114.    Engle, *Sex Education*, 121.
115.    National sex educator, telephone interview with author, 25 June 1997.
116.    Morgan, interview.
117.    Carol Pohli, in "Church Closets and Back Doors: A Feminist View of
        Moral Majority Women," *Feminist Studies* 9, no. 3 (fall 1983): 529–58,
        argues that the move of evangelicals into the political arena introduces
        a different point of view and thereby potentially undermines evangel-
        ical dualistic thinking. A new social and political consciousness might,
        she hypothesized, undercut the totalizing worldview of evangelicals
        and lead to schisms within the Christian Right. So far, however, this
        does not seem to have transpired.
118.    Morgan, interview.
119.    M. M. Bakhtin, *The Dialogic Imagination* (Austin: University of Texas
        Press, 1981), 293.
120.    Morgan, interview.

1.   Debra Haffner and Diane de Mauro, *Winning the Battle: Developing Support for Sexuality and HIV/AIDS Education* (New York: SIECUS, March 1991), see Appendix A.

2.   Brian Wilcox and Jennifer Wyatt, "Adolescent Abstinence Education Programs: A Meta-Analysis" (paper presented at the Joint Meeting of the Society for the Scientific Study of Sexuality and the American Association of Sex Educators, Counselors, and Therapists, Arlington, Va., 16 November 1997).

3.   It is very difficult to determine if a particular sex education program has an impact on reducing teenage sexual behavior or eliminating adolescent pregnancy and childbirth. All of these activities are influenced by a wide range of social factors, such as family background, peer influence, and social disadvantages like poverty, low educational expectations, and dim prospects for the future. It is exceedingly difficult with this many complicated influences to ascertain if an educational program in school had any impact on the child at all. Indeed, according to the most comprehensive and nonpartisan metareviews of such programs, commissioned by the National Campaign to Prevent Teen Pregnancy, "It is not likely that there are any simple, easy-to-implement prevention programs—'magic bullets'—that will substantially change adolescent sexual behavior and pregnancy." See Douglas Kirby, *No Easy Answers: Research Findings on Programs to Reduce Teen Pregnancy* (Washington, D.C.: National Campaign to Prevent Teen Pregnancy, March 1997), 14.

   In addition, there tends to be little funding for program evaluation and often no staff expertise in evaluation methodologies. As a result, many studies are very poorly designed and executed. The best programs are those that address multiple factors of teen pregnancy including social disadvantages, such as the approach taken by the Children's Aid Society's Adolescent Sexuality and Pregnancy Prevention Program in Harlem. Adolescents in this program receive medical services, tutoring, career planning, employment, sports opportunities, as well as sex education. See Douglas Kirby, *Emerging Answers: Research Findings on Programs to Reduce Teen Pregnancy* (Washington, D.C.: National Campaign to Prevent Teen Pregnancy, May 2001); Kirby, *No Easy Answers;* Michael Carrera et al., "Evaluating a Comprehensive Pregnancy Prevention Program," *FLEducator* (fall 1992): 6.

4.   Dale Kunkel et al., *Sex on TV* (University of California, Santa Barbara,

Henry J. Kaiser Foundation, February 2001). For a critique of sexuality in media, see S. Robert Lichter et al., *The Rude and the Crude: Profanity in Popular Entertainment* (Washington, D.C.: Center for Media and Public Affairs, 1999).

5.  John Santelli et al., "Adolescent Sexual Behavior: Estimates and Trends from Four Nationally Representative Surveys," *Family Planning Perspectives* 32, no. 4 (July–August 2000): 156–65 and 194. This study reviews data from the National Survey of Family Growth, the National Survey of Adolescent Males, the Youth Risk Behavior Survey, and the National Longitudinal Study of Adolescent Health.

6.  Ian Hacking, "Making up People," in *Reconstructing Individualism: Autonomy, Individuality, and the Self in Western Thought,* ed. Thomas C. Heller, Morton Sosna, and David Wellbery (Stanford, Calif.: Stanford University Press, 1986), 223.

7.  Henry Jenkins, ed., *The Children's Culture Reader* (New York: New York University Press, 1998), 2.

8.  Rosalind Petchesky, *Abortion and Woman's Choice* (New York: Longman, 1984); Constance Nathanson, *Dangerous Passage: The Social Control of Sexuality in Women's Adolescence* (Philadelphia: Temple University Press, 1991); and Kristen Luker, *Dubious Conceptions* (Cambridge: Harvard University Press, 1996).

9.  Both Petchesky and Nathanson also note that in the Alan Guttmacher Institute's 1976 pamphlet, "Eleven Million Teenagers: What Can Be Done about the Epidemic of Adolescent Pregnancies in the U.S.," the eleven million referred not to teen pregnancies but to estimates of young women who were sexually active.

10.  Nathanson, *Dangerous Passage*, 47.

11.  The overall U.S. teen pregnancy rate declined 17 percent between 1990 and 1996, from 117 pregnancies per 1,000 women (fifteen to nineteen years old) to 97 per 1,000. See Alan Guttmacher Institute (AGI), "Teenage Pregnancy: Overall Trends and State-by-State Information" (New York: AGI, 1999).

12.  Paul Gibson, "Gay Male and Lesbian Youth Suicide," in ADAMHA, *Report of the Secretary's Task Force on Youth Suicide*, Department of Health and Human Services publication no. ADM 89–1623, vol. 3 (Washington, D.C.: U.S. Government Printing Office, 1989), 110–42.

13.  See, for example, Scott Hershberger and Anthony D'Augelli, "The Impact of Victimization on the Mental Health and Suicidality of Lesbian, Gay, and Bisexual Youths," *Developmental Psychology* 31, no. 1 (1995): 65–74, for a review of data.

14. Hacking, "Making up People."

15. Governor's Commission on Lesbian and Gay Youth, Press Conference, "Making Schools Safe for Gay and Lesbian Youth," Boston, Mass., 30 June 1993.

16. Planned Parenthood Federation of America, "Responsible Sex Education," photocopy in *R.E.A.L. Life: Resources to Promote Sexuality Education*, n.d.

17. Focus on the Family, "A Wolf in Sheep's Clothing: A Special Report" (Colorado Springs, Colo.: Focus on the Family, n.d.).

18. Concerned Women for America (CWA), "Sex Education in American Schools" (Washington, D.C.: CWA, n.d.).

19. National activist, interview with author, New York, 18 October 1994.

20. Local activist, telephone interview with author, 8 November 1994.

21. Janice M. Irvine, "One Generation Post-Stonewall," in *A Queer World*, ed. Martin Duberman (New York: New York University Press, 1997), 572–88.

22. Dianne Berger, telephone interview with author, 25 January 1998.

23. Leslie Kantor, interview with author, New York City, 3 May 1995.

24. For examples, see Nadine Strossen, *Defending Pornography* (New York: New York University Press, 1995).

25. Kathy McCoy and Charles Wibbelsman, *The New Teenage Body Book* (New York: Putnam Press, 1992).

26. Elaine Allegrini, "Outcry Grows over Sex Manual," *The* (Kingston, Mass.) *Enterprise*, October 1990, 1.

27. "Text of Petition Opposing Book," (Quincy, Mass.) *Patriot Ledger*, 3 October 1990, 1.

28. Local activist/school board president, telephone interview with author, 24 February 1992.

29. Jane Lane, "Parents Clash over Opinions of Health Text," *Pembroke Mariner*, 7 November 1990, 4. See also Tiffany Vail, "Parents Argue over School's Use of Sex Text," (Quincy, Mass.) *Patriot Ledger*, 3 October 1990, 1.

30. Lane, "Parents Clash," 4.

31. Local activist/school board president, telephone interview with author, 24 February 1992.

32. Vail, "Parents Argue," 1.

33. Local activist/school board president, telephone interview with author, 24 February 1992.

34. Ibid.

35.  Local activist/school board president, telephone interview with author, 31 January 1991. Following quote from 24 February 1992.

36.  William Kilpatrick, *Why Johnny Can't Tell Right from Wrong: Moral Literacy and the Case for Character Education* (New York: Simon and Schuster, 1992), 66–67.

37.  Don Feder, talk presented at Newton Citizens for Public Education public forum, "What's Wrong with Sex Education Anyway?" Newton, Mass., 31 March 1993.

38.  Local activist, interview with author, New Hampshire, 29 July 1996.

39.  Kantor, interview.

40.  See Nancy Rosenblum, *Obligations of Citizenship and Demands of Faith* (Princeton, N.J.: Princeton University Press, 2000); Stephen Carter, *The Culture of Disbelief* (New York: Basic Books, 1992); and Richard John Neuhaus, *The Naked Public Square* (Grand Rapids, Mich.: William B. Eerdmans, 1984).

41.  Rhys Williams and N. J. Demerath, "Cultural Power: How Underdog Religious and Nonreligious Movements Triumph against Structural Odds," in *Sacred Companies,* ed. N. J. Demerath, Peter Dobkin Hall, Terry Schmitt, and Rhys Williams (New York: Oxford University Press, 1998).

42.  "Christian Group Coaches School Board Candidates," *New York Times,* 14 June 1995, B8.

43.  National activist, interview with author, New York, 18 October 1994.

44.  Mary Douglas, *Risk and Blame: Essays in Cultural Theory* (New York: Routledge, 1992), 46.

45.  Family Research Council, "Condom Roulette," *In Focus* (newsletter), n.d.

46.  Susan Arnold, James Whitman, Cecil Fox, and Michele Cotler-Fox, Scientific Correspondence, "Latex Gloves Not Enough to Exclude Viruses," *Nature,* 1 September 1988, 19.

47.  Kay Stone, telephone conversation with author, 5 March 1998.

48.  Condoms, like most else in life where safety and danger coexist, are not absolutely foolproof. Condoms break, although infrequently, and they may slip off if donned improperly. But their centrality in HIV prevention has prompted heightened scrutiny of condom efficacy through both lab studies and research on HIV transmission rates among discordant couples. Condom manufacturers are held to strict quality standards and condoms are subjected to a battery of tests related to breakage. For example, condoms are consistently found to be effective in studies on discordant couples that track the infection rate

of the uninfected partner based on whether condoms are used. One such study of 124 discordant couples found that over two years not one partner became infected with consistent condom use. The Centers for Disease Control and Prevention has concluded, "Latex condoms are highly effective against the sexual transmission of HIV when used consistently and correctly during sexual intercourse."

See "Background Information on the Morbidity and Mortality Weekly Report: The Effectiveness of Condoms. Update" (Atlanta, Ga.: Centers for Disease Control and Prevention); Erin McNeill et al., eds., *The Latex Condom: Recent Advances, Future Directions* (Research Triangle Park, N.C.: Family Health International, 1998); "A Response to Recent Questions about Latex Condom Effectiveness in Preventing Sexual Transmission of the AIDS Virus" (Seattle, Wash.: Program for Appropriate Technology in Health, Office of Population, U.S. Agency for International Development, January 1994); "Update: Barrier Protection against HIV Infection and Other Sexually Transmitted Diseases," *Morbidity and Mortality Weekly Report* 42, no. 30 (6 August 1993); Isabelle De Vincenzi, "A Longitudinal Study of Human Immunodeficiency Virus Transmission by Heterosexual Partners," *New England Journal of Medicine* 331, no. 6 (11 August 1994): 341–46; Alberto Saracco et al., "Man-to-Woman Sexual Transmission of HIV: Longitudinal Study of 343 Steady Partners of Infected Men," *Journal of Acquired Immune Deficiency Syndromes* 6 (1993): 497–502.

In July 2001, the National Institutes of Health released a controversial report on a review of 138 studies on condom efficacy. The report concluded that condoms were effective at reducing risk of HIV and gonorrhea infection (85 percent for HIV among men who "always" used condoms during sexual intercourse) but said data were "insufficient" regarding condom effectiveness in sexually transmitted diseases such as genital ulcers. The report prompted conservative doctors to call for the resignation of the Centers for Disease Control director. Meanwhile, health care providers distinguished between infections transmitted through the skin and those transmitted by bodily fluids. Bernadine Healy, who headed the National Institutes of Health in the first Bush administration, said, "Just because it doesn't protect against everything doesn't mean it's not effective and useful." See Katie Leishman, "Controversy and Need for Study on Condoms," *UPI Science News*, 27 July 2001; and Ceci Connolly, "Administration Promoting Abstinence," *Washington Post*, 30 July 2001, A1.

49. *What Works: Sexuality Education*, prod. Jeanne Blake, Media Works, 1997, videocassette.

50. Pilgrim Family Institute, "'Safe Sex': The Facts," *Pilgrim Family Citizen*, November 1992 (handout). Emphasis in original.

51. Ibid.

52. Ibid.

53. Ibid.

54. Joe S. McIlhaney, *Sex: What You Don't Know Can Kill You* (Grand Rapids, Mich.: Baker Books, 1997).

55. *No Second Chance*, prod. Jeremiah Films, Project Reality, Golf, Ill., Sex Respect program, videocassette, quoted in *Teaching Fear: The Religious Right's Campaign against Sexuality Education* (Washington, D.C.: People for the American Way, 1996).

56. Blake, *What Works*.

57. Brian Wilcox and Jennifer Wyatt, "Adolescence Abstinence Education Programs: A Meta-Analysis" (paper presented at the Joint Meeting of the Society for the Scientific Study of Sexuality and the American Association of Sex Educators, Counselors, and Therapists, Arlington, Va., 16 November 1997).

58. Douglas Kirby, *Emerging Answers: Research Findings on Programs to Reduce Teen Pregnancy* (Washington, D.C.: National Campaign to Prevent Teen Pregnancy, May 2001); Douglas Kirby, *No Easy Answers: Research Findings on Programs to Reduce Teen Pregnancy* (Washington, D.C.: National Campaign to Prevent Teen Pregnancy, March 1997).

59. David Greenberg, "Teen-AID Sales Fund 'Pro-Life' Facility," *Gainesville* (Florida) *Sun*, 23 February 1992, 1A.

60. Concerned Women for America, *Concerned Women for America News* (newsletter), n.d.

61. Blake, *What Works*.

62. Maura Reynolds, "So-Called San Marcos 'Miracle' Actually May Be Just a Myth," *San Diego Union*, 19 December 1991, B-9.

63. Personal correspondence to Debra Haffner, executive director of SIECUS, by Nancy Bowen, chief, Division of Maternal and Child Health, county of San Diego; also Reynolds, "So-Called San Marcos 'Miracle.'"

64. Bowen, Letter to Debra Haffner.

65. Reynolds, "So-Called San Marcos 'Miracle,'" B-9.

66. Ibid.

67. Blake, *What Works*.

68. Kantor, interview with author, New York City, 16 November 1993.

69. Ibid.

70. Mariamne Whatley and Bonnie Trudell, "Teen-Aid: Another Problematic Sexuality Curriculum," *Journal of Sex Education and Therapy* 4 (1993): 251–71; see also Leslie Kantor, "Scared Chaste? Fear-Based Educational Curricula," *SIECUS Report* (December 1992–January 1993): 1–15; Bonnie Trudell and Mariamne Whatley, "Sex Respect: A Problematic Public School Sexuality Curriculum," *Journal of Sex Education and Therapy* 17, no. 2 (1991): 102–13.

71. Nancy Roach and LeAnna Benn, *Me, My World, My Future* (junior high text) (Spokane, Wash.: Teen-Aid, 1993) 12–13.

72. Leslie Kantor, Letter to Maria Kennedy, corporate counsel to Lehn and Fink Products, 17 August 1994; Maria Kennedy, Letter to Bruce Cook, president, Choosing the Best, Atlanta, Ga., 30 September 1994. Thanks to Kantor for providing me with these letters.

73. Whatley and Trudell, "Teen-Aid," 263.

74. Tim and Beverly LaHaye, *The Act of Marriage* (Grand Rapids, Mich.: Zondervan Publishing, 1976), chaps. 2 and 3.

75. Steve Potter and Nancy Roach, *Sexuality, Commitment, and Family* (senior high text) (Spokane, Wash.: Teen-Aid, 1990). See also Whatley and Trudell, "Teen-Aid," for a critique.

76. Ann Lindberg, "Sex Education Program Will Get Graphic," (St. Petersburg) *Florida Times*, 11 April 1996, 1B.

77. Bruce Cook, *Choosing the Best* (Atlanta, Ga.: Choosing the Best, 1998), 25.

78. James Coughlin, *Facing Reality* (parent-teacher guide) (Golf, Ill.: Project Respect, 1990), 24.

79. Ibid., 89.

80. See Kantor, "Scared Chaste?" for a full critique.

81. Tina Hoff et al., *Sex Education in America* (Menlo Park, Calif.: Henry J. Kaiser Foundation, September 2000). Available on the Internet at www.kff.org/content/2000/3048/SexEd.pdf.

82. Leslie Kantor, interview with author, New York, November 1993.

83. Bonnie Trudell, *Doing Sex Education* (New York: Routledge, 1993).

84. Local activist, interview with author, New York, 6 December 1994.

85. See Mariamne Whatley, "Commentary: Whose Sexuality Is It Anyway?" in *Sexuality and the Curriculum*, ed. James Sears (New York: Teachers College Press, 1992), 78–84. First, teacher-training programs provide inadequate instruction by which future teachers can learn about sexuality or AIDS education. One study of 169 teacher-education programs in the United States found that few of them require students

to take sex education. So most teachers are getting scant foundation in sex education pedagogy. Monica Rodriguez et al., "Teaching Our Teachers to Teach: A SIECUS Study on Training and Preparation for HIV/AIDS Prevention and Sexuality Education" (New York: SIECUS, 1999). This study was based on a review of course catalogs and therefore may be an underestimate if some courses are not mentioned in the catalog.

86. Laura Pappano, "Amid the Uproar, Teachers Back Away from Sex Ed," *Boston Globe*, 23 May 1993, 10.

87. Gayle Rubin, "Thinking Sex: Notes for a Radical Theory of the Politics of Sexuality," in *Pleasure and Danger: Exploring Female Sexuality*, ed. Carole S. Vance (Boston: Routledge and Kegan Paul, 1984), 278.

88. Don Feder, talk presented at Newton Citizens for Public Education public forum, "What's Wrong with Sex Education Anyway?" Newton, Mass., 31 March 1993.

89. Judith Riesman, talk presented at Newton Citizens for Public Education public forum, "What's Wrong with Sex Education Anyway?" Newton, Mass., 31 March 1993.

90. Focus on the Family, "Wolf in Sheep's Clothing."

91. Letter from Scott L. Thomas, administrative counsel of the American Family Association (AFA) Law Center, Tupelo, Mississippi, to Mr. Nolen Cox, of AFA of Georgia, 10 August 1992. Quote from AFA of Georgia, Valdosta, Ga., from Nolen Cox, executive director, to "Sex Education Review Committee member," 1 September 1992.

92. Barbara Huberman, interview with author, Washington, D.C., 28 August 2000; also Leslie Kantor, telephone interview with author, 24 August 2000. Both Huberman and Kantor are sexuality educators with national influence, and each recounted threats she had received and described her knowledge of threats other educators had received.

93. Konstance McKaffree, telephone interview with author, 28 August 1996.

94. Dianne Berger, telephone interview with author, 25 January 1998.

95. Ibid.

96. Ibid.

97. James Davison Hunter, *Before the Shooting Begins* (New York: Free Press, 1994), 50–60.

98. Janet Jones, "The Typical Censorship Scenario," from *What's Left after the Right* (Washington, D.C.: National Education Association, n.d.), reprinted in *Massachusetts Advocacy Kit* (Cambridge: Planned Parenthood League of Massachusetts).

99.  Local activist, interview with author, Massachusetts, 16 March 1993.

100. See Steve LeBlanc, "Sex Ed Foes Tied to Christian Groups," (Waltham, Mass.) *News Tribune*, 28 June 1993, 1; Steve LeBlanc, "Sex Ed Clash Flares: Reports Linking Foes to Christian Right Spark Debate; Leader Slams 'Fear Tactics,'" *Newton Graphic*, 1 July 1993, 1; and Rachel Layne, "Politics of Sex Education: National Right-Wing Ties Alleged as Fight Enters Voting Booth," *The Newton TAB*, 29 July 1993, 1.

101. Local activist, interview with author, New York, 2 November 1994.

102. Local activist, interview with author, New Hampshire, 29 July 1996.

103. Local activist, interview with author, Massachusetts, 16 March 1993.

104. *Los Angeles Times*, 22 March 1992, quoted in Boston, *Most Dangerous Man in America*, 91.

105. Louis Bolce, quoted in D. W. Miller, "Striving to Understand the Christian Right," *Chronicle of Higher Education*, 30 June 2000, A17–18.

106. Christian Smith, *American Evangelicalism* (Chicago: University of Chicago Press, 1998).

107. Local activist, interview with author, New Hampshire, 31 July 1996.

108. "Christian Group Coaches School Board Candidates," *New York Times*, 14 June 1995, B8.

109. See James Guth, John Green, Lyman Kellstedt, and Corwin Smidt, "Onward Christian Soldiers: Religious Activist Groups in American Politics," in *Religion and the Culture Wars*, ed. John Green et al. (Lanham, Md.: Rowman and Littlefield, 1996), 62–85.

110. Local activist, interview with author, Massachusetts, 16 November 1993.

111. Local activist, interview with author, New Hampshire, 31 July 1996.

112. Ibid.

113. Smidt et al., "Characteristics of Christian Political Activists," 153.

114. Local activist, interview with author, Massachusetts, 26 May 1993.

115. Julia Lesage, "Christian Coalition Leadership Training," in *Media, Culture, and the Religious Right*, ed. Linda Kintz and Julia Lesage (Minneapolis: University of Minnesota Press, 1998), 312.

116. Local activist, interview with author, New Hampshire, 26 July 1996.

117. Ibid.

118. Ibid.

119. Local activist, interview with author, New Hampshire, 31 July 1996.

120. Local activist, interview with author, New Hampshire, 26 July 1996.

121. Local activist, interview with author, Massachusetts, 31 January 1991.

122. Local activist, telephone interview with author, 26 August 1996.

123. Local activist, interview with author, Massachusetts, 26 May 1993. See also Steve LeBlanc, "Letter Dubs Group as 'Extremists,'" *Newton Graphic*, 29 April 1993. 1; and Rachel Layne, "Groups Rally behind Sex Ed Plans," *The Newton TAB*, 4 April 1993.

124. See Martha Kempner, "1998–99 Sexuality Education Controversies in the United States," *SIECUS Report* 27, no. 6 (August–September 1999): 4–14; and Debra Haffner, "SIECUS at Thirty-Five," *SIECUS Report* 27, no. 4 (April–May 1999): 2–3. Also see Ruth Mayer and Leslie Kantor, "1995–1996 Trends in Opposition to Comprehensive Sexuality Education in Public Schools in the United States," *SIECUS Report* 24, no. 6 (1996): 3–11.

125. Paul Richter and Marlene Cimons, "Clinton Fires Surgeon General over New Flap," *Los Angeles Times*, 10 December 1994, A36.

126. Toni Morrison, *Lecture and Speech of Acceptance, Upon the award of the Nobel Prize for Literature, Delivered in Stockholm on the Seventh of December, Nineteen Hundred and Ninety-Three* (New York: Knopf, 1994), 13, 16.

127. Kantor, interview, November 1993.

## 6. DOING IT WITH WORDS

1. Darlene Hayes-Tharpe and Shari Singer, prods., and Ron Weiner, dir., *The Phil Donahue Show*, WGN Continental Broadcasting Company, 1979.

2. Quoted in Allan Brandt, *No Magic Bullet: A Social History of Venereal Disease in the United States since 1880* (New York: Oxford University Press, 1985), 28.

3. J. L. Austin, *How to Do Things with Words* (Cambridge: Harvard University Press, 1962), 152. These two strategies correspond to Austin's two dimensions of performatives, the perlocutionary and illocutionary, which have been further amplified and debated among scholars. See also Shoshana Felman, *The Literary Speech Act* (Ithaca, N.Y.: Cornell University Press, 1983); Judith Butler, *Excitable Speech: A Politics of the Performative* (New York: Routledge, 1997).

4. The phrase "natural modesty" appears in the literature of countless community debates. It appeared early on in the psychoanalytic attacks on sex education launched by psychiatrist Melvin Anchell referring to traditional Freudian theories of development and a latency period.

5. See Judith Reisman, Edward Eichel, John Court, and J. Gordon Muir,

eds., *Kinsey, Sex, and Fraud: The Indoctrination of a People* (Lafayette, La.: Huntington House, 1990), 117.

6.    Edward Eichel and J. Gordon Muir, "The Kinsey Grand Scheme," in *Kinsey, Sex, and Fraud*, ed. Judith Reisman et al. (Lafayette, La.: Huntington House, 1990), 214.

7.    E. A. Sicilliano, Letter to the Editor, "Newton Schools Would Be Spreading Gospel of Immorality," *Newton Graphic*, 27 January 1993.

8.    Connie Marshner, *Decent Exposure: How to Teach Your Children about Sex* (Brentwood, Tenn.: Wolgemuth and Hyatt, 1988), 34–35.

9.    See evaluations such as Douglas Kirby, *Emerging Answers: Research Findings on Programs to Reduce Teen Pregnancy* (Washington, D.C.: National Campaign to Prevent Teen Pregnancy, May 2001); Douglas Kirby, *No Easy Answers: Research Findings on Programs to Reduce Teen Pregnancy* (Washington, D.C.: National Campaign to Prevent Teen Pregnancy Task Force on Effective Programs and Research, March 1997); also see Anne Grunseit et al., "Sexuality Education and Young People's Sexual Behavior: A Review of Studies," *Journal of Adolescent Research* 12, no. 4 (October 1997): 421–53.

10.   James Townsend, quoted in William Martin, *With God on Our Side: The Rise of the Religious Right in America* (New York: Broadway Books, 1996), 106.

11.   Phyllis Schlafly, ed., *Child Abuse in the Classroom* (Alton, Ill.: Pere Marquette Press, 1984).

12.   Melvin Anchell, "Psychoanalysis vs. Sex Education," *National Review*, 20 June 1986, 38.

13.   Randy Engel, *Sex Education: The Final Plague* (Gaithersburg, Md.: Human Life International), 8.

14.   Gloria Lentz, *Raping Our Children: The Sex Education Scandal* (New Rochelle, N.Y.: Arlington House, 1972).

15.   *The Gay Agenda in Public Education*, The Report, 1993, videocassette (800-462-4700).

16.   For examples, see Austin, *How to Do Things with Words;* and Butler, *Excitable Speech.*

17.   Felman, *Literary Speech Act*, 12.

18.   Catherine MacKinnon, *Only Words* (Cambridge: Harvard University Press, 1993).

19.   Ken Plummer, *Telling Sexual Stories: Power, Change, and Social Worlds* (New York: Routledge, 1995), 35.

20.   See Marc Steinberg, "Tilting the Frame: Considerations on Collective Action Framing from a Discursive Turn," *Theory and Society* 27, no. 6

(December 1988): 845–72. See also M. M. Bakhtin, *Speech Genres and Other Late Essays* (Austin: University of Texas Press, 1986).

21. James Kincaid, *Erotic Innocence: The Culture of Child Molesting* (Durham, N.C.: Duke University Press, 1998), 35.

22. Linda Gordon, *Heroes of Their Own Lives* (New York: Penguin Books, 1988).

23. Philip Jenkins, *Moral Panic* (New Haven, Conn.: Yale University Press, 1998), 119.

24. See Kincaid, *Erotic Innocence*, chap. 3. For example, in 1985, although the FBI investigated fifty-three cases of stranger kidnappings, the Center for Missing and Exploited Children claimed there were four thousand to twenty thousand such kidnappings annually. The media inflated the number to fifty thousand (p. 78). And Health and Human Services director Donna Shalala announced that "child abuse and neglect nearly doubled in the U.S. between 1968 and 1993," while there was actually a decline in cases that were investigated (p. 79).

25. See Anne Higonnet, *Pictures of Innocence* (London: Thames and Hudson, 1998).

26. Kincaid, *Erotic Innocence*, 2.

27. Ibid.

28. Richard Delgado and Jean Stefanck, *Must We Defend Nazis?* (New York: New York University Press, 1997).

29. Mari Matsuda et al., eds., *Words That Wound: Critical Race Theory, Assaultive Speech, and the First Amendment* (Boulder, Colo.: Westview Press, 1993), 1.

30. MacKinnon, *Only Words*, 68.

31. See Carole S. Vance, *Pleasure and Danger: Exploring Female Sexuality* (Boston: Routledge and Kegan Paul, 1984), especially the Introduction and Afterword. See also Lisa Duggan and Nan Hunter, *Sex Wars: Sexual Dissent and Political Culture* (New York: Routledge, 1995).

32. See, for example, Kate Ellis et al., eds., *Caught Looking: Feminism, Pornography, and Censorship* (East Haven, Conn.: Long River Books, 1986); and Varda Burstyn, ed., *Women against Censorship* (Vancouver, British Columbia: Douglas and McIntyre, 1985).

33. Donileen Loseke, *Thinking about Social Problems* (New York: Aldine De Gruyter, 1999).

34. Michael McGee, "Twenty Years, 1979–1999, The Education Department," Planned Parenthood Federation of America, unpublished document, October 1999.

35. Eleanor Howe, telephone interview with author, 10 March 1997.

36. In McGee, "Twenty Years."

37. Judith Riesman at "What's Wrong with Sex Education Anyway?" A forum sponsored by Newton Citizens for Public Education, Newton, Mass., 31 March 1993.

38. Local activist, interview with author, New Hampshire, 26 July 1996.

39. Dolores Ayling, in *Why Parents Should Object to the Children of the Rainbow, HIV K–6 Curricula,* Concerned Parents for Educational Accountability (718-891-2582), n.d., videocassette.

40. Ibid.

41. See Grunseit et al., "Sexuality Education"; and Kirby, *Emerging Answers* and *No Easy Answers.* All are metanalyses of a wide range of program evaluations.

42. Butler, *Excitable Speech*, 125.

## 7. THE PASSIONS OF CULTURE WARS

1. Rachel Layne, "The First Step," *The Newton TAB*, 18 May 1993, 31. Also, field notes from Newton School Board Meeting, 10 May 1993.

2. Patricia Mangan and Helen Kennedy, "Parents Sparring over Sex Ed in Newton," *Boston Herald*, 13 January 1993, 1.

3. Local activist, telephone conversation with author, 1 April 1993.

4. See, for example, Newton Citizens for Public Education (NCPE) letter headed, "Protest McCarthyist Tactics," n.d. It says, in part, "NCPE is inspired to use this as an opportunity to protest a resurgence of 'McCarthyism'—cries of guilt by association—now launched against Christians instead of communists."

5. Local activist, interview with author, New York, 1 November 1994.

6. Debates on the social construction of emotions run parallel to those on the social construction of sexuality. From this point of view, emotions are best understood as social, not individual. Sociologists differ on the role of the body: a "weak" constructionist position argues that bodily reactions occur which are then interpreted as emotions, while a "strong" constructionist position argues that bodies react in response to social cues. From either position, emotions are not simply instinctual gut reactions we spontaneously display in appropriate circumstances. We learn what sociologist Arlie Hochschild calls "feeling rules," which are social guidelines that define the expectations of a situation. We engage in emotion management to produce feelings suitable to the definition of the situation. We know, for example, the conventions of feeling that are appropriate for rituals such as funerals as well as for

everyday settings such as the workplace. And we produce suitable feelings. If we do not—for example, by laughing at a funeral—we (and others) are aware of and often uncomfortable with the disparity. This is not a mechanistic process in which feelings are faked or superficially performed. Rather, Hochschild argues that adults have considerable capacity to manage their emotions, and in a complex process of negotiation and microaction that she calls "deep acting," the individual can evoke or suppress internal feelings in order to correspond with emotional conventions. Emotions are inextricably bound up with cognitive meanings and interpretation. See Arlie Russell Hochschild, "Emotion Work, Feeling Rules, and Social Structures," *American Journal of Sociology* 85, no. 3 (1979): 551–75; Arlie Hochschild, *The Managed Heart* (Berkeley: University of California Press, 1983); Susan Shott, "Emotion and Social Life: A Symbolic Interactionist Analysis," *American Journal of Sociology* 84, no. 6 (1979): 1,317–34; Peggy Thoits, "The Sociology of Emotions," *Annual Review of Sociology* 15 (1989): 317–42; Catherine Lutz and Lila Abu-Lughod, eds., *Language and the Politics of Emotion* (Cambridge: Cambridge University Press, 1990); and Deborah Lupton, *The Emotional Self: A Sociocultural Exploration* (Thousand Oaks, Calif.: Sage Publications, 1998). Thanks also to Jack Hewitt for helpful conversations on this topic.

7. See James Jasper, "The Emotions of Protest," *Sociological Forum* 13, no. 3 (1998): 397–424; James Jasper, *The Art of Moral Protest* (Chicago: University of Chicago Press, 1997); Myra Marx Ferree and David Merrill, "Hot Movements, Cold Cognitions: Thinking about Social Movements in Gendered Terms," *Contemporary Sociology* 29, no. 3 (2000): 454–62.

8. See Neil Smelser, *Theory of Collective Behavior* (New York: Free Press of Glencoe, 1963).

9. Ibid.

10. See Mayer Zald and John McCarthy, eds., *Dynamics of Social Movements* (Cambridge, Mass.: Winthrop Publishing, 1979); and Charles Tilly, *From Mobilization to Revolution* (Reading, Mass.: Addison-Wesley, 1978).

11. Stanely Cohen, *Folk Devils and Moral Panics* (London: MacGibbon and Kee, 1972). For an example of positing collective behavior as irrational, see Smelser, *Theory of Collective Behavior;* for an example of how moral theory posits disproportionality of emotional reaction, see Erich Goode and Nachman Ben-Yehuda, *Moral Panics* (Cambridge, Mass.: Blackwell, 1994).

12.	See Jeffrey Weeks, *Sexuality* (London: Tavistock Publications, 1986); Gayle Rubin, "Thinking Sex," in *Pleasure and Danger*, ed. Carole S. Vance (Boston: Routledge and Kegan Paul, 1984), 267–319.

13.	Brian Jones et al., "Toward a Unified Model for Social Problems Theory," quoted in Goode and Ben-Yehuda, *Moral Panics,* 36. For another perspective on the question of disproportionality, see P. A. Waddington, "Mugging as a Moral Panic," *British Journal of Sociology* 37, no. 2 (1986): 245–59.

14.	For review articles, see Thoits, "Sociology of Emotions"; Catherine Lutz, "The Anthropology of Emotions," *Annual Review of Anthropology* 15 (1986): 405–36. See also Lutz and Abu-Lughod, eds., *Language and the Politics of Emotion;* and Kobena Mercer, "Looking for Trouble," in *The Lesbian and Gay Studies Reader*, ed. Henry Abelove et al. (New York: Routledge), 350–59, who discusses "structure of feeling" in reactions to the photography of Robert Mapplethorpe.

15.	Lauren Berlant, *The Queen of America Goes to Washington City* (Durham, N.C.: Duke University Press, 1997).

16.	Linda Kintz, *Between Jesus and the Market* (Durham, N.C.: Duke University Press, 1997).

17.	See Verta Taylor, "Watching for Vibes: Bringing Emotions into the Study of Feminist Organizations," in *Feminist Organizations*, ed. Myra Marx Ferree and Patricia Yancey Martin (Philadelphia: Temple University Press, 1995), 223–33, for a review of this literature.

18.	Carole S. Vance, "Negotiating Sex and Gender in the Attorney General's Commission on Pornography," in *Uncertain Terms: Negotiating Gender in American Culture*, ed. Faye Ginsburg and Anna Lowenhaupt Tsing (Boston: Beacon Press, 1990); Arlene Stein, *The Stranger Next Door* (Beacon Press, 2001).

19.	Jasper, "Emotions of Protest."

20.	Emotions would seemingly be central to James Davidson Hunter's work, since, especially in *Before the Shooting Begins* (New York: Free Press, 1994), 148, he suggests the potential for violence in the culture wars over abortion. However, his treatment of emotions recalls the work of earlier theorists who dismissed feelings as irrational. For example, Hunter worries that without formal, cognitive moral schemas, "all we have left are our emotions" and then public debate "becomes an exercise in emoting toward one another." Moreover, among sociologists, there has been a debate about whether "culture wars" even exist. See Hunter, *Before the Shooting Begins;* James Davison Hunter, *Culture Wars: The Struggle to Define America* (New York: Basic Books, 1991);

and Rhys Williams, ed., *Cultural Wars in American Politics* (New York: Aldine De Gruyter, 1997).

21. Samuel R. Delany, "The Rhetoric of Sex, the Discourse of Desire," in *Heterotopia: Postmodern Utopia and the Body Politic*, ed. Tobin Siebers (Ann Arbor: University of Michigan Press, 1994), 239.

22. Hochschild, "Emotion Work, Feeling Rules." Hochschild makes a similar argument about ideology, which she says is constituted both by framing rules and feeling rules. Mary Katzenstein, however, argues that discursive politics are over cognitive meanings. See Mary Katzenstein, *Faithful and Fearless* (Princeton, N.J.: Princeton University Press, 1998).

23. See Deborah Lupton, *The Emotional Self* (Thousand Oaks, Calif.: Sage Publications, 1998).

24. Hochschild, *Managed Heart*.

25. Hochschild, "Emotion Work, Feeling Rules," 561.

26. Ibid.

27. Judith Butler, *Excitable Speech* (New York: Routledge, 1997), 39.

28. James Kincaid, *Child-Loving: The Erotic Child and Victorian Culture* (New York: Routledge, 1992), 7.

29. Alex Ross, "Concert Rage," *The New Yorker*, 26 March 2001, 34.

30. Peter Stearns, *American Cool: Constructing a Twentieth-Century Emotional Style* (New York: New York University Press, 1994).

31. Joanna Weiss, "The Players in a Rinkside Tragedy," *Boston Globe,* 11 July 2000, A1.

32. Local activist, interview with author, New York, 19 October 1994.

33. Jean Hardisty, "Constructing Homophobia," *The Public Eye,* March 1993, 1–13.

34. *Ballot Measure 9,* prod. and dir. Heather MacDonald, Oregon Tape Project, 1994.

35. Local activist, interview with author, New York, 31 October 1994.

35. Ibid.

37. Local activist, interview with author, New York, 2 November 1994.

38. Local activist, interview with author, Massachusetts, 26 May 1993.

39. Ibid.

40. Stuart Hall et al., *Policing the Crisis* (Basingsstoke, England: Macmillian Education, 1978).

41. Quoted in Peter Golding and Philip Elliot, "News Value and News Production," in *Media Studies*, 2d ed., ed. Paul Marris and Sue Thornham (New York: New York University Press, 1999), 633.

42. Sarah Kellogg, "Quiet Sex Ed Hearings Disappoint Those Looking for Fiery Condemnation," *Grand Rapids, MI, Press,* 6 December 1995.

43.   Local activist, interview with author, New Hampshire, 31 July 1996.

44.   William Gamson, *Talking Politics* (New York: Cambridge University Press, 1992).

45.   Sam Dillon, "AIDS Curriculum: Fighting Words," *New York Times,* 24 October 1994, B1.

46.   Louise Phillips described this in an interview with the author, Staten Island, New York, 2 November 1994. She said that her colleague, Erica Zurer, had called Phillips to explain that journalist Sam Dillon had taken her words out of context: "She did say I was a killer, but her context was that I was a killer in terms of the work that I had put in . . . and his connection was that she was a killer. She said, 'I don't speak that way. I would not say that about anybody.' So, I said, 'Well, thank you for saying that. I'm still vicious but I'm not a killer, right?' So, in that way being that it was the *New York Times* . . . , I guess I should be grateful for what was written, that it wasn't worse."

47.   Colin Gordon, ed., *Power/Knowledge: Selected Interviews and Other Writings, 1972–1977 by Michel Foucault* (New York: Pantheon Books, 1980), 186.

48.   In addition, in the early nineties, a fund-raising letter sent out by the evangelical American Family Association featured reproductions of supposedly reprehensible homoerotic art and promised to send more copies to those who mailed contributions. See "Target Smut" (Los Angeles, Calif.: Citizens for Decent Literature); Marjorie Hein, *Sex, Sin, and Blasphemy* (New York: New Press, 1993), 145; and Nadine Strossen, *Defending Pornography* (New York: New York University Press, 1995).

49.   Tiffany Vail, "Parents Argue over School's Use of Sex Text," (Quincy, Mass.) *Patriot Ledger,* 3 October 1990, 1.

50.   Carole S. Vance, p. 126.

51.   Robert Putnam, "Bowling Alone: America's Declining Social Capital," *Journal of Democracy* 6, no. 1 (1995): 65–78; see also Robert Putnam, *Bowling Alone: Civic Disengagement in America* (New York: Simon and Schuster, 2000).

52.   Kay Lehman Schlozman, Sidney Verba, and Henry Brady, "Civic Participation and the Equality Problem," in *Civic Engagement in American Democracy,* ed. Theda Skocpol and Morris Fiorina (Washington, D.C.: Brookings Institute Press, 1999), 427–60.

53.   Amy E. Ansell, "The Color of America's Culture Wars," in *Unraveling*

the *Right*, ed. Amy E. Ansell (Boulder, Colo.: Westview Press, 1998), 173–91.

54. See Jean Hardisty, *Mobilizing Resentment* (Boston: Beacon Press, 1999), for a discussion of the Christian Right's leadership. Thanks also to Leslie Kantor for a discussion on this topic.

55. See Donna Minkowitz, "Wrong Side of the Rainbow," *The Nation* 256, no. 25 (June 1993): 901–4.

56. *Children of the Rainbow: First Grade* (New York: Board of Education of the City of New York, 1991). See also Janice M. Irvine, "One Generation Post-Stonewall," in *A Queer World*, ed. Martin Duberman (New York: New York University Press, 1997), 572–88.

57. William Gamson, *Talking Politics*, 36.

58. Jonathan Kozol, *Savage Inequalities* (New York: Harper Perennial, 1991).

59. Ibid., 4.

60. Emanuel Tobier, "Schooling in New York City," in *City Schools: Lessons from New York*, ed. Diane Ravitch and Joseph Viteritti (Baltimore, Md.: Johns Hopkins University Press, 2000), 36.

61. Andy Humm, interview with author, New York City, 27 September 1994.

62. Angela Dillard, *Guess Who's Coming to Dinner Now?* (New York: New York University Press, 2001).

63. Local activist, interview with author, New York, 1 November 1994.

64. See Cindy Patton, "Tremble, Hetero Swine!" in *Fear of a Queer Planet: Queer Politics and Social Theory*, ed. Michael Warner (Minneapolis: University of Minnesota Press, 1993), 143–77, for a discussion of this passage and the reciprocal discourses of the Christian Right and the lesbian and gay rights movement.

65. See Irvine, "One Generation Post-Stonewall," 575.

66. "The Rainbow Curriculum," *60 Minutes* 25, no. 28 (transcript of the show that aired on 4 April 1993).

67. National activist, interview with author, New York, 18 October 1994.

68. Laura D'Angelo, "Repercussions Continue after School Board Vote," *Staten Island Sunday Advance*, 6 September 1992.

69. Quoted in Tony Hiss, "The End of the Rainbow," *The New Yorker*, 12 April 1993, 51.

70. N'Tanya Lee, Don Murphy, and Lisa North, "Sexuality, Multicultural Education, and the New York City Public Schools," *Radical Teacher* 45 (winter 1994): 12–16.

71. Local activist, interview with author, New York, 31 January 1995.

72. Lee, Murphy, and North, "Sexuality, Multicultural Education."

73. Local activist, interview with author, New York, 14 November 1994.

74. Local activist, interview with author, New York, 31 January 1995.

75. Cited in Hiss, "End of the Rainbow."

76. Dillon, "AIDS Curriculum."

77. Hiss, "End of the Rainbow," 43.

78. Local activist, interview with author, New York, 6 December 1994.

79. Marc Steinberg, "Tilting the Frame: Considerations on Collective Action Framing from a Discursive Turn," *Theory and Society* 27, no. 6 (December 1988): 17.

80. Jasper, *Art of Moral Protest*, 356.

81. See Joshua Gamson, *Freaks Talk Back* (Chicago: University of Chicago Press, 1998), 109–25.

82. Local activist, interview with author, New York, 2 November 1994.

83. Ibid.

84. Local activist, interview with author, New Hampshire, 29 July 1996.

85. Local activist, interview with author, New Hampshire, 19 July 1996.

86. Local activist, interview with author, New Hampshire, 31 July 1996.

87. Merrimack School District, "Prohibition of Alternate Lifestyle Instruction," Policy 6540, August 1995, Merrimack, N.H.

88. Local activist, interview with author, New Hampshire, 29 July 1996.

89. Tamara Lush, "Merrimack Teachers, Parents File Lawsuit over Policy on 'Gays,'" *Manchester Union Leader*, 16 February 1996, A4.

90. Statement of Mary Bonauto, esquire, Gay and Lesbian Advocates and Defenders, Boston, Mass., 15 February 1996 (photocopy).

91. Chris Ager, Letter to the Editor, *Merrimack Village Crier*, 1 August 1995.

92. Local activist, interview with author, New Hampshire, 29 July 1996.

93. Jeffrey Merritt, "Many Students Say Gay Policy Unwelcome," *Nashua Telegraph*, 31 August 1995, 1.

94. Jeffrey Merritt, "Opponents of Gay Policy Plead with Board to Rescind Vote," *Nashua Telegraph*, 6 September 1995, 1.

95. Jeffrey Merritt, "Homosexual Policy Triggers Lawsuit," *Nashua Telegraph*, 16 February 1996, 1.

96. See Don Botsch, "Meanwhile in the Parking Lot," *Merrimack Village Crier*, 22 August 1995; and Jeffrey Merritt, "Enforcement of Gay Policy Stirs Concern," *Nashua Telegraph*, 16 August 1995, 1.

97. Merritt, "Enforcement of Gay Policy," 1.

98. Local activist, interview with author, New Hampshire, 29 July 1996.

99. Local activist, interview with author, New Hampshire, 31 July 1996.

1. Stefani Kipenec, "Baptists Call for Boycott of Disney," *Boston Globe*, 19 June 1997, A3.

2. Nat Hentoff, "The War against Gays and Lesbians," *Village Voice*, 24 November 1998, 38.

3. Ruth Mayer, "1996–97 Trends in Opposition to Comprehensive Sexuality Education in Public Schools in the United States," *SIECUS Report* 25, no. 4 (August–September 1997): 20–26.

4. See Lauren Berlant, *The Queen of America Goes to Washington City* (Durham, N.C.: Duke University Press, 1997), 17.

5. Mary Douglas, *Purity and Danger* (London: Routledge, 1966), 133.

6. See Jeffrey Moran, *Teaching Sex* (Cambridge: Harvard University Press, 2000).

7. Berlant, *Queen of America*.

8. Corwin Smidt et al., "The Characteristics of Christian Political Activists: An Interest Group Analysis," in *Christian Political Activism at the Crossroads*, ed. William R. Stevenson Jr. (Lanham, Md.: University Press of America, 1994), 159.

9. Alan Yang, *From Wrongs to Rights* (Washington, D.C.: National Gay and Lesbian Task Force, n.d.).

10. Alan Wolfe, *One Nation, After All* (New York: Viking Penguin, 1998), 79.

11. Clyde Wilcox and Robin Wolpert, "Gay Rights in the Public Sphere: Public Opinion on Gay and Lesbian Equality," in *The Politics of Gay Rights*, ed. Craig Rimmerman, Kenneth Wald, and Clyde Wilcox (Chicago: University of Chicago Press, 2000), 415.

12. Yang, *From Wrongs to Rights*.

13. Ibid.

14. See Edward O. Laumann et al., *The Social Organization of Sexuality: Sexual Practices in the United States* (Chicago: University of Chicago Press, 1994).

15. Michel Foucault, "On the Genealogy of Ethics," in *Michel Foucault: Beyond Structuralism and Hermeneutics*, 2d ed., ed. H. Dreyfus and P. Rabinow (Chicago: University of Chicago Press, 1983), 238.

16. Wilcox and Wolpert, "Gay Rights."

17. Kevin Jennings, interview with author, Boston, 7 November 1994.

18. Al Ferreira, interview with author, Cambridge, Massachusetts, 12 May 1993.

19. Janice M. Irvine, "One Generation Post-Stonewall," in *A Queer World*,

ed. Martin Duberman (New York: New York University Press, 1997), 572–88.

20. In this chapter I am not discussing HIV/AIDS education in public schools, in which there is occasionally a limited discussion of sexual behaviors that are risky (for example, anal sex) regardless of the partner's gender. Rather, here I focus on the types of programs which are most typically initiated by lesbian and gay education reformers, such as diversity programs and anti-bias, anti-violence, and anti-risk programs.

21. Mayer, "1996–97 Trends."

22. Local and national activist, interview with author, New York, 18 October 1994.

23. Andy Humm, interview with author, New York City, 27 September 1994.

24. Local activist, interview with author, New York, 31 October 1994.

25. Tim and Beverly LaHaye, *The Act of Marriage* (Grand Rapids, Mich.: Zondervan Publishing, 1976), 279.

26. John Shotter and Michael Billig, "A Bakhtinian Psychology: From out of the Heads of Individuals and into the Dialogues between Them," in *Bakhtin and the Human Sciences*, ed. Michael Bell and Michael Gardiner (Thousand Oaks, Calif.: Sage Publications, 1998), 16.

27. Tom Stebbins, *Friendship Evangelism by the Book* (Camp Hill, Pa.: Christian Publications, 1995).

28. Flo Conway and Jim Siegelman, *Snapping: America's Epidemic of Sudden Personality Change* (Philadelphia: J. B. Lippincott Company, 1978).

29. See, for example, Simon LeVay, *The Sexual Brain* (Cambridge: MIT Press, 1993); and Dean Hamer, *The Science of Desire* (New York: Simon and Schuster, 1994).

30. Steven Epstein, "Gay Politics, Ethnic Identity: The Limits of Social Constructionism," *Socialist Review* 17, nos. 3 and 4 (May–August 1987): 24.

31. Eve K. Sedgwick, *Epistemology of the Closet* (Berkeley: University of California Press, 1990).

32. Local activist, interview with author, New York, 31 October 1994.

33. New York City Public Schools, *Children of the Rainbow* (New York City Board of Education, 1991), 372.

34. Local activist, interview with author, New York, 2 November 1994.

35. Local activist, interview with author, New York, 15 November 1994.

36. Local activist, interview with author, New York, 2 November 1994.

37. Jerry Falwell, "America Is Losing the War against Homosexuals" (fundraising letter to membership) (Lynchburg, Va.: Moral Majority, 1983).

38. Morton Kondracke, "Anita Bryant Is Mad about Gays," *New Republic*, 7 May 1977, 14.

39. Amber Hollibaugh, "Sexuality and the State," *Socialist Review* 9, no. 3 (May–June 1979): 55–72.

40. Bev[erly] LaHaye, Letter to Members (appearing in the CWA newsletter) (Concerned Women for America, May 1992).

41. Local activist, interview with author, New York, 1 November 1994.

42. Local activist, interview with author, Massachusetts, 27 October 1994.

43. See Jean Hardisty, *Mobilizing Resentment* (Boston: Beacon Press, 1999).

44. William Consiglio, *Homosexual No More* (Wheaton, Ill.: Victor Books, 1991), 87.

45. Ibid.

46. See "Challenging the Ex-Gay Movement," December 1998, p. 18, and Surina Khan, "Calculated Compassion: How the Ex-Gay Movement Serves the Right's Attack on Democracy," October 1998 (both booklets were published by Political Research Associates in Somerville, Mass.).

47. The following is from "Calculated Compassion" and personal communication with Surina Khan, who was at that time at Political Research Associates in Somerville, Mass.

48. See Hardisty, *Mobilizing Resentment*.

49. Wolfe, *One Nation*, 77.

50. Frank Rich, "Has Jerry Falwell Seen the Light?" *New York Times*, 6 November 1999, 17.

51. "Calculated Compassion," 1.

52. This discussion of moral shocks draws on James Jasper, *The Art of Moral Protest* (Chicago: University of Chicago Press, 1997); and James Jasper, "The Emotions of Protest: Affective and Reactive Emotions in and around Social Movements," *Sociological Forum* 13, no. 3 (1998): 397–424.

53. William Miller, *The Anatomy of Disgust* (Cambridge: Harvard University Press, 1997), xi.

54. David Colker, "Anti-Gay Video Highlights Church's Agenda," *Los Angeles Times*, 22 February 1993, 1.

55. *The Gay Agenda*, The Report, 1992, videocassette.

56. Frederick Clarkson, "The Anti-Gay Nineties," *Freedom Writer* 10, no. 2 (March–April 1993): 1–3; also see Miller, *Anatomy of Disgust*.

57.     *Ballot Measure 9*, prod. and dir. Heather MacDonald, Oregon Tape Project, 1994, videocassette.

58.     Clarkson, "Anti-Gay Nineties."

59.     Paul Cameron, telephone conversation with author, 9 November 1994.

60.     Paul Cameron, telephone conversation with author, 5 March 1998.

61.     National activist, interview with author, New York, 18 October 1994.

62.     Statement of the resolution of the American Sociological Association, 1985. For a full review of Paul Cameron's history in relation to professional organizations such as the APA and ASA, see http://psychology.ucdavis.edu/rainbow/html/facts_cameron_sheet.html.

63.     Gregory M. Herek, "Bad Science in the Service of Stigma: A Critique of the Cameron Group's Survey Studies," in *Stigma and Sexual Orientation*, ed. Gregory Herek (Thousand Oaks, Calif.: Sage Publications, 1998), 225.

64.     David Colker, "Statistics in 'Gay Agenda' Questioned," *Los Angeles Times,* 22 February 1993. See also Sara Diamond, "The Antigay Agenda," in *Not by Politics Alone* (New York: Guilford Press, 1998); Jennifer Terry, *An American Obsession* (Chicago: University of Chicago Press, 1999); and Hardisty, *Mobilizing Resentment,* 121.

65.     See "Anti-Gay Adviser Stirs Controversy," *San Francisco Chronicle*, 19 August 1985, 7; "Dannemeyer Blast," *Washington Times*, 3 February 1988.

66.     Paul Cameron, William Playfair, and Stephen Wellum, "The Longevity of Homosexuals: Before and after the AIDS Epidemic," *Omega: Journal of Death and Dying* 29, no. 3 (1994): 249–72.

67.     One significant methodological error in this study is that Cameron used data from a convenience sample to generalize the population at large. There are important differences between the obituaries in major city newspapers and the obituaries in gay newspapers. While city newspapers routinely include comprehensive sections for death notices and obituaries, gay newspapers do not. Gay newspapers typically began to run obituaries after the onset of the AIDS epidemic and, unlike the death notices section in city newspapers, do not print a representative sample of the community. For a range of reasons, many gay men and lesbians do not have their obituaries printed in gay newspapers. This makes it impossible to accurately compare city newspapers with gay newspapers. For more details on methodological problems with Cameron's gay obituary study, see http://psychology.ucdavis.edu/rainbow/html/facts_cameron_ obit.html.

68.     Tim LaHaye, telephone interview with author, 19 May 1997.

69. Local activist, telephone interview with author, New Hampshire, 26 August 1996.

70. Miller, *Anatomy of Disgust*, 9.

71. Jasper, *Art of Moral Protest*.

72. Mainstream abortion opponents like the National Right to Life Committee were joined in the eighties by more militant groups such as Operation Rescue and Lambs of Christ. Anti-abortion strategies intensified throughout the nineties. In his book on how to close abortion clinics, veteran anti-abortion activist Joseph Scheidler advised the use of "inflammatory rhetoric" such as "holocaust" to describe abortion, "abortuary" and "death camp" in relation to clinics, and "'fornication' for sex outside of marriage, [and] 'adultery' for 'having an affair.'" Regarding criticism of his advice that the display of certain images was sensational, Scheidler claimed, "Pictures of dead babies are 'emotional.' They are supposed to be." The first clinic bombing occurred in 1982. By 2001, there had been forty such bombings. In the early nineties, a mobilization called No Place to Hide (NPH) targeted physicians who performed abortions. NPH publicly eschewed violence; it advocated displaying "wanted posters" with the addresses of doctors so that activists could picket their homes. The first murder occurred in 1993, when Dr. David Gunn of Pensacola, Florida, was shot three times in the back outside a clinic. By 2001, there had been seven murders of clinic doctors and staff. The National Abortion Federation had compiled 3,031 acts of disruption between 1977 and 2001, which along with murder and attempted murder (seventeen attempts) included such incidents as arson, bombings, assault, anthrax threats, and vandalism. While many anti-abortion organizations condemned the violence, some of the more militant direct action groups did not, such as the leader of Missionaries to the Preborn, who said that Dr. Gunn's murder had saved "human beings who were scheduled for execution."

Meanwhile, the highly publicized grotesque murders of two gay men in the late nineties—Matthew Shepard, who was beaten and tied to a fence, and Billy Jack Gaither, who was beaten with an ax handle and set on fire—made visible anti-gay violence. In an important turn, the killings prompted widespread public speculation about whether the Christian Right's rhetoric might contribute to a climate of hatred. Matthew's mother, Judy Shepard, wrote a letter that was sent out to high school counselors saying, "I believe that my son was killed because somehow, somewhere, his killers learned that the lives of gay people are not as worthy of respect, dignity and honor as the lives of other people." There is certainly no simple causal relationship between speech and violence. And, unlike with anti-abortion violence, the murderers of Shepard and Gaither had no explicit connection to right-wing organizations. But as the number of anti-gay murders doubled from fourteen in 1997 to thirty-three in 1998, some people, including some in the Christian Right, began to think its inflammatory rhetoric might implicitly condone violence. See Joseph M. Scheidler, *Closed: Ninety-Nine Ways to Stop Abortion*, updated edition (Rockford, Ill.: Tan Books and Publishers, 1993), 194, 198; Statistics compiled by the National Abortion Federation, 1755 Massachusetts Avenue, N.W., Washington, D.C. 20036; see also Patricia Baird-Windle and Eleanor Bader, *Targets of Hatred: Anti-Abortion Terrorism* (New York: Palgrave, 2001); Sara Diamond, *Not by Politics Alone* (New York: Guilford Press, 1998), 145; Tom Cole, "The Crusade of a Former Homosexual," *Cincinnati Enquirer*, 26 November 1999, A22; and National Coalition of Anti-Violence Programs Fifth Annual Report, cited in Chuck Colbert, "Keeping Track of Anti-Gay Hate," New America News Service, 27 May 1999.

73.    Cal Thomas and Ed Dobson, *Blinded by Might: Can the Religious Right Save America?* (Grand Rapids, Mich.: Zondervan Publishing, 1999), 81. Once-prominent Christian Right leader Jerry Falwell, whose persistent anti-gay message was described by one United Methodist minister as "close to spiritual violence," admitted to being "strident" in his language. Noting that "words can lead to actions," Falwell acknowledged potential consequences of "reckless and dangerous language" and promised to avoid characterizations that might be seen as "sanctioning hate or antagonism against homosexuals." For example, he stopped using the term "abomination" in relation to gay people. The criticism this prompted from others in the Christian Right, who had collectively refused any responsibility for Shepard's death, suggested less than unanimous support for Falwell's promised reforms. And Falwell himself had already lost credibility because of a series of public embarrassments such as remarks about the Jewish anti-christ and the claim that Teletubby Tinky Winky was gay. See Shannon Brennan, "Falwell, White Open Dialogue on Acceptance," (Lynchburg, Va.) *News & Advance*, 24 October 1999, A1; Rich, "Has Jerry."

74.    Leroy Aarons, *Prayers for Bobby* (New York: Harper Collins, 1995), 191.

75.    See John D'Emilio, *Sexual Politics, Sexual Communities* (Chicago: University of Chicago Press, 1983); Andrew Sullivan, ed., *Same-Sex Mar-*

*riage: Pro and Con* (New York: Vintage Books, 1997); and Michael Warner, *The Trouble with Normal* (New York: Free Press, 1999).

76. Warner, *Trouble with Normal,* 40.

77. Local teacher, interview with author, New York, 6 December 1994.

78. Jennings, interview.

79. Hollibaugh, "Sexuality and the State."

80. David Goodstein, "Fighting the Briggs Brigade," *The Advocate,* 14 June 1978.

81. Hollibaugh, "Sexuality and the State," 66.

82. Anne Roiphe, "Promoting Gayness? No—Just Basic Decency," *New York Observer,* 11 January 1992.

83. Activists themselves did not necessarily believe that sexuality was inborn and fixed. Some would tell me they believed sexual identity was constructed and yet show me a letter or other document in which they had argued that children could not be harmed by gay-related programs because their sexuality was biologically determined.

84. Donna Minkowitz, "Recruit, Recruit, Recruit," *The Advocate,* 29 December 1992, 17; Donna Minkowitz, "Kids 'R' Us," *Village Voice,* 15 September 1992, 30.

85. Local activist, interview with author, New York, 2 November 1994.

86. Dolores Ayling, in *Why Parents Should Object to the Children of the Rainbow, HIV K–6 Curricula,* Concerned Parents for Educational Accountability, n.d., videocassette.

87. Brucer Bawer, *A Place at the Table* (New York: Poseidon Press, 1993), 179.

88. Donna Minkowitz, telephone interview with author, 22 August 1995. See also Minkowitz, "Recruit."

89. Suzanna Danuta Walters, "Who Let the Dogs Out?" *Images: A Journal of the Gay & Lesbian Alliance against Defamation* (summer 2001): 5.

90. Leslie Kantor, interview with author, New York City, 19 August 1997.

## 9. IF ASKED, DON'T TELL: A FINAL COMMENT

1. Paul Weyrich et al., "Is the Religious Right Finished? An Insider's Conversation," *Christianity Today,* 6 September 1999, 43–59. See also Cal Thomas and Ed Dobson, *Blinded by Might: Can the Religious Right Save America?* (Grand Rapids, Mich.: Zondervan Publishing, 1999).

2. Frank Rich, "Pig vs. Prig," *New York Times,* 23 September 1998, A29.

3. Henry J. Kaiser Foundation, *Sex Education in America: A Series of National Surveys of Students, Parents, Teachers, and Principals* (Menlo Park, Calif.: Henry J. Kaiser Foundation, 2000).

4. David Landry, Lisa Kaeser, and Cory Richards, "Abstinence Promotion and the Provision of Information about Contraception in Public School District Sexuality Education Policies," *Family Planning Perspectives* 31, no. 6 (November–December 1999): 280–86.

5. Kaiser Foundation, *Sex Education in America*.

6. Martha Kempner, telephone conversation with author, 21 June 2001.

7. Martha Kempner, "Sexuality Education Is Debated as Restrictive Programs Gain Popularity," *SIECUS Report* 28, no. 6 (August–September 2000): 12. Also, Kempner, telephone conversation.

8. Leslie Kantor, telephone conversation with author, 24 August 2000; Barbara Huberman, interview with author, Washington, D.C., 28 August 2000; Kempner, "Sexuality Education Is Debated."

9. Monica Rodriguez et al., *Teaching Our Teachers to Teach: A SIECUS Study on Training and Preparation for HIV/AIDS Prevention and Sexuality Education* (New York: SIECUS 1999). This study was based on a review of course catalogs and therefore may be an underestimate if some courses are not mentioned in the catalogs.

10. Jacqueline Darroch, David Landry, and Susheela Singh, "Changing Emphases in Sexuality Education in U.S. Public Secondary Schools, 1988–1999," *Family Planning Perspectives* 32, no. 5 (September–October 2000): 204–11.

11. Martha Quillin, "Franklin Schools Slice Sex-Ed Chapters out of Health Books," (North Carolina) *News and Observer*, 25 September 1997, 1.

12. Marjorie Kauth-Karjala, "Abortion References to Be Torn from Van Buren School Texts," Belleville, Michigan (1998).

13. Irma Lemus, "Schools Remove Sex Ed Videos," *Burbank Leader*, 29–30 April 2000, weekend section, 2.

14. Kempner, "Sexuality Education Is Debated," 12.

15. Tom Gorman, "Hemet Schools Scrap Sex Education over Suit," *Los Angeles Times*, 9 March 1995, A3.

16. Robin Franzen, "Too Much Knowledge," *Oregonian*, 17 May 1996, B2.

17. Kaiser Foundation, *Sex Education in America*.

18. Quoted in Franzen, "Too Much Knowledge."

19. Don Boekelheide, "On the Front Line of the War on Teen Pregnancy," *Charlotte Observer*, 6 March 1996, 15A.

20. Ann Lindberg, "Sex Education Program Will Get Graphic," (St. Petersburg) *Florida Times*, 11 April 1996, 1B.

21. In Section 510(b) of Title V of the Social Security Act, Public Law 104–193, "abstinence education" is defined as an approach which: "a.

has as its exclusive purpose teaching the social, psychological, and health gains to be realized by abstaining from sexual activity; b. teaches abstinence from sexual activity outside marriage as the expected standard for all school-age children; c. teaches that abstinence from sexual activity is the only certain way to avoid out-of-wedlock pregnancy, sexually transmitted diseases, and other associated health problems; d. teaches that a mutually faithful monogamous relationship in the context of marriage is the expected standard of sexual activity; e. teaches that sexual activity outside of the context of marriage is likely to have harmful psychological and physical effects; f. teaches that bearing children out-of-wedlock is likely to have harmful consequences for the child, the child's parents, and society; g. teaches young people how to reject sexual advances and how alcohol and drug use increase vulnerability to sexual advances; h. teaches the importance of attaining self-sufficiency before gaining in sexual activity."

22.  S. Williams, "Abstinence Becomes a Business," *Milwaukee Journal Sentinel*, 9 October 2000, 1A.

23.  Ceci Connolly, "Administration Promoting Abstinence," *Washington Post*, 30 July 2001, A1.

24.  Focus on the Family, 19 March 2001 article, described in William Smith, "Where Is U.S. Health and Human Services Secretary Thompson on the Issues?" *SIECUS Report* 29, no. 3 (February–March 2001): 36.

25.  Carolyn B. Maloney, U.S. Representative (D-N.Y.), "Sex Education for the Young," editorial, *Washington Post*, 7 August 2001, A14.

26.  Connolly, "Administration Promoting."

27.  Ibid.; Sharon Lerner, "An Orgy of Abstinence," *Village Voice*, 1–7 August 2001. Thanks also to William Smith for discussion on this topic.

28.  National Coalition Against Censorship (NCAC), "Abstinence-Only Education: A Joint Statement," NCAC, New York, winter 2000–2001. See also Gary Simson and Erika Sussman, "Keeping the Sex in Sex Education: The First Amendment's Religion Clauses and the Sex Education Debate," *Southern California Review of Law and Women's Studies* 9, no. 2 (spring 2000): 265–97. Thanks to Joan Bertin for a discussion of these issues.

29.  Kaiser Foundation, "Sex Education in America."

30.  See Judith Butler, *Excitable Speech* (New York: Routledge, 1997), for an analysis of implicit and explicit censorship.

31.  Michael McGee, "Twenty Years, 1979–1999, The Education Department" (Planned Parenthood Federation of America, 1999, photocopy).

32.  Kaiser Foundation, *Sex Education in America;* Hickman-Brown Public

Opinion Research Survey, March 1999, Commissioned by SIECUS and Advocates for Youth. Hickman-Brown surveyed 1,050 adults nationwide in February–March 1999. See also "The Thirtieth Annual Phi Delta Kappa/Gallup Poll of the Public's Attitudes toward the Public Schools," *Phi Delta Kappan* September 1998, 54; and Henry J. Kaiser Family Foundation, *National Survey of Public Secondary School Principals: The Politics of Sex Education* (Menlo Park, Calif.: Henry J. Kaiser Family Foundation, December 1999).

33. National Abortion Rights Action League (NARAL), *Who Decides?* 9th ed. (Washington, D.C.: NARAL Foundation, 2000).

34. Susan Wilson, "The Abstinence Stress Test" (photocopy). My thanks to Susan Wilson for discussion and information.

35. David Satcher, "The Surgeon General's Call to Action to Promote Sexual Health," 28 June 2001. On the call for Satcher to resign, see James Gerstenzang, "Satcher's Sex Report Puts Bush in Hot Seat," *Los Angeles Times,* 30 June 2001, 18.

36. William Smith, telephone interview with author, 21 June 2001.

37. Douglas Kirby, *No Easy Answers: Research Findings on Programs to Reduce Teen Pregnancy* (Washington, D.C.: National Campaign to Prevent Teen Pregnancy Task Force on Effective Programs and Research, March 1997); Brian Wilcox and Jennifer Wyatt, "Adolescent Abstinence Education Programs: A Meta-Analysis" (paper presented at the Joint Meeting of the Society for the Scientific Study of Sexuality and the American Association of Sex Educators, Counselors, and Therapists, Arlington, Va., 16 November 1997).

38. Douglas Kirby, *Emerging Answers: Research Findings on Programs to Reduce Teen Pregnancy* (Washington, D.C.: National Campaign to Prevent Teen Pregnancy, May 2001), 88.

39. Elayne Bennett's Best Friends program withdrew its anticipated participation from the evaluation procedure. Huberman, interview; Brian Wilcox, telephone conversation with author, 19 September 2000.

40. Judith Levine, *Harmful to Minors: The Perils of Protecting Children from Sex* (Minneapolis: University of Minnesota Press, 2002), 116.

41. Michel Foucault warns us about the regulatory power of sexual discourse, while Wendy Brown reminds us that silence is a practice that can help us escape regulation. Michel Foucault, *The History of Sexuality, Vol. 1: An Introduction* (New York: Random House, 1978); Wendy Brown, "Freedom's Silences," in *Censorship and Silencing: Practices of Cultural Regulation*, ed. Robert Post (Los Angeles: Getty Research Institute Publications, 1998), 313–27.

42. Butler, *Excitable Speech*.

43. David Shribman, "A Shift in Culture, Presidency," *Boston Globe*, 1 February 1998, A29.

44. Ibid.

45. Ibid.

46. Joseph Kahn, "For Nation, a Debate on Sexual Boundaries," *Boston Globe*, 13 September 1998, A20.

47. "The Pill and the Pupil," *Newsweek*, 24 July 1967, 72.

48. Linda Matchan and Alison Bass, "For Parents, Difficult Discussions Seen in Store," *Boston Globe*, 12 September 1998, A2.

49. Garry Trudeau, "Doonesbury," *Boston Globe*, 10 February 1998.


ON METHODS AND TERMINOLOGY

1. The actual identities of these local activists are irrelevant in my arguments, and I have chosen to identify them simply by home state and date of interview, except for a few cases which were widely publicized.

2. Although her discussion does not focus on public education, see Cindy Patton, *Fatal Advice: How Safe-Sex Education Went Wrong* (Durham, N.C.: Duke University Press, 1996).

3. Nancy Ammerman, "North American Protestant Fundamentalism," in *Fundamentalisms Observed*, ed. Martin E. Marty and R. Scott Appleby (Chicago: University of Chicago Press, 1991), 1–65.

4. Christian Smith, *American Evangelicalism* (Chicago: University of Chicago Press, 1998).

Carter, President Jimmy, 63; and White House Conference on Families, 68

Catholic sex education curricula, 97–103

censorship in sex education programs, 124–25, 189–90, 192–93

Centers for Disease Control and Prevention (CDC), 115, 116

child abuse, 135–36; and legislation, 135

*Children of the Rainbow* teachers guide, 115, 154–58, 160–62, 170, 172–73

*Choosing the Best* sex education curriculum, 120, 121

Christian Coalition: entry into local politics, 72, 126–28; growth of, 71. *See also* Christian Right

Christian Crusade: in opposition to sex education, 44, 48–49, 56, 62; publications, 46. *See also* Hargis, Reverand Billy James

Christian Right: affiliation with ex-gay movement, 175–76; affiliation with other religions, 129–30; coalition with pro-family movement, 74–75; engagement in sex education debates, 11–12; infiltration of local politics, 71–72, 194–95; opposition to gay education reform, 167, 171–72, 173–74; opposition to SIECUS, 27–28, 42–43; rise during 1970s, 63–80; sexual politics of, 49–52, 61–62; sexual publications, 81, 82; sexualization of Christian evangelicalism, 81–106; use of depravity narratives, 58, 76; use of language, 64, 148–49; use of Scripture, 74–75,

78. *See also* Christian Coalition; pro-family movement

Clinton, President William: influence of impeachment on American sexual culture, 2, 186, 187, 196

community-level opposition to sex education, 43–44, 46–49, 141–43

Concerned Women for America: affiliations, 71, 126, 175; endorsement of AFLA, 101; opposition to SIECUS, 110–11. *See also* LaHaye, Beverly

contraception, as sex education topic, 5, 6, 8, 20, 116–17; and controversy over condom use, 116–17, 240–41 n. 48

Denton, Senator Jeremiah Denton, as cosponsor of AFLA, 90–91, 93, 96

depravity narratives, 54–58, 73, 111–14; and exploitation of racial anxieties, 55–56; and sexual stigmatization, 56–57

Drake, Gordon, as Director of Education for Christian Crusade, 46, 47, 51, 55, 56, 59–60

Elders, Surgeon General Joycelyn, 1, 14, 50, 197

emotional aspect of sex education conflicts, 143–64, 249–50 n. 6, 251 n. 19

emotional molestation, 135–40

evangelical religious groups. *See* Christian Right

ex-gay movement, 174–76. *See also* gay education reform

*Facing Reality,* 121

Ku Klux Klan, 49, 67, 74

Reed, Ralph, 71, 125, 128. *See also* Christian Coalition

Riesman, Judith: opposition to sex education programs, 123, 132, 138, 150–51

Robertson, Pat, 76, 165. *See also* Christian Coalition

*Roe v. Wade*, 19, 34, 88

Romantic child, 13–14, 33, 197, 198

Rubin, Isadore: and accusations of communist affiliation, 52; as SIECUS board member, 32. *See also* anti-communism, as propaganda tool of Christian Right

St. Margaret's Hospital sex education curriculum, 97–98, 100–101

San Marcos "miracle", 118–19. *See also* Teen-Aid sex education curriculum

Schlafly, Phyllis, 40, 68, 133; and opposition to ERA, 67

Schulz, Esther, as first SIECUS education director, 37–38, 43, 61. *See also* SIECUS

Section 510(b), 102, 190–91, 192–93, 194. *See also* abstinence-only programs

Sex Information and Education Council of the United States (SIECUS), 188, 192; criticisms of, 73, 110–11, 123; emphasis on science and health, 25–26, 27; history of, 17–34, 215 n. 2; inception of, 22–29; as model for comprehensive sex education, 6–7, 211 n. 17; 1960s efforts, 36–40; opposition to by religious conservatives, 27–28; purpose of, 25; and sex education opponents, 50–53, 55–56; and sexual speech, 29–33, 131; as single-issue organization, 71; strategies for advocacy of sex education, 119–20, 121; support of gay rights, 166; as target of depravity narratives, 114; ties to religious groups, 23–24. *See also* Calderone, Mary

Sex Respect curriculum, 100, 117–18, 121, 194

sexual culture in the 1960s, 18–22, 33–34; and guidelines for school sex education programs 38–39; and sex education conflicts, 35–62

sexual language, 13, 190; and public expression of, 36–37, 196–98; of sexual movement, 10–11

sexual speech, 195–97; and claims against, 136–40; and inherent power of, 131–34

sexual revolution, 19, 20, 36, 42, 69

single-issue oppositional groups, 41; as seeds of the New Right, 41

Starr Report, 2, 196

stigmatization of sex education, 111–24, 195

Teen-Aid sex education curriculum, 69, 101–2, 118–19, 120, 121, 194

teen pregnancy, as sex education issue, 109–11, 237 n. 3

White House Conference on Families, 66; as target for pro-family movement, 68

Williams, Sally, 18, 38, 40, 124, 215 n. 6. *See also* Anaheim sex education program

Text: 10/13 Adobe Garamond
Display: Gill Sans Book
Compositor: BookMatters, Berkeley
Printer and Binder: Thomson-Shore, Inc.